Patient Reported Outcomes in Rheumatic Diseases

Editors

JENNIFER L. BARTON
PATRICIA KATZ

RHEUMATIC DISEASE CLINICS OF NORTH AMERICA

www.rheumatic.theclinics.com

Consulting Editor
MICHAEL H. WEISMAN

May 2016 • Volume 42 • Number 2

ELSEVIER

1600 John F. Kennedy Boulevard • Suite 1800 • Philadelphia, Pennsylvania, 19103-2899
http://www.theclinics.com

RHEUMATIC DISEASE CLINICS OF NORTH AMERICA Volume 42, Number 2
May 2016 ISSN 0889-857X, ISBN 13: 978-0-323-44523-8

Editor: Jennifer Flynn-Briggs
Developmental Editor: Casey Jackson

Rheumatic Disease Clinics of North America (ISSN 0889-857X) is published quarterly by Elsevier Inc., 360 Park Avenue South, New York, NY 10010-1710. Months of issue are February, May, August, and November. Business and editorial offices: 1600 John F. Kennedy Boulevard, Suite 1800, Philadelphia, PA 19103-2899. Periodicals postage paid at New York, NY and additional mailing offices. Subscription prices are USD 335.00 per year for US individuals, USD 634.00 per year for US institutions, USD 100.00 per year for US students and residents, USD 395.00 per year for Canadian individuals, USD 791.00 per year for Canadian institutions, USD 465.00 per year for international individuals, USD 791.00 per year for international institutions, and USD 230.00 per year for Canadian and foreign students/residents. To receive student/resident rate, orders must be accompanied by name of affiliated institution, date of term, and the *signature* of program/residency coordinator on institution letterhead. Orders will be billed at individual rate until proof of status received. Foreign air speed delivery is included in all *Clinics* subscription prices. All prices are subject to change without notice. **POSTMASTER:** Send address changes to *Rheumatic Disease Clinics of North America,* Elsevier Health Sciences Division, Subscription Customer Service, 3251 Riverport Lane, Maryland Heights, MO 63043. **Customer Service: 1-800-654-2452 (US and Canada). From outside of the US and Canada: 314-447-8871. Fax: 314-447-8029. For print support, e-mail: JournalsCustomerService-usa@elsevier.com. For online support, e-mail: JournalsOnline Support-usa@elsevier.com.**

Reprints. For copies of 100 or more of articles in this publication, please contact the Commercial Reprints Department, Elsevier Inc., 360 Park Avenue South, New York, New York, 10010-1710; Tel.: +1-212-633-3874, Fax: +1-212-633-3820, and E-mail: reprints@elsevier.com.

Rheumatic Disease Clinics of North America is covered in *MEDLINE/PubMed (Index Medicus), Current Contents/Clinical Medicine, Science Citation Index, ISI/BIOMED,* and *EMBASE/Excerpta Medica.*

Contributors

CONSULTING EDITOR

MICHAEL H. WEISMAN, MD
Cedars-Sinai Chair and Director, Division of Rheumatology, Professor of Medicine, Cedars-Sinai Medical Center; Distinguished Professor, David Geffen School of Medicine at UCLA, Los Angeles, California

EDITORS

JENNIFER L. BARTON, MD
Assistant Professor of Medicine, Oregon Health and Science University; Rheumatology Attending, VA Portland Health Care System, Portland, Oregon

PATRICIA KATZ, PhD
Professor of Medicine, University of California, San Francisco, San Francisco, California

AUTHORS

LEIGH F. CALLAHAN, PhD
Mary Link Briggs Distinguished Professor of Medicine and Professor of Social Medicine and Orthopaedics, Thurston Arthritis Research Center, University of North Carolina, Chapel Hill, Chapel Hill, North Carolina

LIRON CAPLAN, MD, PhD
Associate Professor of Medicine, Veterans Affairs Medical Center (VAMC), Denver, Colorado; University of Colorado School of Medicine, Aurora, Colorado

AIMEE O. HERSH, MD
Assistant Professor, Pediatric Rheumatology, University of Utah, Salt Lake City, Utah

JOEL M. HIRSH, MD
Division of Rheumatology, Associate Professor, Department of Medicine, Denver Health, University of Colorado Denver School of Medicine, Denver, Colorado

ANNA L. KRATZ, PhD
Assistant Professor, Department of Physical Medicine and Rehabilitation, University of Michigan, Ann Arbor, Michigan

MARY MAHIEU, MD
Division of Rheumatology, Department of Medicine, Northwestern University Feinberg School of Medicine, Chicago, Illinois

HIRAL MASTER, DPT, MPH
Department of Physical Therapy, University of Delaware, Newark, Delaware

KALEB MICHAUD, PhD
Associate Professor, University of Nebraska Medical Center, Omaha, Nebraska; Co-Director, National Data Bank for Rheumatic Diseases, Wichita, Kansas

DEREK T. NHAN, BS, BA
Veterans Affairs Medical Center (VAMC), Denver, Colorado; University of Colorado School of Medicine, Aurora, Colorado

ALEXIS OGDIE, MD, MSCE
Assistant Professor of Medicine and Epidemiology, Division of Rheumatology, Center for Clinical Epidemiology and Biostatistics, Perelman School of Medicine, University of Pennsylvania, Philadelphia, Pennsylvania

ANA-MARIA ORBAI, MD, MHS
Assistant Professor of Medicine, Division of Rheumatology, Johns Hopkins University, Baltimore, Maryland

RUSSELL E. PELLAR, BESc
Faculty of Medicine, Saint Joseph's Health Care, Schulich School of Medicine and Dentistry, University of Western Ontario, London, Ontario, Canada

JANET ELIZABETH POPE, MD, MPH, FRCPC
University of Western Ontario; Professor of Medicine, Division Head, Rheumatology, Department of Medicine, St. Joseph's Health Care, London, Ontario, Canada

ROSALIND RAMSEY-GOLDMAN, MD, DrPH
Professor of Medicine, Division of Rheumatology, Department of Medicine, Northwestern University Feinberg School of Medicine, Chicago, Illinois

PARISSA K. SALIMIAN, BA
Clinical Research Coordinator, Division of Developmental Medicine, Boston Children's Hospital, Boston, Massachusetts

THERESA M. TINGEY, B Arts Sc
Faculty of Medicine, Saint Joseph's Health Care, Schulich School of Medicine and Dentistry, University of Western Ontario, London, Ontario, Canada

LILIAN H.D. VAN TUYL, MSc, PhD, MBA
Amsterdam Rheumatology and Immunology Center, VU University Medical Center, Amsterdam, The Netherlands

ELIZABETH R. WAHL, MD
Fellow, VA Quality Scholars Program, Division of Rheumatology, San Francisco Veterans Affairs Medical Center, San Francisco, California

ELISSA R. WEITZMAN, ScD, MSc
Assistant Professor, Division of Adolescent/Young Adult Medicine, Boston Children's Hospital; Department of Pediatrics, Harvard Medical School; Computational Health Informatics Program, Boston Children's Hospital, Boston, Massachusetts

DANIEL K. WHITE, PT, ScD, MSc
Department of Physical Therapy, University of Delaware, Newark, Delaware

DAVID A. WILLIAMS, PhD
Professor, Departments of Anesthesiology, Medicine, Psychiatry, and Psychology, University of Michigan, Ann Arbor, Michigan

JAMES P. WITTER, MD, PhD, FACR
Chief Science Officer PROMIS and PEPR, Medical Officer/Program Director, Rheumatic Diseases Clinical Program, National Institute of Arthritis and Musculoskeletal and Skin Diseases, Bethesda, Maryland

JINOOS YAZDANY, MD, MPH
Associate Professor, Division of Rheumatology, Department of Internal Medicine, University of California, San Francisco, San Francisco, California

SUSAN YOUNT, PhD
Associate Professor, Department of Medicine Social Sciences, Northwestern University Feinberg School of Medicine, Chicago, Illinois

Contents

Foreword: Patient-Reported Outcomes in Rheumatic Diseases xiii

Michael H. Weisman

Preface: The Patient Experience: Patient-Reported Outcomes in Rheumatology xv

Jennifer L. Barton and Patricia Katz

The History of Patient-Reported Outcomes in Rheumatology 205

Leigh F. Callahan

The rheumatology community began incorporating patient-reported outcomes in the early 1980s, helping shift the care of chronic diseases from a narrower biomedical model to a broader biopsychosocial model of health. Early efforts were focused primarily in clinical trials and clinical research, but over the last decade there has been increasing use in routine rheumatology clinical care. More than 250 valid and reliable scales to assess domains of importance to patients with rheumatic conditions have been developed. The approach to measurement continues to be refined. Rheumatology has much to be proud of in contributions to the important field of patient-reported outcomes.

Patient-Reported Outcomes in Rheumatoid Arthritis 219

Lilian H.D. van Tuyl and Kaleb Michaud

Patient-reported outcomes (PROs) and their measures have a long and important history for determining the status and treatment of patients with rheumatoid arthritis (RA). This article describes the history and evolution of PROs for RA and the current state of the field, with key examples of accepted and widely used measures, and offers some reflection on the roles of PROs for the study and management of RA.

Patient-Reported Measures of Physical Function in Knee Osteoarthritis 239

Daniel K. White and Hiral Master

Knee osteoarthritis is a common cause of an array of functional limitations in older adults, and the accurate assessment of such limitations is critical for practicing clinicians and scientists. Patient-reported measures are a valuable resource to track the type and severity of limitation, although the psychometric performance of each instrument should be thoroughly evaluated before adoption. This article reviews the validity, reliability, sensitivity to change, and responsiveness of 3 patient-reported measures of physical function: the Western Ontario and McMaster Universities Osteoarthritis Index, the Knee Injury and Osteoarthritis Outcome Score, and the Patient Reported Outcomes Measurement Information System Physical Function scale.

Patient-Reported Outcomes in Systemic Lupus Erythematosus **253**

Mary Mahieu, Susan Yount, and Rosalind Ramsey-Goldman

Successful management of complex conditions such as systemic lupus erythematosus (SLE) and comorbid conditions benefit from patient-reported outcomes (PRO). Measuring health-related quality of life with PROs provides SLE patients with an opportunity to participate in their treatment and to facilitate better communication with the multidisciplinary team involved in their care. Health outcomes research has produced well-validated instruments that can be used across diseases; others have been specifically developed for SLE. The use of generic and SLE-specific PROs depends on needs, including population monitoring, treatment decision making, clinical trials research, and for evaluating and comparing the effect of therapies.

Patient-Reported Outcomes in Psoriatic Arthritis **265**

Ana-Maria Orbai and Alexis Ogdie

Patient-reported outcome (PRO) measures are an important component to assessing disease impact and therapy response in patients with psoriatic arthritis (PsA). Overall, there are few PsA-specific PROs. Most PROs used in PsA are borrowed from other diseases (eg, rheumatoid arthritis and ankylosing spondylitis) or general population PROs. PROs are used in PsA clinical trials and in the clinical management of PsA. In this review, we discuss the most commonly used PRO in PsA, including their inclusion in composite measures. Future studies may be helpful to determine the best performing PROs in patients with PsA.

Patient-Reported Outcomes in Axial Spondyloarthritis **285**

Derek T. Nhan and Liron Caplan

Axial spondyloarthritis (axSpA), a subtype of spondyloarthritis, is a debilitating inflammatory condition involving the spinal and sacroiliac joints, contributing to a significant diminution in quality of life. Historically, characterization of patient outcomes in axSpA has been a challenge due to the lack of data from longitudinal epidemiologic studies and the nonspecific nature of inflammatory laboratory markers to monitor disease activity. In this review, measures developed to address these clinical domains are discussed and compared, of which 3 are commonly used in diagnosis and therapeutic planning. Provider data regarding utilization of these measures are also included to clarify current clinical practice trends.

Patient-Reported Outcome Measures in Systemic Sclerosis (Scleroderma) **301**

Russell E. Pellar, Theresa M. Tingey, and Janet Elizabeth Pope

Scleroderma (systemic sclerosis) is a rare autoimmune connective tissue disease that can damage multiple organs and reduce quality of life. Patient-reported outcome measures capture the patient's perspective. Some measures are specific to systemic sclerosis and others are general. Patient-reported outcomes in systemic sclerosis are important to aid in understanding the impact of systemic sclerosis on patients.

Patient-Reported Outcomes and Fibromyalgia **317**

David A. Williams and Anna L. Kratz

Fibromyalgia (FM) is classified as a chronic pain condition accompanied by symptoms of fatigue, sleep problems, problems with cognition, negative mood, limited functional status, and the presence of other chronic overlapping pain conditions. Comprehensive assessment of all of these components can be challenging. This paper provides an overview of patient-reported approaches that can be taken to assess FM in the contexts of diagnosis, symptom monitoring, phenotyping/characterization, and for purposes of clinical trials.

Using Patient-Reported Outcome Measures to Capture the Patient's Voice in Research and Care of Juvenile Idiopathic Arthritis **333**

Aimee O. Hersh, Parissa K. Salimian, and Elissa R. Weitzman

Patient-reported outcome (PRO) measures provide a valuable window into how patients with juvenile idiopathic arthritis and their parents perceive their functioning, quality of life, and medication side effects in the context of their disease and treatment. Momentum behind adoption of PRO measures is increasing as these patient-relevant tools capture information pertinent to taking a patient-centered approach to health care and research. This article reviews the clinical and research utility of obtaining PROs across domains applicable to the experience of juvenile idiopathic arthritis and summarizes available self-report and parent-proxy PRO measures. Current challenges and limitations of PRO usage are discussed.

The Challenge and Opportunity of Capturing Patient Reported Measures of Rheumatoid Arthritis Disease Activity in Vulnerable Populations with Limited Health Literacy and Limited English Proficiency **347**

Joel M. Hirsh

Limited health literacy and limited English proficiency are widely prevalent and contribute to rheumatoid arthritis (RA) health care disparities. The RA Patient Global Assessment of Disease Activity often introduces complexity to the health care encounters of patients and research subjects with limited health literacy and limited English proficiency. Important work is being done to ensure that patient-reported outcomes are validated and appropriate for diverse and vulnerable populations.

Challenges and Opportunities in Using Patient-reported Outcomes in Quality Measurement in Rheumatology **363**

Elizabeth R. Wahl and Jinoos Yazdany

Use of patient-reported outcome measures (PROs) in rheumatology research is widespread, but use of PRO data to evaluate the quality of rheumatologic care delivered is less well established. This article reviews the use of PROs in assessing health care quality, and highlights challenges and opportunities specific to their use in rheumatology quality measurement. It first explores other countries' experiences collecting and evaluating national PRO data to assess quality of care. It describes the current use of PROs as quality measures in rheumatology, and frames an agenda for future work supporting development of meaningful quality measures based on PROs.

The Promise of Patient-Reported Outcomes Measurement Information System—Turning Theory into Reality: A Uniform Approach to Patient-Reported Outcomes Across Rheumatic Diseases **377**

James P. Witter

PROMIS, the Patient-Reported Outcomes Measurement Information System, is opening new possibilities to explore and learn how patient (or proxy) self-report of core symptoms and health-related quality of life can meaningfully advance clinical research and patient care. PROMIS leverages Item Response Theory to agnostically assess, across diseases and conditions or clinical settings, numerous universally applicable core "domains" of health (symptoms and functioning) from the patient perspective. Importantly, PROMIS is enabling the testing and adoption of computerized adaptive testing, which holds great potential to minimize patient burden while maximizing accuracy.

Index **395**

RHEUMATIC DISEASE CLINICS OF NORTH AMERICA

FORTHCOMING ISSUES

August 2016
Sjogren's Disease
Hal Scofield, *Editor*

November 2016
Imaging in Rheumatic Diseases
Pamela F. Weiss, *Editor*

February 2017
Infection and Malignancy in Rheumatic Diseases
Kevin Winthrop and Leonard Calabrese, *Editors*

RECENT ISSUES

February 2016
Corticosteroids
Marcy B. Bolster, *Editor*

November 2015
Psoriatic Arthritis
Christopher T. Ritchlin, *Editor*

August 2015
Scleroderma
Maureen D. Mayes, *Editor*

Foreword

Patient-Reported Outcomes in Rheumatic Diseases

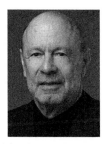

Michael H. Weisman, MD
Consulting Editor

Barton and Katz have assembled an issue that will be a standard reference for the near future. Their experts show clearly the value of patient-reported outcomes (PROs) in SLE precisely because the disease is extraordinarily complex, and hence, patient input is especially relevant. Similar issues are in play for psoriatic arthritis, since what patients think is important may vary widely from physician assessment. Nowhere could the impact of disease be more potentially devastating than in systemic sclerosis, where patient experience must be paramount. Juvenile arthritis is a special case because of the need to understand the patients, parents, and parent-proxy perspective approach to appraisals of health care decision-making. A very thoughtful article describing the issues of literacy and English proficiency on health outcomes gives some important insights into the challenges of health care disparities. The impact of patient-reported outcomes in the arena of quality assessment is discussed, keeping in mind the challenges posed in the United States by the variability of information technology infrastructures and the diversity of our patient populations. Clearly, the burden of fibromyalgia and knee OA are best captured by PROs, and for rheumatoid arthritis, the PRO has had an almost unchallenged high-ranking status as a meaningful assessment of the impact of this disease. In recent years, PROs are becoming an important aspect of axial spondyloarthritis following the lead of our European colleagues, who have used quite rigorous methodologies to categorize the patient experience with this common chronic disease. PROMIS, or patient-reported outcomes measurement information system, standardizes the collection of universally relevant domains of health and disease into one instrument that can capture outcomes across diseases and clinical settings—a major research advance that is bearing fruit as we speak.

Rheum Dis Clin N Am 42 (2016) xiii–xiv
http://dx.doi.org/10.1016/j.rdc.2016.02.002 rheumatic.theclinics.com

Finally, the evolution of PROs in Rheumatology from its controversial research applications in the beginning to their evolution as part of routine care is discussed with great thoughtfulness.

Michael H. Weisman, MD
Division of Rheumatology
Cedars-Sinai Medical Center
David Geffen School of Medicine at UCLA
8700 Beverly Boulevard
Los Angeles, CA 90024, USA

E-mail address:
Michael.Weisman@cshs.org

Preface

The Patient Experience: Patient-Reported Outcomes in Rheumatology

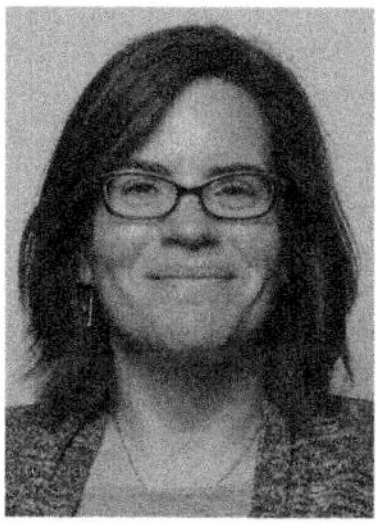
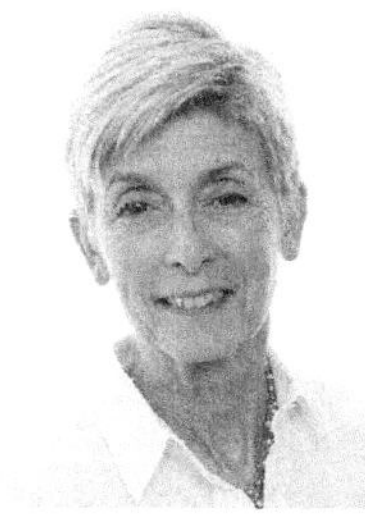

Jennifer L. Barton, MD   Patricia Katz, PhD
Editors

Historically, measurement of disease activity and response to therapy in the rheumatic diseases has presented significant challenges to clinicians, researchers, and patients. Disease-specific and generic instruments utilized in rheumatology have progressed over time and increasingly (although not entirely) reflect what matter to patients. Rheumatology has relied on patient-reported outcomes (PROs) perhaps more heavily than other subspecialties, as we lack specific biomarkers or gold standards such as blood pressure or hemoglobin A1c to track disease. Given the chronicity of disease and its impact on patient quality of life, work productivity, morbidity, and mortality, arriving at accurate, consistent, and feasible outcome measures for clinical practice and clinical trials is imperative. The patient experience has increasingly been recognized as central to the mission of rheumatology to achieve high-quality, high-value care.

In this issue of the *Rheumatic Disease Clinics of North America*, our contributors provide a wide-ranging view of PROs' development and use in rheumatology. First, we present a review of the history of PROs in rheumatology using the Health Assessment Questionnaire as an example, followed by articles on disease-specific selection and use of PROs (including rheumatoid arthritis, lupus, psoriatic arthritis, ankylosing spondylitis, scleroderma, fibromyalgia, juvenile idiopathic arthritis, and osteoarthritis). Each of these disease-specific articles discusses relevant PRO domains and provides suggestions for instruments to assess those domains.

The final three articles address several broad topics relevant to assessment of PROs in rheumatology. As disparities in process and outcomes in the rheumatic diseases persist despite advances in treatment and treatment strategies, it is important to ensure that PROs accurately reflect the experience of all patients, including those who are most vulnerable to poorer outcomes: those with limited health literacy and limited English language proficiency. Hirsh highlights the challenges of using measures

Rheum Dis Clin N Am 42 (2016) xv–xvi
http://dx.doi.org/10.1016/j.rdc.2016.02.001   rheumatic.theclinics.com
0889-857X/16/$ – see front matter

that were not developed with input from diverse populations of patients with rheumatic disease who may face barriers to communication.

Exciting progress has been made in the field of PROs in terms of technology and the use of computer- adapted testing and item response theory under the guidance of the NIH-funded Patient-Reported Outcomes Measurement Information System, or PROMIS. In the article by Wahl and Yazdany, an exploration of the intersection between quality measures and PROs is presented, and the importance of PROs to delivering quality of care to rheumatology patients worldwide is discussed. In the final article by Witter, the background of PROMIS, the technology utilized, the use of PROMIS measures in rheumatology clinical practice as well as research, and the promise of PROMIS to "enable precision, person-centered medicine" in the future.

Over the past two decades, in addition to tremendous progress in the treatment and strategies of rheumatic diseases, the field of PROs has advanced. The patient experience lies at the center of rheumatologic care. It is hoped that the standardization of PROs, their incorporation into routine practice, and quality metrics will move the field of rheumatology closer to its goal of providing high-quality, equitable care to all, in ways that matter most to patients.

We appreciate the generous contributions to this issue from authors who are experts in the field and drivers of innovation in rheumatology.

Jennifer L. Barton, MD
Oregon Health & Science University
VA Portland Health Care System
3710 SW US Veterans Road
Portland, OR 97239, USA

Patricia Katz, PhD
University of California, San Francisco
3333 California Street
Suite 270
San Francisco, CA 94143, USA

E-mail addresses:
bartoje@ohsu.edu (J.L. Barton)
patti.katz@ucsf.edu (P. Katz)

The History of Patient-Reported Outcomes in Rheumatology

Leigh F. Callahan, PhD

KEYWORDS

• Patient-reported outcomes • Health Assessment Questionnaire
• Arthritis Impact Measurement Scales • Rheumatic diseases • Rheumatology
• Health status assessment • Self-report measures

KEY POINTS

- Historically, rheumatology researchers and clinicians have been at the forefront of patient-reported outcomes assessment and changing the paradigm from a narrower biomedical model to a broader biopsychosocial model of health.
- The Health Assessment Questionnaire and the Arthritis Impact Measurement Scales were published in 1980 as the foundation patient-reported outcome scales in rheumatology.
- More than 250 instruments are available for measuring outcomes of importance to patients with rheumatic diseases, including functional incapacity, disability, pain, fatigue, depression, anxiety, perceived helplessness, self-efficacy, sleep disruptions, work limitations, and social role participation.
- The approach for patient-reported outcome measurement is moving from classic test theory to modern psychometric theory and the Patient Reported Outcome Measurement Information System offers opportunities for rheumatology.
- The initial use of patient-reported outcomes measures in rheumatology was in the research arena, but strong efforts were made over the last 15 to 20 years to promote their value in routine clinical care to assess, monitor, and predict outcomes, such as work disability, costs, and mortality and assess new therapies in clinical trials.

INTRODUCTION

Chronic diseases require measurement for diagnosis and management. As noted by Lord Kelvin in the 19th century, "When you cannot measure it, when you cannot express it in numbers, you have scarcely, in your thoughts, advanced to the stage of science, whatever the matter may be." Measurement in arthritis and rheumatic

---

No conflicts of interest.

Department of Medicine, Thurston Arthritis Research Center, University of North Carolina, Chapel Hill, 3330 Thurston Building, CB 7280, Chapel Hill, NC 27599, USA
E-mail address: Leigh_Callahan@med.unc.edu

Rheum Dis Clin N Am 42 (2016) 205–217
http://dx.doi.org/10.1016/j.rdc.2016.01.012 **rheumatic.theclinics.com**
0889-857X/16/$ – see front matter

diseases initially focused on radiographic changes, tender or swollen joints, erythrocyte sedimentation rate, grip strength, morning stiffness, and the subjective global assessment by a physician of a patient's status. In 1949, the American Rheumatism Association Functional Classification was proposed by Steinbrocker's committee to assess functional status in patients with rheumatoid arthritis (RA).[1] Physicians classified RA patients' function into 1 of 4 categories: (1) complete functional capacity, (2) functional capacity adequate to conduct normal activities, (3) functional capacity adequate to perform few or none, and (4) largely or wholly incapacitated.[1] This classification was the first attempt to quantify and measure functional incapacity or disability, the final common pathway of uncontrolled arthritis and many rheumatic and musculoskeletal conditions.[2]

In the 1970s, individuals interested in measuring health status outcomes noted that in chronic disease, outcome must be more sensitive and include physical, mental, and social functioning of the patient.[3,4] In rheumatic diseases, many of the outcomes of importance to the patient are best assessed through self-report. In addition to functional incapacity or disability, these outcomes include pain, fatigue, depression, anxiety, perceived helplessness, self-efficacy, sleep disruptions, work limitations, and social role participation.[5,6] As noted in the introductions to the 2003 and 2011 *Arthritis Care and Research* special issues on patient outcomes in rheumatology, historically, rheumatology researchers have been at the forefront of patient-reported outcomes assessment.[5,7] This article reviews the beginnings of patient-reported outcome assessment in rheumatic diseases, the breadth of patient-reported outcome measures and instruments available today, refinements of the patient-reported outcomes measurement approach, and efforts that have been made to incorporate patient-reported measures as a standard of assessment in clinical research including clinical trials and in routine rheumatologic clinical care.

THE BEGINNING OF PATIENT-REPORTED OUTCOMES IN RHEUMATIC DISEASES

In the February 1980 issue of *Arthritis and Rheumatism*, 2 seminal articles were published back to back.[8,9] Fries and colleagues[8] published, Measurement of Patient Outcome in Arthritis, and Meenan and colleagues[9] published Measuring Health Status in Arthritis: The Arthritis Impact Measurement Scales. Both articles described multidimensional self-report questionnaires designed to assess outcomes in patients with rheumatic disease. The article by Fries and colleagues[8] presented a structure for the representation of patient outcome represented by 5 separate dimensions: death, discomfort, disability, drug (therapeutic) toxicity, and dollar cost. Each dimension represented an outcome directly related to patient welfare, and the dimensions could be performed at interview or by patient questionnaire.[8] The patient-reported Health Assessment Questionnaire (HAQ) disability index, sometimes referred to as the *HAQ DI, original, or legacy HAQ,* evaluates difficulty in performing activities of daily living over the past week in 8 categories (dressing and grooming, arising, eating, walking, hygiene, reaching, gripping, and errands and chores). Twenty specific activities are assessed on a 4-point Likert scale from without difficulty to unable to do. Thirteen additional questions assess the use of assistive devices, and 8 additional questions assess help received from others.

The Arthritis Impact Measurement Scales (AIMS) assess physical, emotional, and social well being.[9] Mobility, physical activity, dexterity, social role, social activity, activities of daily living, pain, depression, and anxiety were all part of the original AIMS, which was a combination of previously studied and newly developed (at the time) health status scales. The 2 previously tested measures that the AIMS instrument was built on were Bush's Index of Well-Being[10] and the Rand Health Insurance Study batteries.[11] The AIMS instrument had 46 questions in the 9 groups noted above. For items that permitted a range of response levels, options ranged from never to always on a 6-point Likert scale.[9]

Both the original HAQ and AIMS spawned several derivations including the modified Stanford Health Assessment Questionnaire (MHAQ),[12] the HAQ II,[13] the multidimensional HAQ (MDHAQ),[14] the Rheumatoid Arthritis–HAQ, a difficult 8-item HAQ (DHAQ), and a rescored 20-item HAQ[15] and the Improved HAQ[16] from the HAQ.[17] For the AIMS, there is the original version, and expanded version (AIMS2),[18] a short-form of the AIMS2 (AIMS2-SF),[19] a child version,[20] and a version for the elderly (Geri-AIMS).[21] The AIMS has been translated into many languages including Spanish, Italian, Portuguese, French, Canadian French, Dutch, Swedish, Turkish, Norwegian, Greek, Chinese, Japanese, Russian, and Persian[22] and the HAQ, MHAQ, and MDHAQ into more than 60 languages and dialects.[17,23]

James Fries, MD, a founding father and leader in this specialty for almost 40 years, reflected on the early years and milestones for measurement in rheumatology in a video created for an Association of Rheumatology Health Professionals' Distinguished Lecture delivered by Teresa Brady, PhD. He noted that in the beginning the "obvious criticism to patient-oriented measures was that they were soft—scientists need to retain attention to hard measures like erythrocyte sedimentation rate." He also emphasized that social scientists developed the methods for validating these measures and stated, "...if patient reported measures were well-crafted, they had better measurement characteristics than the so called hard measures." He commented that rheumatologists were clinicians of chronic disease more than other subspecialties, contributing to their leadership in the patient-reported outcome movement. And, he stated that by "getting these measures... accepted as valid ... people almost didn't notice that their thinking had shifted from a narrower medical model to a broader psychosocial model of health and illness."

MEASURES AVAILABLE FOR ASSESSING PATIENT-REPORTED OUTCOMES IN RHEUMATIC DISEASE

After the HAQ and AIMS established the groundwork for patient-reported outcome measurement in rheumatic diseases, the field expanded exponentially. In addition to the derivations, updates, enhancements, and modifications to the HAQ and AIMS, many measures assessing a range of domains important to patients with rheumatic diseases were developed. There were also more scales targeted to specific rheumatic disease diagnoses. In 1992, a special issue of *Arthritis Care and Research (AC&R)* on health status assessment included a review of 9 measures. In 2003, a special issue of *AC&R* on patient outcomes in rheumatology included a review of 108 measures.[7] Most recently, an *AC&R* special issue in 2011 reviewed 250 measures in 4 domains.[5] The primary domains included pathology and symptoms, function, health status and quality of life, and psychological.[5] The summaries of the various measures presented in the reviews of instruments represented in the 4 domains include information on how to obtain, administer, and score the instruments, with references to the primary articles. Relevant psychometric property data of the scales are also presented. All measures in the issue have been determined to be valid and reliable and have been used extensively in rheumatology. Although quite exhaustive and comprehensive, the issue did not include all measures that were developed and used in rheumatology.

The measures reviewed in the domain of pathology and symptoms include instruments for rheumatoid arthritis,[17,24] adult and pediatric systemic lupus erythematosus,[25,26] ankylosing spondylitis,[27] gout,[28] psoriatic arthritis,[29] fibromyalgia,[30] systemic sclerosis (scleroderma),[31] adult and juvenile dermatomyositis, polymyositis, inclusion body myositis,[32] low back pain,[33] and various joints affected with osteoarthritis including the shoulder,[34] hand,[35] hip,[36] knee,[37] and foot.[38] Symptom measures of adult and pediatric pain,[39,40] fatigue,[41] and sleep[42] are also reviewed. These symptom measures include some disease-specific instruments and measures that are appropriate for a range of rheumatic diseases.

In the review of measures in the function domain, general functional status measures for adults and children that are valid in disease-specific and across several rheumatic diseases are included.[43,44] Also under this domain, patient-reported measures of disability,[22] social function and participation,[45] and work disability and productivity[46] are covered. Health status and quality-of-life measures also include adult and pediatric surveys for general health status[47,48] and disease-specific instruments.[49–52]

The psychological measures reviewed in this issue include measures of depression and depressive symptoms,[53] anxiety measures,[54] and measures of self-efficacy.[55] Other psychological measures used in rheumatic diseases that are not reviewed in the issue include perceived helplessness and the multidimensional health locus of control scales.[56–60]

REFINEMENTS OF THE PATIENT-REPORTED OUTCOME MEASUREMENT APPROACH

The scales assessing patient-reported outcomes in rheumatology from the early 1980s until around 2005 were developed and tested using classic test theory (CTT).[61] Instruments developed with CTT require administering all items of the scale, even though only some of the items may be appropriate for that particular patient's underlying illness experience. For example, some items are too high for individuals who are severely disabled (eg, can you walk a mile for a person in a wheel chair) and some items are too low for individuals with minimal disability (eg, can you get up and down from a chair for a person who is able to jog a few miles a day).[61] Item response theory (IRT), often referred to as *modern psychometric theory*, models the association between items designed to measure some latent construct, or trait, underlying an illness experience and the construct.[61,62] Examples of latent constructs include common symptoms of rheumatic diseases, such as pain, fatigue, and stiffness. A radiograph or laboratory test cannot be used to evaluate these symptoms, which are certainly experienced by people with arthritis. Patient-reported items that are scaled and scored measure these constructs indirectly. IRT methods make it possible to estimate a person's level of a trait with any subset of items appropriate for the person selected from a larger item bank, allowing for efficiency, especially when administered through computerized adaptive tests.[62]

In late 2004, the National Institutes of Health initiated a multicenter cooperative group referred to as *the Patient-Reported Outcomes Measurement Information System* (PROMIS).[63] The goal of PROMIS was to build and validate common, accessible item banks to measure key symptoms and health concepts applicable to a range of chronic conditions, including rheumatic diseases. The effort was designed to enable efficient and interpretable clinical practice and clinical trial applications of patient-reported outcomes.[63]

PROMIS developed measures of self-reported health within a domain hierarchy that included self-reported health, physical health, mental health, and social health.[61] Although all of the domains are relevant to rheumatic diseases, the physical health domain was particularly relevant, as it included physical function, pain, and fatigue.[61] In PROMIS, the term *physical function* rather than *disability* was preferred.[16,64]

Physical function represents the ability to perform activities of daily living, including instrumental activities. A PROMIS physical function item bank of 124 items was created and can be administered using computerized adaptive tests.[61] PROMIS has also developed several static short forms including a 20-item PROMIS HAQ, which corresponds to the HAQ-DI. The PROMIS HAQ differs from the HAQ-DI in 2 ways. The PROMIS HAQ does not have the 1-week timeframe for an individual to reference their physical function and it also has an added response option from the original 4 responses. An additional choice of "with a little difficulty" has been added.[16]

PROMIS and the use of IRT offer the ability to assess patients with differing medical conditions at various levels of impairments (both at the highest and lowest trait levels) with more precision and efficiency. The track record of rheumatology as the subspecialty that led patient-reported outcomes suggests that rheumatology will embrace the opportunity offered by this measurement advance.

PATIENT-REPORTED OUTCOME MEASURES IN ROUTINE RHEUMATOLOGIC CLINICAL CARE AND CLINICAL TRIALS

The initial use of patient-reported outcome measures was in the research arena, including clinical trials. Only a few rheumatologists were using patient questionnaires in routine clinical care in the 1980s and early 1990s. The 2 individuals who not only made substantial contributions to the development of patient self-reported questionnaires and their use in research but also led the charge to incorporate these measures into routine rheumatologic clinical care are Theodore Pincus, MD, and Frederick Wolfe, MD. In 1991, the 2 published an editorial in the *Journal of Rheumatology* titled, "Standard self-report questionnaires in routine clinical and research practice—an opportunity for patients and physicians."[65] This article expressed a tireless commitment since the early 1980s to promote the use of patient-reported measures through publications, workshops, and one-on-one communication throughout rheumatology worldwide.

In May 1995, Dr Wolfe was guest editor of an issue of *Rheumatic Disease Clinics of North America* titled *Data Collection and Analysis*. He noted in the preface to the issue that it was "meant to serve as a manual for research within the longitudinal setting of the clinic where patient care is administered."[66] The issue covered outcomes and disease factors that rheumatologists treating within the broad bio-psycho-social model are concerned with, including pain, function, psychological status, radiographic damage, laboratory measures, physical examination components, costs, and mortality. Dr Pincus authored the lead article in the issue titled, Why should rheumatologists collect patient self-report questionnaires in routine rheumatologic care?[67] He summarized the evidence for their use noting that they are: highly reliable; correlated significantly with data from traditional joint counts, radiographs, laboratory tests, and physical function measures; predictive of morbidity and mortality; able to detect change in status in clinical trials; document long-term outcomes; offer measurable insights into psychosocial problems; and provide sensitive and simple methods for monitoring inexpensively.[67] He has expanded the evidence since then, promoting the value of the measures in quality of care, treating to target, predicting mortality, and providing value in clinical trials in addition to adding to the support for their use in routine clinical care.[68–88] Dr Pincus has "viewed quantitative measurement of patient status in routine care of patients with rheumatic diseases more as a continuous quality improvement activity, rather than as a research activity, with evolution of use of the HAQ to a 2-page multi-dimensional health global estimate of status, the 3 RA core data set measures consolidated into a RAPID3 (routine assessment of patient index data) score, as well as queries concerning sleep, anxiety depression, symptom checklist (review of systems and screen for distress and depression), change in status, exercise status, and recent medical history".[89]

SUMMARY

Rheumatic diseases are chronic conditions in which patients experience functional declines; symptoms of pain, fatigue, and stiffness; challenges in work productivity and social roles; and psychosocial issues and distress. All of these aspects of disease are best captured through patient self-report. For the past 35 years, rheumatology has led the way in chronic diseases for the development, evaluation, and use of patient-reported outcome measures in research, routine clinical care, and clinical trials. Patient-reported outcome measurement continues to evolve and the acceptance of the measures routinely is still not where it needs to be, but much has been accomplished.

ACKNOWLEDGMENTS

The author thanks Teresa Brady, PhD, for sharing the videos from her Association of Rheumatology Health Professionals' Distinguished Lecture.

REFERENCES

1. Steinbrocker O, Traeger CH, Batterman RC. Therapeutic criteria in rheumatoid arthritis. J Am Med Assoc 1949;140(8):659–62.
2. Liang MH, Jette AM. Measuring functional ability in chronic arthritis: a critical review. Arthritis Rheum 1981;24(1):80–6.
3. Ware JE Jr. Scales for measuring general health perceptions. Health Serv Res 1976;11(4):396–415.
4. Gilson BS, Gilson JS, Bergner M, et al. The sickness impact profile. Development of an outcome measure of health care. Am J Public Health 1975;65(12):1304–10.
5. Katz PP. Introduction to special issue: patient outcomes in rheumatology, 2011. Arthritis Care Res 2011;63(Suppl 11):S1–3.
6. Golightly YM, Allen KD, Nyrop KA, et al. Patient-reported outcomes to initiate a provider-patient dialog for the management of hip and knee osteoarthritis. Semin Arthritis Rheum 2015;45(2):123–31.
7. Katz PP. Introduction to special patient outcomes in rheumatology issue of Arthritis Care & Research. Arthritis Care Res 2003;49(S5):S1–4.
8. Fries JF, Spitz P, Kraines RG, et al. Measurement of patient outcome in arthritis. Arthritis Rheum 1980;23(2):137–45.
9. Meenan RF, Gertman PM, Mason JH. Measuring health status in arthritis. The arthritis impact measurement scales. Arthritis Rheum 1980;23(2):146–52.
10. Patrick DL, Bush JW, Chen MM. Toward an operational definition of health. J Health Soc Behav 1973;14(1):6–23.
11. Brook RH, Ware JE Jr, Davies-Avery A, et al. Overview of adult health measures fielded in Rand's health insurance study. Med Care 1979;17(7 Suppl):iii–x, 1–131.
12. Pincus T, Summey JA, Soraci SA Jr, et al. Assessment of patient satisfaction in activities of daily living using a modified Stanford Health Assessment Questionnaire. Arthritis Rheum 1983;26(11):1346–53.
13. Wolfe F, Michaud K, Pincus T. Development and validation of the health assessment questionnaire II: a revised version of the health assessment questionnaire. Arthritis Rheum 2004;50(10):3296–305.

14. Pincus T, Swearingen C, Wolfe F. Toward a multidimensional Health Assessment Questionnaire (MDHAQ): assessment of advanced activities of daily living and psychological status in the patient-friendly health assessment questionnaire format. Arthritis Rheum 1999;42(10):2220–30.
15. Wolfe F. Which HAQ is best? A comparison of the HAQ, MHAQ and RA-HAQ, a difficult 8 item HAQ (DHAQ), and a rescored 20 item HAQ (HAQ20): analyses in 2,491 rheumatoid arthritis patients following leflunomide initiation. J Rheumatol 2001;28(5):982–9.
16. Fries JF, Cella D, Rose M, et al. Progress in assessing physical function in arthritis: PROMIS short forms and computerized adaptive testing. J Rheumatol 2009;36(9):2061–6.
17. Maska L, Anderson J, Michaud K. Measures of functional status and quality of life in rheumatoid arthritis: Health Assessment Questionnaire Disability Index (HAQ), Modified Health Assessment Questionnaire (MHAQ), Multidimensional Health Assessment Questionnaire (MDHAQ), Health Assessment Questionnaire II (HAQ-II), Improved Health Assessment Questionnaire (Improved HAQ), and Rheumatoid Arthritis Quality of Life (RAQoL). Arthritis Care Res 2011;63(Suppl 11):S4–13.
18. Meenan RF, Mason JH, Anderson JJ, et al. AIMS2. The content and properties of a revised and expanded Arthritis Impact Measurement Scales Health Status Questionnaire. Arthritis Rheum 1992;35(1):1–10.
19. Guillemin F, Coste J, Pouchot J, et al. The AIMS2-SF: a short form of the Arthritis Impact Measurement Scales 2. French Quality of Life in Rheumatology Group. Arthritis Rheum 1997;40(7):1267–74.
20. Coulton CJ, Zborowsky E, Lipton J, et al. Assessment of the reliability and validity of the arthritis impact measurement scales for children with juvenile arthritis. Arthritis Rheum 1987;30(7):819–24.
21. Hughes SL, Edelman P, Chang RW, et al. The GERI-AIMS. Reliability and validity of the arthritis impact measurement scales adapted for elderly respondents. Arthritis Rheum 1991;34(7):856–65.
22. Gignac MA, Cao X, McAlpine J, et al. Measures of disability: Arthritis Impact Measurement Scales 2 (AIMS2), Arthritis Impact Measurement Scales 2-Short Form (AIMS2-SF), The Organization for Economic Cooperation and Development (OECD) Long-Term Disability (LTD) Questionnaire, EQ-5D, World Health Organization Disability Assessment Schedule II (WHODASII), Late-Life Function and Disability Instrument (LLFDI), and Late-Life Function and Disability Instrument-Abbreviated Version (LLFDI-Abbreviated). Arthritis Care Res 2011;63(Suppl 11):S308–24.
23. Bruce B, Fries JF. The Stanford Health Assessment Questionnaire: dimensions and practical applications. Health Qual Life Outcomes 2003;1:20.
24. Anderson JK, Zimmerman L, Caplan L, et al. Measures of rheumatoid arthritis disease activity: Patient (PtGA) and Provider (PrGA) Global Assessment of Disease Activity, Disease Activity Score (DAS) and Disease Activity Score with 28-Joint Counts (DAS28), Simplified Disease Activity Index (SDAI), Clinical Disease Activity Index (CDAI), Patient Activity Score (PAS) and Patient Activity Score-II (PASII), Routine Assessment of Patient Index Data (RAPID), Rheumatoid Arthritis Disease Activity Index (RADAI) and Rheumatoid Arthritis Disease Activity Index-5 (RADAI-5), Chronic Arthritis Systemic Index (CASI), Patient-Based Disease Activity Score With ESR (PDAS1) and Patient-Based Disease Activity Score without ESR (PDAS2), and Mean Overall Index for Rheumatoid Arthritis (MOI-RA). Arthritis Care Res 2011;63(Suppl 11):S14–36.

25. Romero-Diaz J, Isenberg D, Ramsey-Goldman R. Measures of adult systemic lupus erythematosus: updated version of British Isles Lupus Assessment Group (BILAG 2004), European Consensus Lupus Activity Measurements (ECLAM), Systemic Lupus Activity Measure, Revised (SLAM-R), Systemic Lupus Activity Questionnaire for Population Studies (SLAQ), Systemic Lupus Erythematosus Disease Activity Index 2000 (SLEDAI-2K), and Systemic Lupus International Collaborating Clinics/American College of Rheumatology Damage Index (SDI). Arthritis Care Res 2011;63(Suppl 11):S37–46.
26. Lattanzi B, Consolaro A, Solari N, et al. Measures of disease activity and damage in pediatric systemic lupus erythematosus: British Isles Lupus Assessment Group (BILAG), European Consensus Lupus Activity Measurement (ECLAM), Systemic Lupus Activity Measure (SLAM), Systemic Lupus Erythematosus Disease Activity Index (SLEDAI), Physician's Global Assessment of Disease Activity (MD Global), and Systemic Lupus International Collaborating Clinics/American College of Rheumatology Damage Index (SLICC/ACR DI; SDI). Arthritis Care Res 2011; 63(Suppl 11):S112–7.
27. Zochling J. Measures of symptoms and disease status in ankylosing spondylitis: Ankylosing Spondylitis Disease Activity Score (ASDAS), Ankylosing Spondylitis Quality of Life Scale (ASQoL), Bath Ankylosing Spondylitis Disease Activity Index (BASDAI), Bath Ankylosing Spondylitis Functional Index (BASFI), Bath Ankylosing Spondylitis Global Score (BAS-G), Bath Ankylosing Spondylitis Metrology Index (BASMI), Dougados Functional Index (DFI), and Health Assessment Questionnaire for the Spondylarthropathies (HAQ-S). Arthritis Care Res 2011;63(Suppl 11):S47–58.
28. Taylor WJ. Gout measures: Gout Assessment Questionnaire (GAQ, GAQ2.0), and physical measurement of tophi. Arthritis Care Res 2011;63(Suppl 11):S59–63.
29. Mease PJ. Measures of psoriatic arthritis: Tender and Swollen Joint Assessment, Psoriasis Area and Severity Index (PASI), Nail Psoriasis Severity Index (NAPSI), Modified Nail Psoriasis Severity Index (mNAPSI), Mander/Newcastle Enthesitis Index (MEI), Leeds Enthesitis Index (LEI), Spondyloarthritis Research Consortium of Canada (SPARCC), Maastricht Ankylosing Spondylitis Enthesis Score (MASES), Leeds Dactylitis Index (LDI), Patient Global for Psoriatic Arthritis, Dermatology Life Quality Index (DLQI), Psoriatic Arthritis Quality of Life (PsA-QOL), Functional Assessment of Chronic Illness Therapy-Fatigue (FACIT-F), Psoriatic Arthritis Response Criteria (PsARC), Psoriatic Arthritis Joint Activity Index (PsAJAI), Disease Activity in Psoriatic Arthritis (DAPSA), and Composite Psoriatic Disease Activity Index (CPDAI). Arthritis Care Res 2011;63(Suppl 11):S64–85.
30. Williams DA, Arnold LM. Measures of fibromyalgia: Fibromyalgia Impact Questionnaire (FIQ), Brief Pain Inventory (BPI), Multidimensional Fatigue Inventory (MFI-20), Medical Outcomes Study (MOS) Sleep Scale, and Multiple Ability Self-Report Questionnaire (MASQ). Arthritis Care Res 2011;63(Suppl 11):S86–97.
31. Pope J. Measures of systemic sclerosis (scleroderma): Health Assessment Questionnaire (HAQ) and Scleroderma HAQ (SHAQ), physician- and patient-rated global assessments, Symptom Burden Index (SBI), University of California, Los Angeles, Scleroderma Clinical Trials Consortium Gastrointestinal Scale (UCLA SCTC GIT) 2.0, Baseline Dyspnea Index (BDI) and Transition Dyspnea Index (TDI) (Mahler's Index), Cambridge Pulmonary Hypertension Outcome Review (CAMPHOR), and Raynaud's Condition Score (RCS). Arthritis Care Res 2011; 63(Suppl 11):S98–111.
32. Rider LG, Werth VP, Huber AM, et al. Measures of adult and juvenile dermatomyositis, polymyositis, and inclusion body myositis: Physician and Patient/Parent

Global Activity, Manual Muscle Testing (MMT), Health Assessment Questionnaire (HAQ)/Childhood Health Assessment Questionnaire (C-HAQ), Childhood Myositis Assessment Scale (CMAS), Myositis Disease Activity Assessment Tool (MDAAT), Disease Activity Score (DAS), Short Form 36 (SF-36), Child Health Questionnaire (CHQ), physician global damage, Myositis Damage Index (MDI), Quantitative Muscle Testing (QMT), Myositis Functional Index-2 (FI-2), Myositis Activities Profile (MAP), Inclusion Body Myositis Functional Rating Scale (IBMFRS), Cutaneous Dermatomyositis Disease Area and Severity Index (CDASI), Cutaneous Assessment Tool (CAT), Dermatomyositis Skin Severity Index (DSSI), Skindex, and Dermatology Life Quality Index (DLQI). Arthritis Care Res 2011;63(Suppl 11):S118–57.

33. Smeets R, Koke A, Lin CW, et al. Measures of function in low back pain/disorders: Low Back Pain Rating Scale (LBPRS), Oswestry Disability Index (ODI), Progressive Isoinertial Lifting Evaluation (PILE), Quebec Back Pain Disability Scale (QBPDS), and Roland-Morris Disability Questionnaire (RDQ). Arthritis Care Res 2011;63(Suppl 11):S158–73.
34. Angst F, Schwyzer HK, Aeschlimann A, et al. Measures of adult shoulder function: Disabilities of the Arm, Shoulder, and Hand Questionnaire (DASH) and its short version (QuickDASH), Shoulder Pain and Disability Index (SPADI), American Shoulder and Elbow Surgeons (ASES) Society standardized shoulder assessment form, Constant (Murley) Score (CS), Simple Shoulder Test (SST), Oxford Shoulder Score (OSS), Shoulder Disability Questionnaire (SDQ), and Western Ontario Shoulder Instability Index (WOSI). Arthritis Care Res 2011;63(Suppl 11):S174–88.
35. Poole JL. Measures of hand function: Arthritis Hand Function Test (AHFT), Australian Canadian Osteoarthritis Hand Index (AUSCAN), Cochin Hand Function Scale, Functional Index for Hand Osteoarthritis (FIHOA), Grip Ability Test (GAT), Jebsen Hand Function Test (JHFT), and Michigan Hand Outcomes Questionnaire (MHQ). Arthritis Care Res 2011;63(Suppl 11):S189–99.
36. Nilsdotter A, Bremander A. Measures of hip function and symptoms: Harris Hip Score (HHS), Hip Disability and Osteoarthritis Outcome Score (HOOS), Oxford Hip Score (OHS), Lequesne Index of Severity for Osteoarthritis of the Hip (LISOH), and American Academy of Orthopedic Surgeons (AAOS) Hip and Knee Questionnaire. Arthritis Care Res 2011;63(Suppl 11):S200–7.
37. Collins NJ, Misra D, Felson DT, et al. Measures of knee function: International Knee Documentation Committee (IKDC) Subjective Knee Evaluation Form, Knee Injury and Osteoarthritis Outcome Score (KOOS), Knee Injury and Osteoarthritis Outcome Score Physical Function Short Form (KOOS-PS), Knee Outcome Survey Activities of Daily Living Scale (KOS-ADL), Lysholm Knee Scoring Scale, Oxford Knee Score (OKS), Western Ontario and McMaster Universities Osteoarthritis Index (WOMAC), Activity Rating Scale (ARS), and Tegner Activity Score (TAS). Arthritis Care Res 2011;63(Suppl 11):S208–28.
38. Riskowski JL, Hagedorn TJ, Hannan MT. Measures of foot function, foot health, and foot pain: American Academy of Orthopedic Surgeons Lower Limb Outcomes Assessment: Foot and Ankle Module (AAOS-FAM), Bristol Foot Score (BFS), Revised Foot Function Index (FFI-R), Foot Health Status Questionnaire (FHSQ), Manchester Foot Pain and Disability Index (MFPDI), Podiatric Health Questionnaire (PHQ), and Rowan Foot Pain Assessment (ROFPAQ). Arthritis Care Res 2011;63(Suppl 11):S229–39.
39. Hawker GA, Mian S, Kendzerska T, et al. Measures of adult pain: Visual Analog Scale for Pain (VAS Pain), Numeric Rating Scale for Pain (NRS Pain), McGill

Pain Questionnaire (MPQ), Short-Form McGill Pain Questionnaire (SF-MPQ), Chronic Pain Grade Scale (CPGS), Short Form-36 Bodily Pain Scale (SF-36 BPS), and Measure of Intermittent and Constant Osteoarthritis Pain (ICOAP). Arthritis Care Res 2011;63(Suppl 11):S240–52.

40. Lootens CC, Rapoff MA. Measures of pediatric pain: 21-numbered circle Visual Analog Scale (VAS), E-Ouch Electronic Pain Diary, Oucher, Pain Behavior Observation Method, Pediatric Pain Assessment Tool (PPAT), and Pediatric Pain Questionnaire (PPQ). Arthritis Care Res 2011;63(Suppl 11):S253–62.
41. Hewlett S, Dures E, Almeida C. Measures of fatigue: Bristol Rheumatoid Arthritis Fatigue Multi-Dimensional Questionnaire (BRAF MDQ), Bristol Rheumatoid Arthritis Fatigue Numerical Rating Scales (BRAF NRS) for severity, effect, and coping, Chalder Fatigue Questionnaire (CFQ), Checklist Individual Strength (CIS20R and CIS8R), Fatigue Severity Scale (FSS), Functional Assessment Chronic Illness Therapy (Fatigue) (FACIT-F), Multi-Dimensional Assessment of Fatigue (MAF), Multi-Dimensional Fatigue Inventory (MFI), Pediatric Quality Of Life (PedsQL) Multi-Dimensional Fatigue Scale, Profile of Fatigue (ProF), Short Form 36 Vitality Subscale (SF-36 VT), and Visual Analog Scales (VAS). Arthritis Care Res 2011;63(Suppl 11):S263–86.
42. Omachi TA. Measures of sleep in rheumatologic diseases: Epworth Sleepiness Scale (ESS), Functional Outcome of Sleep Questionnaire (FOSQ), Insomnia Severity Index (ISI), and Pittsburgh Sleep Quality Index (PSQI). Arthritis Care Res 2011;63(Suppl 11):S287–96.
43. White DK, Wilson JC, Keysor JJ. Measures of adult general functional status: SF-36 Physical Functioning Subscale (PF-10), Health Assessment Questionnaire (HAQ), Modified Health Assessment Questionnaire (MHAQ), Katz Index of Independence in activities of daily living, Functional Independence Measure (FIM), and Osteoarthritis-Function-Computer Adaptive Test (OA-Function-CAT). Arthritis Care Res 2011;63(Suppl 11):S297–307.
44. Klepper SE. Measures of pediatric function: Child Health Assessment Questionnaire (C-HAQ), Juvenile Arthritis Functional Assessment Scale (JAFAS), Pediatric Outcomes Data Collection Instrument (PODCI), and Activities Scale for Kids (ASK). Arthritis Care Res 2011;63(Suppl 11):S371–82.
45. Wilkie R, Jordan JL, Muller S, et al. Measures of social function and participation in musculoskeletal populations: Impact on Participation and Autonomy (IPA), Keele Assessment of Participation (KAP), Participation Measure for Post-Acute Care (PM-PAC), Participation Objective, Participation Subjective (POPS), Rating of Perceived Participation (ROPP), and The Participation Scale. Arthritis Care Res 2011;63(Suppl 11):S325–36.
46. Tang K, Beaton DE, Boonen A, et al. Measures of work disability and productivity: Rheumatoid Arthritis Specific Work Productivity Survey (WPS-RA), Workplace Activity Limitations Scale (WALS), Work Instability Scale for Rheumatoid Arthritis (RA-WIS), Work Limitations Questionnaire (WLQ), and Work Productivity and Activity Impairment Questionnaire (WPAI). Arthritis Care Res 2011;63(Suppl 11): S337–49.
47. Busija L, Pausenberger E, Haines TP, et al. Adult measures of general health and health-related quality of life: Medical Outcomes Study Short Form 36-Item (SF-36) and Short Form 12-Item (SF-12) Health Surveys, Nottingham Health Profile (NHP), Sickness Impact Profile (SIP), Medical Outcomes Study Short Form 6D (SF-6D), Health Utilities Index Mark 3 (HUI3), Quality of Well-Being Scale (QWB), and Assessment of Quality of Life (AQoL). Arthritis Care Res 2011;63(Suppl 11): S383–412.

48. Hullmann SE, Ryan JL, Ramsey RR, et al. Measures of general pediatric quality of life: Child Health Questionnaire (CHQ), DISABKIDS Chronic Generic Measure (DCGM), KINDL-R, Pediatric Quality of Life Inventory (PedsQL) 4.0 Generic Core Scales, and Quality of My Life Questionnaire (QoML). Arthritis Care Res 2011;63(Suppl 11):S420–30.
49. Yazdany J. Health-related quality of life measurement in adult systemic lupus erythematosus: Lupus Quality of Life (LupusQoL), Systemic Lupus Erythematosus-Specific Quality of Life Questionnaire (SLEQOL), and Systemic Lupus Erythematosus Quality of Life Questionnaire (L-QoL). Arthritis Care Res 2011;63(Suppl 11):S413–9.
50. Flowers SR, Kashikar-Zuck S. Measures of juvenile fibromyalgia: Functional Disability Inventory (FDI), Modified Fibromyalgia Impact Questionnaire-Child Version (MFIQ-C), and Pediatric Quality of Life Inventory (PedsQL) 3.0 Rheumatology Module Pain and Hurt Scale. Arthritis Care Res 2011;63(Suppl 11):S431–7.
51. Carle AC, Dewitt EM, Seid M. Measures of health status and quality of life in juvenile rheumatoid arthritis: Pediatric Quality of Life Inventory (PedsQL) Rheumatology Module 3.0, Juvenile Arthritis Quality of Life Questionnaire (JAQQ), Paediatric Rheumatology Quality of Life Scale (PRQL), and Childhood Arthritis Health Profile (CAHP). Arthritis Care Res 2011;63(Suppl 11):S438–45.
52. Hersh A. Measures of health-related quality of life in pediatric systemic lupus erythematosus: Childhood Health Assessment Questionnaire (C-HAQ), Child Health Questionnaire (CHQ), Pediatric Quality of Life Inventory Generic Core Module (PedsQL-GC), Pediatric Quality of Life Inventory Rheumatology Module (PedsQL-RM), and Simple Measure of Impact of Lupus Erythematosus in Youngsters (SMILEY). Arthritis Care Res 2011;63(Suppl 11):S446–53.
53. Smarr KL, Keefer AL. Measures of depression and depressive symptoms: Beck Depression Inventory-II (BDI-II), Center for Epidemiologic Studies Depression Scale (CES-D), Geriatric Depression Scale (GDS), Hospital Anxiety and Depression Scale (HADS), and Patient Health Questionnaire-9 (PHQ-9). Arthritis Care Res 2011;63(Suppl 11):S454–66.
54. Julian LJ. Measures of anxiety: State-Trait Anxiety Inventory (STAI), Beck Anxiety Inventory (BAI), and Hospital Anxiety and Depression Scale-Anxiety (HADS-A). Arthritis Care Res 2011;63(Suppl 11):S467–72.
55. Brady TJ. Measures of self-efficacy: Arthritis Self-Efficacy Scale (ASES), Arthritis Self-Efficacy Scale-8 Item (ASES-8), Children's Arthritis Self-Efficacy Scale (CASE), Chronic Disease Self-Efficacy Scale (CDSES), Parent's Arthritis Self-Efficacy Scale (PASE), and Rheumatoid Arthritis Self-Efficacy Scale (RASE). Arthritis Care Res 2011;63(Suppl 11):S473–85.
56. Nicassio PM, Wallston KA, Callahan LF, et al. The measurement of helplessness in rheumatoid arthritis. The development of the arthritis helplessness index. J Rheumatol 1985;12(3):462–7.
57. Callahan LF, Brooks RH, Pincus T. Further analysis of learned helplessness in rheumatoid arthritis using a "Rheumatology Attitudes Index". J Rheumatol 1988;15(3):418–26.
58. DeVellis RF, Callahan LF. A brief measure of helplessness in rheumatic disease: the helplessness subscale of the Rheumatology Attitudes Index. J Rheumatol 1993;20(5):866–9.
59. Wallston KA, Wallston BS, DeVellis R. Development of the Multidimensional Health Locus of Control (MHLC) scales. Health Educ Monogr 1978;6(2):160–70.
60. Wallston KA, Stein MJ, Smith CA. Form C of the MHLC scales: a condition-specific measure of locus of control. J Pers Assess 1994;63(3):534–53.

61. Khanna D, Krishnan E, Dewitt EM, et al. The future of measuring patient-reported outcomes in rheumatology: Patient-Reported Outcomes Measurement Information System (PROMIS). Arthritis Care Res 2011;63(Suppl 11):S486–90.
62. Hill CD, Edwards MC, Thissen D, et al. Practical issues in the application of item response theory: a demonstration using items from the pediatric quality of life inventory (PedsQL) 4.0 generic core scales. Med Care 2007;45(5 Suppl 1):S39–47.
63. Cella D, Yount S, Rothrock N, et al. The Patient-Reported Outcomes Measurement Information System (PROMIS): progress of an NIH Roadmap cooperative group during its first two years. Med Care 2007;45(5 Suppl 1):S3–11.
64. Fries JF, Krishnan E, Bruce B. Items, instruments, crosswalks, and PROMIS. J Rheumatol 2009;36(6):1093–5.
65. Wolfe F, Pincus T. Standard self-report questionnaires in routine clinical and research practice–an opportunity for patients and rheumatologists. J Rheumatol 1991;18(5):643–6.
66. Wolfe F. Preface to data collection and analysis. Rheum Dis Clin North Am 1995; 21(2):xi–xii.
67. Pincus T. Why should rheumatologists collect patient self-report questionnaires in routine rheumatologic care? Rheum Dis Clin North Am 1995;21(2):271–319.
68. Pincus T, Sokka T. Quantitative clinical assessment in busy rheumatology settings: the value of short patient questionnaires. J Rheumatol 2008;35(7):1235–7.
69. Pincus T, Bergman MJ, Yazici Y, et al. An index of only patient-reported outcome measures, routine assessment of patient index data 3 (RAPID3), in two abatacept clinical trials: similar results to disease activity score (DAS28) and other RAPID indices that include physician-reported measures. Rheumatology (Oxford) 2008;47(3):345–9.
70. Pincus T, Amara I, Segurado OG, et al. Relative efficiencies of physician/assessor global estimates and patient questionnaire measures are similar to or greater than joint counts to distinguish adalimumab from control treatments in rheumatoid arthritis clinical trials. J Rheumatol 2008;35(2):201–5.
71. Pincus T, Yazici Y, Swearingen CJ. Quality control of a medical history: improving accuracy with patient participation, supported by a four-page version of the multidimensional health assessment questionnaire (MDHAQ). Rheum Dis Clin North Am 2009;35(4):851–60, xi.
72. Pincus T, Yazici Y, Bergman MJ. Patient questionnaires in rheumatoid arthritis: advantages and limitations as a quantitative, standardized scientific medical history. Rheum Dis Clin North Am 2009;35(4):735–43, vii.
73. Pincus T. Are patient questionnaire scores as "scientific" as laboratory tests for rheumatology clinical care? Bull NYU Hosp Jt Dis 2010;68(2):130–9.
74. Pincus T, Yazici Y, Castrejon I. Pragmatic and scientific advantages of MDHAQ/RAPID3 completion by all patients at all visits in routine clinical care. Bull NYU Hosp Jt Dis 2012;70(Suppl 1):30–6.
75. Castrejon I, Pincus T. Patient self-report outcomes to guide a treat-to-target strategy in clinical trials and usual clinical care of rheumatoid arthritis. Clin Exp Rheumatol 2012;30(4 Suppl 73):S50–5.
76. Pincus T, Gibson KA, Berthelot JM. Is a patient questionnaire without a joint examination as undesirable as a joint examination without a patient questionnaire? J Rheumatol 2014;41(4):619–21.
77. Pincus T, Castrejon I. Are patient self-report questionnaires as "scientific" as biomarkers in "treat-to-target" and prognosis in rheumatoid arthritis? Curr Pharm Des 2015;21(2):241–56.

78. Pincus T, Strand V, Koch G, et al. An index of the three core data set patient questionnaire measures distinguishes efficacy of active treatment from that of placebo as effectively as the American College of Rheumatology 20% response criteria (ACR20) or the Disease Activity Score (DAS) in a rheumatoid arthritis clinical trial. Arthritis Rheum 2003;48(3):625–30.
79. Pincus T, Sokka T. Quantitative measures for assessing rheumatoid arthritis in clinical trials and clinical care. Best Pract Res Clin Rheumatol 2003;17(5):753–81.
80. Pincus T, Sokka T. Uniform databases in early arthritis: specific measures to complement classification criteria and indices of clinical change. Clin Exp Rheumatol 2003;21(5 Suppl 31):S79–88.
81. Pincus T, Sokka T. Quantitative measures and indices to assess rheumatoid arthritis in clinical trials and clinical care. Rheum Dis Clin North Am 2004;30(4): 725–51, vi.
82. Pincus T, Keysor J, Sokka T, et al. Patient questionnaires and formal education level as prospective predictors of mortality over 10 years in 97% of 1416 patients with rheumatoid arthritis from 15 United States private practices. J Rheumatol 2004;31(2):229–34.
83. Chung C, Escalante A, Pincus T. How many versions and translations of the HAQ and its variants are needed? It doesn't matter-just use one. J Clin Rheumatol 2004;10(3):101–4.
84. Pincus T, Yazici Y, Bergman M. Development of a multi-dimensional health assessment questionnaire (MDHAQ) for the infrastructure of standard clinical care. Clin Exp Rheumatol 2005;23(5 Suppl 39):S19–28.
85. Pincus T, Wolfe F. Patient questionnaires for clinical research and improved standard patient care: is it better to have 80% of the information in 100% of patients or 100% of the information in 5% of patients? J Rheumatol 2005;32(4):575–7.
86. Pincus T, Wang X, Chung C, et al. Patient preference in a crossover clinical trial of patients with osteoarthritis of the knee or hip: face validity of self-report questionnaire ratings. J Rheumatol 2005;32(3):533–9.
87. Pincus T, Sokka T. Complexities in the quantitative assessment of patients with rheumatic diseases in clinical trials and clinical care. Clin Exp Rheumatol 2005; 23(5 Suppl 39):S1–9.
88. Pincus T, Yazici Y, Bergman M. Saving time and improving care with a multidimensional health assessment questionnaire: 10 practical considerations. J Rheumatol 2006;33(3):448–54.
89. Pincus T, Maclean R, Yazici Y, et al. Quantitative measurement of patient status in the regular care of patients with rheumatic diseases over 25 years as a continuous quality improvement activity, rather than traditional research. Clin Exp Rheumatol 2007;25(6 Suppl 47):69–81.

[illegible]

Patient-Reported Outcomes in Rheumatoid Arthritis

Lilian H.D. van Tuyl, MSc, PhD, MBA[a], Kaleb Michaud, PhD[b,c,*]

KEYWORDS

- Rheumatoid arthritis • Patient-reported outcomes • Questionnaires
- Health domains

KEY POINTS

- Patient-reported outcomes (PROs) and their measures have a long and important history for determining the status and treatment of patients with rheumatoid arthritis (RA).
- The most important and commonly studied RA PROs are also core measures: physical function, pain, and patient global assessment.
- This article describes the history and evolution of PROs for RA and the current state of the field, with key examples of accepted and widely used measures, and offers some reflection on the roles of PROs for the study and management of RA.

WHAT ARE PATIENT-REPORTED OUTCOMES AND WHY ARE THEY IMPORTANT?

Characteristics of rheumatoid arthritis (RA) can be divided into those signs and symptoms that are assessed by the patient, and those that are assessed by someone or something other than the patient. In the latter case, the assessments are considered objective measures of disease activity or damage, like acute phase reactants, the swelling of joints, or the erosions on a radiograph of a hand. In cases of signs and symptoms reported directly by the patient, without interpretation of a third person, clinicians speak of patient-reported outcomes (PROs).[1]

The degree of disease activity and response to treatment are traditionally determined by the evaluation of the RA core set or indices derived thereof.[2–8] The core set contains 3 PROs: physical function, pain, and a global assessment of disease activity. These PROs have been found to be at least as important as other physical and biochemical (more objective) measures in assessing baseline disease status, improvement during

[a] Amsterdam Rheumatology and Immunology Center, Department of Rheumatology, VU University Medical Center, PO Box 7057 1007 MB, Amsterdam, The Netherlands; [b] Department of Medicine, University of Nebraska Medical Center, 986270 Nebraska Medical Center, Omaha, NE 68198-6270, USA; [c] National Data Bank for Rheumatic Diseases, 1035 North Emporia, Suite 288, Wichita, KS 67214, USA

* Corresponding author. 986270 Nebraska Medical Center, Omaha, NE 68198-6270.
E-mail address: kmichaud@unmc.edu

Rheum Dis Clin N Am 42 (2016) 219–237
http://dx.doi.org/10.1016/j.rdc.2016.01.010 rheumatic.theclinics.com
0889-857X/16/$ – see front matter

interventions, or prediction of long-term outcome.[9–13] However, several important areas, such as fatigue and sleep quality, have only recently been identified as important to patients and thus potentially core areas for measurement.[14–19]

Patients with RA no longer depend on their physicians to tell them what to do, but increasingly take charge of their care processes and functions as partners in obtaining relevant information. Patients and professionals bring different skills, values, and experiences to research.[20–23]

This article gives an overview on the growth and current value of PRO research in RA, the application of research findings into daily clinical practice, and the gap between PRO research and practice that needs to be filled in the coming years.

HISTORY OF PATIENT-REPORTED OUTCOMES IN RHEUMATOID ARTHRITIS

RA has a rich history of PRO research and still is at the forefront of PRO measure (PROM) development and patient participation in research activities. One of the most characteristic symptoms of RA, pain, was first described as an important outcome at the beginning of the nineteenth century, when therapy for RA was mostly nonpharmacologic, with the exception of salicylates (what are now known as nonsteroidal antiinflammatory drugs) such as ibuprofen and diclofenac, but with a less favorable safety profile[24] and of limited efficacy.

With the introduction of gold compounds in the twentieth century[25,26] and the discovery of the so-called disease-modifying antirheumatic drugs (DMARDs) sulfasalazine and hydroxychloroquine,[27–29] as well as glucocorticoids,[30,31] the development of outcomes in RA research became more and more important. One of the first initiatives in outcome research was that of Steinbrocker and Blazer,[32] who developed the therapeutic score card for RA. This method included the patient global assessment of disease activity, as well as joint tenderness, pain, and functional status. In 1956, Lansbury[33] developed the Systemic Index, the first numerical method to assess and compare disease activity between patients. This index included a measure of duration of morning stiffness, a measure of fatigue (hours after rising before onset of fatigue), grip strength, and pain, which was measured as the number of aspirins required for pain relief.

Development of the Health Assessment Questionnaire (HAQ) in 1980, followed by development of a shorter version, the HAQ Disability Index (HAQ-DI), created a revolution in measurement of functional status in RA that is still in use.[34] Years later, Paulus and colleagues[35] developed the Paulus Criteria, including morning stiffness, joint pain, and the patient global assessment. To harmonize the use of outcome measures across RA clinical trials, the American College of Rheumatology (ACR) established a committee to develop the first RA core set of outcome measures. With support of the first Outcome Measures in Rheumatology (OMERACT) meeting in 1992, consensus was reached, resulting in the ACR core set that includes 3 PROs: pain, patient global assessment of disease activity, and functional status.[3,36]

Although already included in the systemic index of Lansbury,[33] it was not until recently that fatigue was identified as one of the most important problems identified by patients with RA, and it has proved highly reliable, sensitive to change, and an independent determinant of disease activity.[15–19] Although fatigue is not part of the ACR core set, OMERACT endorsed fatigue in their core set[15] in 2006, and the European League Against Rheumatism (EULAR) and ACR recommended reporting fatigue in the domain of disease activity in every RA randomized controlled trial (RCT).[2] Although most clinicians agree that morning stiffness is typical for RA, duration of morning stiffness was excluded from the recent update of both the ACR classification and remission criteria.[37,38] Although the importance of the symptom was acknowledged, it was thought that the instruments to measure it yielded data of insufficient reliability to include stiffness in the criteria. A recent review of patient-oriented measurement instruments that have been developed to assess stiffness in patients with RA identified studies between 1987 and 2010 with instruments limited to duration and severity of morning stiffness found similar insufficient data.[39]

At present, international consensus exists on the importance of measurement and reporting of patients' assessment of disease activity, pain, and physical functioning.

Other promising PRO domains that are currently being studied include flare,[40] remission,[41] stiffness,[42] (work) participation,[43] worker productivity,[44] self-management,[45] sleep,[18] and emotional distress.

USE OF PATIENT-REPORTED OUTCOMES IN DIFFERENT CURRENT SETTINGS

The scientific interest in PROs in recent years has been boosted by societal pressure; patients demand to be an active contributor to their care process, whereas, in contrast, health insurance companies and governments call for transparency of outcomes in order to quantify quality of care delivery because costs are increasing to unsustainable levels. Under the influence of health economist Michael Porter,[46,47] health care delivery is more and more patient centered, with value-adding activities as a main driver for good outcomes.

As a consequence, physicians are faced with the request to add value for patients, but often lack information or tools to measure domains that patients find important. Hospitals struggle to identify a single PRO that is important and meaningful for all the patients who are treated within their facilities. Although PRO research activities have been focused toward identification of patient-important domains and optimizing psychometric properties of domain-specific questionnaires, there is a growing interest in the translation of all this evidence into clinical practice in order to start measuring, comparing, and improving outcomes and making good choices about reducing costs. However, it is unclear whether PROs and the instruments to measure them allow for benchmarking across health care providers.

Quality Indicators

In recent years, there have been several quality improvement initiatives within rheumatology, including the development of quality indicators; by measuring, reporting, and comparing outcomes, health care providers are stimulated to innovate and improve. Quality of care is operationalized by Donabedian,[48] who distinguished structure, process, and outcome of care. Structure describes aspects in the setting in which care is delivered; for example, the setting, staff, and medical equipment. Process denotes the actions of the health care professionals; for example, whether the protocol is followed or whether the treatment is adjusted in case of a more severe disease course. The outcome reflects the effect of the given care in terms of mortality, morbidity, and health status. It is thought that more desirable outcomes are obtained if the structure provides the opportunity to deliver qualified care processes. A quality indicator is a measurable element of practice performance for which there is evidence or consensus that it can be used to assess the quality, and hence change the quality of care provided.[49,50]

There is no single, broadly accepted set of quality indicators for RA, but several groups around the world have made an attempt to develop sets of RA quality indicators.[51–56] These sets, developed by, among others, the National Health Service in the United Kingdom, the European Musculoskeletal Conditions Surveillance and Information Network,[54] the ACR,[51] and the Australian Rheumatoid Association,[55] together contain 82 indicators, with only 9 outcome measures. Remarkably, not even 1 patient was consulted to check whether the chosen indicators were of any relevance to the health care experience. This omission is potentially a major lack of face validity and, in Porter's[46,47] words, might not add value to health care delivery. Of the 9 outcome measures, none were PROs. For example, the measurement of physical functioning is regarded as an indicator, but the value or level of functioning is not included. This omission is odd, because from a patient's perspective it does not create value to know that your level of physical functioning has been measured; value is created when physical functioning is measured over time and actions (like additional physiotherapy) are taken to improve functioning when it lags behind. This perspective has created a shift from process measurement to outcome measurement. However, recent discussions highlight that a good balance between process and outcome measurement is needed to be able to understand quality improvement efforts.[57]

It is evident that there is still a lot of work to be done in quality indicators and the incorporation of patients' perspectives on quality of care. A recent study by Radner and colleagues[58] showed that the situation is not very different for cohorts; in a survey among 25 European registers and clinical cohorts involving patients with RA, only 2 PROs, namely HAQ and patient global assessment, were identified as commonly collected. Other PROs, such as fatigue, were less frequently collected.

Patient-reported Outcomes in Remission

Treatment of RA increasingly targets low disease activity, remission, or even sustained remission.[59–62] The recently developed ACR/EULAR remission criteria contain 1 PRO, the patient global assessment.[63,64] During the development of the criteria, the remission committee evaluated the added value of all core set outcome measures, including the 3 PROs. From this it was learned that the patient global was equally good, if not better, at discriminating active from control treatment. Nevertheless, there has been criticism regarding the need for the patient global to equal 1 or less before a patient is classified as in remission, because comorbidity may influence the level of the patient global; another criticism is that this threshold is too low, because some respondents never use the extremities of a scale, in this case the 0, 1, 9, or 10 on a 10-point numerical rating scale, even if they feel extremely well/extremely bad.[65–67]

With treatment increasingly targeting remission, it is important to understand the patient's perspective on this state. An OMERACT working group in collaboration with EULAR has conducted qualitative research to understand which domains of health significantly contribute to patients' experiences of low disease activity.[41,68,69] This qualitative study, conducted in the Netherlands, Austria, and the United Kingdom, identified 3 major themes of patient-perceived remission:

1. Symptoms such as pain, stiffness, and fatigue are either absent or reduced in intensity
2. The impact of RA on daily life diminishes by having increased independence, the ability to do valued activities, an improved mood, and the ability to cope
3. Leading to a return to normality, including the ability to work, enjoy a family role, and be seen as normal by other people

Patients thought that the concept of remission was most influenced by aging, side effects of medication, comorbidities, accrued damage to joints, and disease duration.

In order to prioritize the many domains in order of importance, patients with RA from the Netherlands, United Kingdom, Austria, Denmark, France, and the United States were asked to complete a survey that contained all 26 domains of remission identified in a qualitative study. Patients were asked to rate domains for importance (not important, important, or essential) to characterize a period of remission, and, if important or essential, whether this domain needs to be less, almost gone, or gone to reflect remission. In addition, respondents were asked to determine their personal top 3 most important/essential domains that characterize remission.

Data from 274 patients with RA were collected. The most mentioned domains in patients' top 3 were pain (67%), fatigue (33%), and independence (19%). Domains that were most frequently rated as essential to characterize a period of remission were pain (60%), being mobile (52%), physical function (51%), being independent (47%), and fatigue (41%). Pain needed to be less (13%), almost gone (42%), or gone (45%) to reflect remission. Similar patterns were seen for fatigue (23%, 40%, and 37%), independence (16%, 31%, and 53%), mobility (16%, 35%, and 49%), and physical functioning (14%, 29%, and 57%).[70]

At present, an international validation study to identify appropriate measurement instruments of these domains in low disease activity is ongoing. The first results will be presented during a special-interest group at OMERACT in 2016. By studying the quantification of the added value of these PROs in defining remission, this could lead to an update of the remission definition.

Patient-reported Disease Activity Scores

In 2012 the ACR Rheumatoid Arthritis Clinical Disease Activity Measures Working Group conducted a systematic review resulting in 63 RA disease activity measures.[71] Of these, only 6 were recommended for clinical use, with 3 being entirely patient-reported: Patient Activity Scale (PAS), PAS-II, and Routine Assessment of Patient Index Data with 3 measures (RAPID3). All 3 of these indices are similar because they are the mean of 3 PROs from the core set: pain, patient global, and functional disability. Their main difference is the respective functional disability tool used: HAQ, HAQ-II, or Multidimensional Health Assessment Questionnaire (MDHAQ).[72] Recent work has shown that RAPID3 remission, which is 3 or less on a scale of 0 to 30, is as strict as the ACR/EULAR remission criteria in the prediction of long-term outcomes.

Other RA activity scores that are completely patient reported but not recommended by the ACR's working group because of either being too new (not enough published data) or not having remission criteria include the Rheumatoid Arthritis Disease Activity Index (RADAI) and Rheumatoid Arthritis Index of Disease Activity (RAID).[73–75] The RADAI is older and includes 6 Likert scales on arthritis activity, pain, stiffness, stiffness duration, global health, joint swelling, and joint tenderness. The RAID is the patient-derived score to capture the impact of RA on daily life. It includes visual analog scales for 7 domains: pain, functional disability assessment, fatigue, sleep, physical well-being, emotional well-being, and coping. This score was developed in close collaboration between patients and professionals, has been validated in different settings, and is freely available in 67 languages and dialects from the developer's Web site. Although the instrument is not in use as a disease activity score, cutoff state values have been proposed.[76]

SPECIFIC PATIENT-REPORTED OUTCOME MEASURES BY DOMAINS IN RHEUMATOID ARTHRITIS

As shown in **Fig. 1**, the RA core set measures contain 3 PRO domains: physical function, pain, and a patient global assessment of disease activity.[77] Although several PRO indices using measures in these domains have qualities similar to or superior to other core set measures,[10,12,78–80] each is also important to address individually because there is no clear consensus on which measures to use.

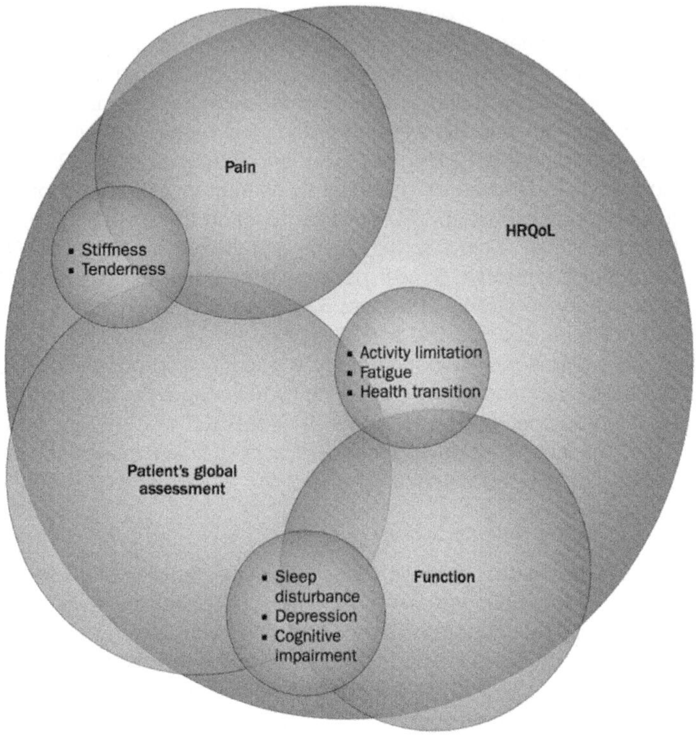

Fig. 1. Relationships between PROs in RA and other rheumatic diseases. Considerable overlap exists between the broad concept of health-related quality of life (HRQoL) and more specific domains (eg, pain, function, patient global assessment). In addition, these domains overlap with the 3 most important PROs in all rheumatic diseases: pain, function, and patient global assessment. HRQoL, health-related quality of life. (*From* van Tuyl LH, Boers M. Patient-reported outcomes in core domain sets for rheumatic diseases. Nat Rev Rheumatol 2015;11(12):710; with permission.)

Physical Function

The physical function domain has a myriad of PROMs. The original core set stated that, "Any patient self-assessment instrument which has been validated, has reliability, has been proven in RA trials to be sensitive to change, and which measures physical function in RA patients is acceptable." They recommended the Arthritis Impact Measurement Scales (AIMS), HAQ, and a few others that have seen much less use in rheumatology during the past 20 years.[36] The AIMS and subsequent AIMS2 had more than 60 items and covered several health domains in addition to physical function,[81,82] which made them difficult to implement outside of clinical trials.[83] Although the original long HAQ also contained additional nondisability items, its short form, the HAQ Disability Index, became the gold standard for use in clinical trials and clinics for decades.[34] With 20 Likert items and 21 questions about devices, the HAQ was similarly difficult for rheumatologists to use consistently in the clinical workplace as pressure mounted on reducing patient wait times and simplifying scoring.[84]

The first major change to the HAQ was the modified HAQ (MHAQ), which used a single item from each of the 8 dimensions in the HAQ and simplified scoring by taking the average item value.[85] Because of large floor effect issues with the MHAQ,[86]

Pincus and colleagues[87] added 2 difficult items, playing sports and walking 2 miles, to the MHAQ to create the 10-item Multidimensional HAQ (MDHAQ). Using Item Response Theory (IRT), a quantitative method that assesses item properties and information content, Wolfe and colleagues[88] developed the HAQ-II, a 10-item measure that used 5 legacy items from the HAQ and 5 new items to efficiently reproduce the original 41-item HAQ. One issue with having so many similar measures was that some confused the HAQ, MHAQ, MDHAQ, HAQ-II, and so forth as being interchangeable, although clinicians now better understand their important differences.[86,88,89]

Expanding this use of IRT, the US National Institutes of Health developed the Patient Reported Outcomes Measurement Information System (PROMIS),[90] which has created a series of physical function measures for general use. These measures include physical function 10-item (PF-10) and 20-item (PF-20) measures that have been shown to be effective in patients with RA.[91] **Fig. 2** shows the comparison of information content (measured by standard error) and physical function (theta) in the HAQ, PROMIS PF-10 and PF-20, and other measures. Of note is how well the HAQ performs in patients with the worst physical function and how the PROMIS measures perform better in patients with the best physical function.[91] As expectations for patients with RA have improved since the HAQ was first developed to measure disability (or worse physical functioning), there has been growing interest in incorporating these newer PROMIS physical functioning measures into rheumatology studies. In addition, PROMIS has developed a computerized adaptive test (CAT) for physical

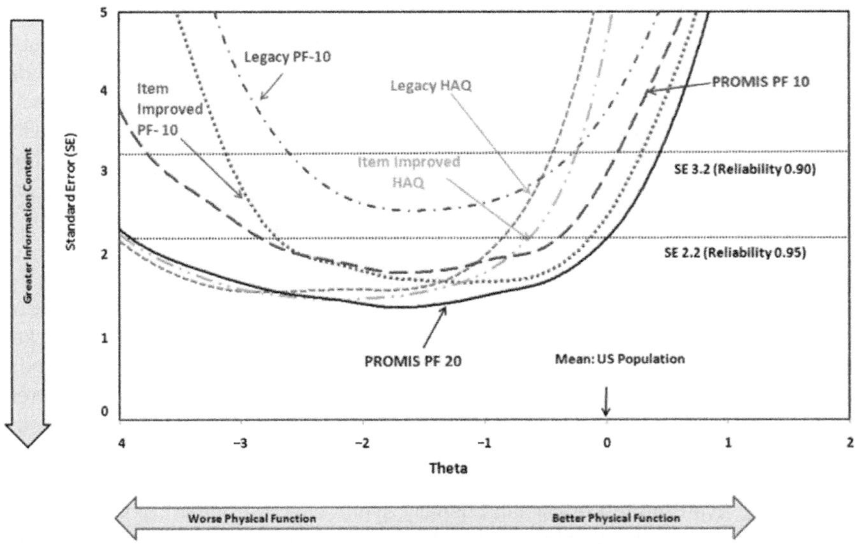

Fig. 2. Comparison of select physical function PROMs. Physical function, or theta on the horizontal scale, is mapped against sensitivity/reliability, or standard error on the vertical scale. A better measure has a greater breadth of physical function ability and greater depth in sensitivity. The PROMIS PF-20 is the most sensitive, maintaining a reliability of 0.95 over more than 4 SDs. The HAQ (or Legacy HAQ) has good sensitivity in areas of poorer function appropriate for historical RA, but is worse for patients with RA with physical function closer to mean US population levels, resulting in a larger floor effect. (*From* Fries JF, Krishnan E, Rose M, et al. Improved responsiveness and reduced sample size requirements of PROMIS physical function scales with item response theory. Arthritis Res Ther 2011;13(5):R147; with permission.)

function that requires an electronic interface but can provide similar results to the PROMIS PF-10 in only 4 to 5 items.

Pain

Pain is one of the most common PROMs and, through general quality improvement needs since the late 1990s, it has mostly become established as the fifth vital sign, although its general utility in the clinic is unclear.[92,93] Although the primary vital sign measure of pain is a numerical or verbal rating scale with a range of 0 to 10, pain in RA is often measured on a 10-cm visual analog scale (VAS) between anchors of 0 (no pain) and 100 (unbearable pain, severe pain, worst imaginable/possible pain, and so forth). Studies in patients with RA and other patients with chronic pain have shown that differences of 5 points or less (out of 100) are negligible compared with minimal clinically important differences, and some clinicians have resorted to 11-point and 21-point numeric rating scales, especially as forms became machine readable. For example, Wolfe and Michaud[94] found that a generally acceptable level of pain in 12,090 patients with RA was less than or equal to 20 and a minimal clinically important improvement (MCII) of 11. Tubach and colleagues[95] found from 358 international patients with RA that their pain MCII was 15 absolute points or a relative 20% improvement. This finding is similar to reviews of other chronic pain conditions[95,96]; depending on the baseline amount of pain, the MCII may similarly change (eg, 20, 25, and 30 for least, average, and worst pain baseline).[97]

Limitations of measuring pain through a single item are not recent, and some clinicians have proposed using additional items in the clinic and in trials.[98,99] The Rheumatoid Arthritis Pain Scale (RAPS) is the only RA-specific pain PRO measure and has 24 items.[100] The Regional Pain Scale (RPS) examines the extent of bodily pain through its 19-item measure, and helps identify concomitant fibromyalgia.[101] Many investigators report pain values as subscales of larger health-related quality-of-life measures such as the Short-form 36 (SF-36) and AIMS.[102,103] In addition, PROMIS has 2 pain dimensions, pain intensity and pain interference, with CAT and short-form measures providing reliable results in patients with RA.[104]

Patient Global

Patient global assessment of disease activity, or patient global, is a simple and important measure, but controversial in its interpretation.[105] Physicians have always asked patients how they are doing and have often used the answer to help guide their medical decisions. Confusion arises in determining how much of the patient's current health problems can be assigned to their RA, and whether comorbidities, treatment side effects, and other health problems that may or may not be RA related should be included so that patient global is similar to the patient global assessment of general health.[106,107] Even though physicians usually synthesize the patient global measure when determining their own physician global assessment of RA activity, these measures often disagree in meaningful ways.[108,109] The ACR/EULAR remission guidelines recommended the following wording: "For patient global assessment, 'Considering all of the ways your arthritis has affected you, how do you feel your arthritis is today?' (anchors: very well–very poor)."[63] Subsequent studies have shown that patient global is the measure most likely to prevent a patient from achieving a score that indicates remission.[66,67] Future work is needed to determine how to separate the impact of comorbidities and mood disorders; how to test psychometric changes for patients who avoid selecting the VAS anchors; and how sociolinguistic changes, including time windows, affect this outcome measure.

Additional Patient-reported Outcome Domains

Although much of the RA PRO research literature has focused on the 3 core measures mentioned earlier, there are a variety of others to consider, as **Fig. 1** shows. A systematic review of PROs in RA clinical trials found 63 PROMs covering 14 domains of health.[110] Fatigue, sleep, and depression are discussed later, and readers are invited to investigate further the several other PRO domains, including work/productivity, coping, well-being, and general quality of life.

Although the high prevalence of fatigue in RA was established early on,[111,112] there are a variety of ways of measuring it.[113] In their 2007 systematic review, Hewlett and colleagues[114] found 23 different fatigue scales used by patients with RA, but only 6 provided evidence of reasonable validation. Arguments have been made for a validated multidimensional fatigue scale for RA trials at the same time increasing the use of a fatigue VAS in the rheumatology clinic.[115] Because most studies have used a single VAS to measure fatigue with a wide variety of anchors,[114] when analyzed, the MCII have been found to be smaller than pain at 10 (out of 100).[17,116] In trying to understand the pathways on how to improve fatigue for patients with RA, studies found that improving pain, function, and depression had the greatest impacts.[117–119] Outside of DMARD treatment, exercise has been shown to have a significant effect on improving fatigue.[120,121]

Often connected with fatigue, sleep disturbances are increased in RA and have important associations with disease activity, pain, and overall quality of life.[122–126] Because patients emphasized the importance of quality sleep, there was a transition from polysomnography studies on small groups[122–124] to using sleep PROs on larger groups.[19,127] A 2009 review found 45 sleep questionnaire instruments covering 14 domains of sleep and recommended 4 for testing in future RA clinical trials: Athens Insomnia Scale, Medical Outcome Study (MOS) Sleep Measure, Pittsburgh Sleep Diary, and Women's Health Initiative Insomnia Rating Scale.[128] However, the most commonly used in trials have been simpler items measuring frequency of sleep disturbances, quality of sleep, and sleep VAS.[110] This trend changed during 2 RCTs for abatacept when the MOS sleep questionnaire was used and validated.[129] Other observational studies have additionally helped validate sleep PROMs and have shown their association with RA activity,[19,129] and the minimal clinically important difference (MCID) was lower for the sleep VAS at 6 (out of 100).[17]

Although depression is increased in RA compared with healthy controls, it does not seem to be increased compared with chronic diseases with similar pain levels.[130,131] The prevalence of depression is associated with younger age and the screening tool used, with levels ranging from 15% for the Hospital Anxiety and Depression Scale (HADS) to 39% for the Patient Health Questionnaire (PHQ-9).[132] In RA treatment clinical trials there have been at least 3 PRO tools used to measure depression: Beck Depression Inventory (BDI), HADS, and Mental Health Inventory (MHI) depression subscale.[133] Observational studies have shown a strong association of pain extent, fatigue, ethnicity, and low socioeconomic status with self-reported depression or PHQ-9.[134–136] Even with the large overlap with other domains, there seems to be an independent temporal impact of depression symptoms with RA activity.[137] Although there are several depression PRO questionnaires validated in patients with RA, it is not clear which, if any, are feasible, practical, and helpful for treating RA in the clinic.

THE FUTURE

Even with the more than 30 specific examples of PROs used by patients with RA in this article and in **Table 1**, there are many more available and being developed.

Table 1
Examples of PRO measures (PROMs) in RA by health domain

	Domain	PROMs
ACR core measures	Physical function	HAQ, HAQ-II, MDHAQ, AIMS2, PROMIS PF-10, PF-20, and PF-CAT
	Pain	VAS, NRS, RAPS, RPS, PROMIS pain intensity and pain interference
	Global assessment	VAS, NRS
Potential core measure candidates	Fatigue	VAS, NRS, MAF, SF-36 vitality, FACITFS, PMS, BRAF NRS
	Stiffness	Morning stiffness duration, severity
	Flares	Patient reported flare, worsening, and treatment change
Multidimensional RA activity measures		PAS, PAS-II, RAPID-3, RADAI, RAID
Others	Sleep	VAS, NRS, AIS, MOS Sleep Measure, Pittsburgh Sleep Diary, WHI Insomnia Rating Scale
	Depression	HADS, PHQ-8/9, BDI, MHI
	Work	WLQ, WALS, SPS-6, EWPS, RA WIS, disability/work status

Abbreviations: AIS, Athens Insomnia Scale; BRAF, Bristol Rheumatoid Arthritis Fatigue; EWPS, Endicott Work Productivity Scale; FACITFS, Functional Assessment of Chronic Illness Therapy Fatigue Scale; MAF, Multidimensional Assessment of Fatigue scale; NRS, Numerical Rating Scale; PMS, Profile of Mood States; SPS-6, 6-item Stanford Presenteeism Scale; WALS, Workplace Activity Limitations Scale; WHI, Women's Health Initiative; WIS, Work Instability Scale; WLQ, Work Limitations Questionnaire.

The authors recommend browsing (and contributing to) the online EULAR Outcome Measures Library (http://oml.eular.org), which, at the time of this writing, had 28 indices used in RA.[138] There are several measures for each of the primary health domains that are important to patients with RA and their treatment. In order to interpret research using these measures, there is a need for additional studies that allow for improved comparison and interpretation of various measures on the same health domain scale (see **Fig. 2** for the example of physical function). For example, depending on the specific item and method used to collect the pain 0 to 10 score, a study with a mean pain score of 3 and another with 4 may not be different.[139] In addition, it is important for research conducted with PROs to provide consistent and detailed information on the items used; MDHAQ is not the same PROM as HAQ, just as patient global assessment of RA severity is not the same as patient global assessment of health. Having these measures in a standardized PROM library is useful and should allow for more comparisons across studies.

Similarly, PROMs used in research studies are rarely also used in clinical care. Noting what are feasible to measure in the clinic setting along with being reliable and sensitive is a necessity, because rheumatologists are increasingly required to collect PRO domains. When standardized and consistent, these data can be combined with those of rheumatology clinics throughout the country for large-scale quality improvement research. The ACR's RISE (Rheumatology Informatics System for Effectiveness) registry already has data on more than a million rheumatology patient visits, and early analysis shows a variety of PROMs used for patients with RA and around half of early participants collecting physical function PRO.[140]

The future of PROMs in RA is uncertain, because the use of specific technologies at the individual level and in the clinic and research may result in a movement away from the paper questionnaire and more toward the CAT. PROMIS has developed several CAT PROMs in domains important to RA, and these are generic so that a score from a patient with RA can be placed on the same index and comparison with a patient who does not have RA. Similar to our general quality-of-life PROMs, this may allow for greater context of the burden of RA with that of other conditions, but studies are still needed to show when changes in these PROMs should affect treatment decisions. No matter what new PROMs are developed, it is clear that PROs will continue to be an important part of the care and study of RA.

REFERENCES

1. US Department of Health and Human Services FDA Center for Drug Evaluation and Research, US Department of Health and Human Services FDA Center for Biologics Evaluation and Research, US Department of Health and Human Services FDA Center for Devices and Radiological Health. Guidance for industry: patient-reported outcome measures: use in medical product development to support labeling claims: draft guidance. Health Qual Life Outcomes 2006;4:79.
2. Aletaha D, Landewe R, Karonitsch T, et al. Reporting disease activity in clinical trials of patients with rheumatoid arthritis: EULAR/ACR collaborative recommendations. Ann Rheum Dis 2008;67(10):1360–4.
3. Boers M, Tugwell P, Felson DT, et al. World Health Organization and International League of Associations for rheumatology core endpoints for symptom modifying antirheumatic drugs in rheumatoid arthritis clinical trials. J Rheumatol Suppl 1994;41:86–9.
4. Felson DT, Anderson JJ, Boers M, et al. American College of Rheumatology. Preliminary definition of improvement in rheumatoid arthritis. Arthritis Rheum 1995;38(6):727–35.
5. Maiden N, Capell HA, Madhok R, et al. Does social disadvantage contribute to the excess mortality in rheumatoid arthritis patients? Ann Rheum Dis 1999;58(9): 525–9.
6. Prevoo ML, van 't Hof MA, Kuper HH, et al. Modified disease activity scores that include twenty-eight-joint counts. Development and validation in a prospective longitudinal study of patients with rheumatoid arthritis. Arthritis Rheum 1995; 38(1):44–8.
7. Smolen JS, Breedveld FC, Schiff MH, et al. A simplified disease activity index for rheumatoid arthritis for use in clinical practice. Rheumatology (Oxford) 2003; 42(2):244–57.
8. van der Heijde DM, van 't Hof M, van Riel PL, et al. Development of a disease activity score based on judgment in clinical practice by rheumatologists. J Rheumatol 1993;20(3):579–81.
9. Minnock P, Kirwan J, Bresnihan B. Fatigue is a reliable, sensitive and unique outcome measure in rheumatoid arthritis. Rheumatology (Oxford) 2009;48(12): 1533–6.
10. Pincus T, Amara I, Segurado OG, et al. Relative efficiencies of physician/ assessor global estimates and patient questionnaire measures are similar to or greater than joint counts to distinguish adalimumab from control treatments in rheumatoid arthritis clinical trials. J Rheumatol 2008;35(2):201–5.
11. Pincus T, Callahan LF, Sale WG, et al. Severe functional declines, work disability, and increased mortality in seventy-five rheumatoid arthritis patients studied over nine years. Arthritis Rheum 1984;27(8):864–72.

12. Pincus T, Chung C, Segurado OG, et al. An index of patient reported outcomes (PRO-Index) discriminates effectively between active and control treatment in 4 clinical trials of adalimumab in rheumatoid arthritis. J Rheumatol 2006; 33(11):2146–52.
13. Sokka T, Hakkinen A, Krishnan E, et al. Similar prediction of mortality by the health assessment questionnaire in patients with rheumatoid arthritis and the general population. Ann Rheum Dis 2004;63(5):494–7.
14. Hewlett S, Carr M, Ryan S, et al. Outcomes generated by patients with rheumatoid arthritis: how important are they? Musculoskelet Care 2005;3(3):131–42.
15. Kirwan JR, Minnock P, Adebajo A, et al. Patient perspective: fatigue as a recommended patient centered outcome measure in rheumatoid arthritis. J Rheumatol 2007;34(5):1174–7.
16. Nicklin J, Cramp F, Kirwan J, et al. Collaboration with patients in the design of patient-reported outcome measures: capturing the experience of fatigue in rheumatoid arthritis. Arthritis Care Res (Hoboken) 2010;62(11):1552–8.
17. Wells G, Li T, Maxwell L, et al. Determining the minimal clinically important differences in activity, fatigue, and sleep quality in patients with rheumatoid arthritis. J Rheumatol 2007;34(2):280–9.
18. Wells G, Li T, Maxwell L, et al. Responsiveness of patient reported outcomes including fatigue, sleep quality, activity limitation, and quality of life following treatment with abatacept for rheumatoid arthritis. Ann Rheum Dis 2008;67(2): 260–5.
19. Wolfe F, Michaud K, Li T. Sleep disturbance in patients with rheumatoid arthritis: evaluation by medical outcomes study and visual analog sleep scales. J Rheumatol 2006;33(10):1942–51.
20. Higgins PD, Schwartz M, Mapili J, et al. Patient defined dichotomous end points for remission and clinical improvement in ulcerative colitis. Gut 2005;54(6): 782–8.
21. Kirwan JR, Newman S, Tugwell PS, et al. Progress on incorporating the patient perspective in outcome assessment in rheumatology and the emergence of life impact measures at OMERACT 9. J Rheumatol 2009;36(9):2071–6.
22. Peyrin-Biroulet L. What is the patient's perspective: how important are patient-reported outcomes, quality of life and disability? Dig Dis 2010;28(3):463–71.
23. Spoorenberg A, van TA, Landewe R, et al. Measuring disease activity in ankylosing spondylitis: patient and physician have different perspectives. Rheumatology (Oxford) 2005;44(6):789–95.
24. Moreland LW, Russell AS, Paulus HE. Management of rheumatoid arthritis: the historical context. J Rheumatol 2001;28(6):1431–52.
25. Forestier J. L'Aurothiopie dans les rheumatisme chronique. Ann Med Interne (Paris) 1929;53:323–7.
26. Kean WF, Forestier F, Kassam Y, et al. The history of gold therapy in rheumatoid disease. Semin Arthritis Rheum 1985;14(3):180–6.
27. Bagnall AW. The value of chloroquine in rheumatoid disease: a four-year study of continuous therapy. Can Med Assoc J 1957;77(3):182–94.
28. Landewe RB, Boers M, Verhoeven AC, et al. COBRA combination therapy in patients with early rheumatoid arthritis: long-term structural benefits of a brief intervention. Arthritis Rheum 2002;46(2):347–56.
29. Sinclair R, Duthie J. Salazopyrin in the treatment of rheumatoid arthritis. Ann Rheum Dis 1949;8(3):226.

30. Barnes A, Smith HL, Slocumb CH, et al. Effect of cortisone and corticotropin (ACTH) on the acute phase of rheumatic fever; further observations. AMA Am J Dis Child 1951;82(4):397–425.
31. Hench P, Slocumb C, Barnes A, et al. The effect of a hormone of the adrenal cortex, 17-hydroxy-11-dehydrocorticosterone (compound E), on the acute phase of rheumatic fevers. Proceedings of the Staff Meetings of the Mayo Clinic 1949;24:277–97. Available at: http://www.ncbi.nlm.nih.gov/pubmed/18118071.
32. Steinbrocker O, Blazer A. A therapeutic score card for rheumatoid arthritis; a standardized method of appraising results of treatment. N Engl J Med 1946;235:501–6.
33. Lansbury J. Numerical method of evaluating the status of rheumatoid arthritis. Ann Rheum Dis 1958;17(1):101–7.
34. Bruce B, Fries JF. The Stanford Health Assessment Questionnaire: a review of its history, issues, progress, and documentation. J Rheumatol 2003;30(1):167–78.
35. Paulus HE, Egger MJ, Ward JR, et al. Analysis of improvement in individual rheumatoid arthritis patients treated with disease-modifying antirheumatic drugs, based on the findings in patients treated with placebo. The Cooperative Systematic Studies of Rheumatic Diseases Group. Arthritis Rheum 1990;33(4):477–84.
36. Felson DT, Anderson JJ, Boers M, et al. The American College of Rheumatology preliminary core set of disease activity measures for rheumatoid arthritis clinical trials. The Committee on Outcome Measures in Rheumatoid Arthritis Clinical Trials. Arthritis Rheum 1993;36(6):729–40.
37. Arnett FC, Edworthy SM, Bloch DA, et al. The American Rheumatism Association 1987 revised criteria for the classification of rheumatoid arthritis. Arthritis Rheum 1988;31(3):315–24.
38. Pinals RS, Masi AT, Larsen RA. Preliminary criteria for clinical remission in rheumatoid arthritis. Arthritis Rheum 1981;24(10):1308–15.
39. van Tuyl LH, Lems WF, Boers M. Measurement of stiffness in patients with rheumatoid arthritis in low disease activity or remission: a systematic review. BMC Musculoskelet Disord 2014;15:28.
40. Lie E, Woodworth TG, Christensen R, et al. Validation of OMERACT preliminary rheumatoid arthritis flare domains in the NOR-DMARD study. Ann Rheum Dis 2014;73(10):1781–7.
41. van Tuyl LH, Hewlett S, Sadlonova M, et al. The patient perspective on remission in rheumatoid arthritis: 'You've got limits, but you're back to being you again'. Ann Rheum Dis 2015;74(6):1004–10.
42. Orbai AM, Smith KC, Bartlett SJ, et al. "Stiffness has different meanings, I think, to everyone". examining stiffness from the perspective of people living with rheumatoid arthritis. Arthritis Care Res (Hoboken) 2014;66(11):1662–72.
43. Hoving JL, van Zwieten MC, van der Meer M, et al. Work participation and arthritis: a systematic overview of challenges, adaptations and opportunities for interventions. Rheumatology (Oxford) 2013;52(7):1254–64.
44. Tang K, Boonen A, Verstappen SM, et al. Worker productivity outcome measures: OMERACT filter evidence and agenda for future research. J Rheumatol 2014;41(1):165–76.
45. Flurey CA, Morris M, Richards P, et al. It's like a juggling act: rheumatoid arthritis patient perspectives on daily life and flare while on current treatment regimes. Rheumatology (Oxford) 2014;53(4):696–703.
46. Porter ME. A strategy for health care reform–toward a value-based system. N Engl J Med 2009;361(2):109–12.

47. Porter ME. What is value in health care? N Engl J Med 2010;363(26):2477–81.
48. Donabedian A. The quality of care. How can it be assessed? JAMA 1988; 260(12):1743–8.
49. Committee on Quality of Health Care in America, Institute of Medicine. Crossing the quality chasm. a new health system for the 21st century. Washington, DC: National Academy Press; 2001. Available at: http://www.ncbi.nlm.nih.gov/books/NBK222273/.
50. Nash D, Clarke J, Skoufalos A, et al. Conceptualizations and definitions of quality. Health care quality: the clinician's primer. 2012. Available at: http://net.acpe.org/Current_Materials/Quality/2012_Fall_Quality/Quality_Pre-work_Fall_2012/Nash Book_chap2367911.pdf.
51. National Committee for Quality Assurance (NCQA), Physician Consortium for Performance Improvement (PCPI), American College of Rheumatology (ACR). Rheumatoid arthritis: physician performance measurement set. American Medical Association and National Committee for Quality Assurance; 2008. Available at: http://rheumatoidarthritis.semarthritisrheumatism.com/Content/PDFs/RR-NCQA-Arthritis.pdf.
52. MacLean CH, Saag KG, Solomon DH, et al. Measuring quality in arthritis care: methods for developing the Arthritis Foundation's quality indicator set. Arthritis Rheum 2004;51(2):193–202.
53. Navarro-Compan V, Smolen JS, Huizinga TW, et al. Quality indicators in rheumatoid arthritis: results from the METEOR database. Rheumatology (Oxford) 2015; 54(9):1630–9.
54. Petersson IF, Strombeck B, Andersen L, et al. Development of healthcare quality indicators for rheumatoid arthritis in Europe: the eumusc.net project. Ann Rheum Dis 2014;73(5):906–8.
55. Australian Institute of Health and Welfare. National indicators for monitoring osteoarthritis, rheumatoid arthritis and osteoporosis. Canberra: Australian Institute of Health and Welfare; 2006. Available at: http://www.aihw.gov.au/publication-detail/?id=6442467905.
56. van Hulst LT, Fransen J, den Broeder AA, et al. Development of quality indicators for monitoring of the disease course in rheumatoid arthritis. Ann Rheum Dis 2009;68(12):1805–10.
57. Bilimoria KY. Facilitating quality improvement: pushing the pendulum back toward process measures. JAMA 2015;314(13):1333–4.
58. Radner H, Dixon W, Hyrich K, et al. Consistency and utility of data items across European rheumatoid arthritis clinical cohorts and registers. Arthritis Care Res (Hoboken) 2015;67(9):1219–29.
59. Smolen JS, Aletaha D, Bijlsma JW, et al. Treating rheumatoid arthritis to target: recommendations of an international task force. Ann Rheum Dis 2010;69(4): 631–7.
60. Sokka T, Hetland ML, Makinen H, et al. Remission and rheumatoid arthritis: Data on patients receiving usual care in twenty-four countries. Arthritis Rheum 2008; 58(9):2642–51.
61. van Tuyl LH, Lems WF, Voskuyl AE, et al. Tight control and intensified COBRA combination treatment in early rheumatoid arthritis: 90% remission in a pilot trial. Ann Rheum Dis 2008;67(11):1574–7.
62. Wells GA, Boers M, Shea B, et al. Minimal disease activity for rheumatoid arthritis: a preliminary definition. J Rheumatol 2005;32(10):2016–24.

63. Felson DT, Smolen JS, Wells G, et al. American College of Rheumatology/European League Against Rheumatism provisional definition of remission in rheumatoid arthritis for clinical trials. Arthritis Rheum 2011;63(3):573–86.
64. van Tuyl LH, Vlad SC, Felson DT, et al. Defining remission in rheumatoid arthritis: results of an initial American College of Rheumatology/European League Against Rheumatism consensus conference. Arthritis Rheum 2009;61(5): 704–10.
65. Inanc N, Yilmaz-Oner S, Can M, et al. The role of depression, anxiety, fatigue, and fibromyalgia on the evaluation of the remission status in patients with rheumatoid arthritis. J Rheumatol 2014;41(9):1755–60.
66. Masri KR, Shaver TS, Shahouri SH, et al. Validity and reliability problems with patient global as a component of the ACR/EULAR remission criteria as used in clinical practice. J Rheumatol 2012;39(6):1139–45.
67. Studenic P, Smolen JS, Aletaha D. Near misses of ACR/EULAR criteria for remission: effects of patient global assessment in Boolean and index-based definitions. Ann Rheum Dis 2012;71(10):1702–5.
68. van Tuyl LH, Sadlonova M, Davis B, et al. Remission in rheumatoid arthritis: working toward incorporation of the patient perspective at OMERACT 12. J Rheumatol 2016;43(1):203–7.
69. van Tuyl LH, Smolen JS, Wells GA, et al. Patient perspective on remission in rheumatoid arthritis. J Rheumatol 2011;38(8):1735–8.
70. van Tuyl LH, Sadlonova M, Hewlett S, et al. The patient perspective on absence of disease activity in rheumatoid arthritis: a survey to identify key domains of patient perceived remission. Ann Rheum Dis 2015;74(Suppl 2):435.433–436.
71. Anderson J, Caplan L, Yazdany J, et al. Rheumatoid arthritis disease activity measures: American College of Rheumatology recommendations for use in clinical practice. Arthritis Care Res 2012;64(5):640–7.
72. Anderson JK, Zimmerman L, Caplan L, et al. Measures of rheumatoid arthritis disease activity: Patient (PtGA) and Provider (PrGA) Global Assessment of Disease Activity, Disease Activity Score (DAS) and Disease Activity Score With 28-Joint Counts (DAS28), Simplified Disease Activity Index (SDAI), Clinical Disease Activity Index (CDAI), Patient Activity Score (PAS) and Patient Activity Score-II (PASII), Routine Assessment of Patient Index Data (RAPID), Rheumatoid Arthritis Disease Activity Index (RADAI) and Rheumatoid Arthritis Disease Activity Index-5 (RADAI-5), Chronic Arthritis Systemic Index (CASI), Patient-Based Disease Activity Score With ESR (PDAS1) and Patient-Based Disease Activity Score Without ESR (PDAS2), and Mean Overall Index for Rheumatoid Arthritis (MOI-RA). Arthritis Care Res (Hoboken) 2011;63(Suppl 11):S14–36.
73. Gossec L, Dougados M, Rincheval N, et al. Elaboration of the preliminary Rheumatoid Arthritis Impact of Disease (RAID) score: a EULAR initiative. Ann Rheum Dis 2009;68(11):1680–5.
74. Gossec L, Paternotte S, Aanerud GJ, et al. Finalisation and validation of the rheumatoid arthritis impact of disease score, a patient-derived composite measure of impact of rheumatoid arthritis: a EULAR initiative. Ann Rheum Dis 2011; 70(6):935–42.
75. Leeb BF, Haindl PM, Maktari A, et al. Patient-centered rheumatoid arthritis disease activity assessment by a modified RADAI. J Rheumatol 2008;35(7): 1294–9.
76. Dougados M, Brault Y, Logeart I, et al. Defining cut-off values for disease activity states and improvement scores for patient-reported outcomes: the example of

the Rheumatoid Arthritis Impact of Disease (RAID). Arthritis Res Ther 2012; 14(3):R129.

77. van Tuyl LH, Boers M. Patient-reported outcomes in core domain sets for rheumatic diseases. Nat Rev Rheumatol 2015;11(12):705–12.
78. Wolfe F, Michaud K, Pincus T. A composite disease activity scale for clinical practice, observational studies, and clinical trials: the patient activity scale (PAS/PAS-II). J Rheumatol 2005;32(12):2410–5.
79. Pincus T, Swearingen CJ, Bergman M, et al. RAPID3 (Routine Assessment of Patient Index Data 3), a rheumatoid arthritis index without formal joint counts for routine care: proposed severity categories compared to disease activity score and clinical disease activity index categories. J Rheumatol 2008;35(11): 2136–47.
80. Pincus T, Swearingen CJ, Bergman MJ, et al. RAPID3 (Routine Assessment of Patient Index Data) on an MDHAQ (Multidimensional Health Assessment Questionnaire): Agreement with DAS28 (Disease Activity Score) and CDAI (Clinical Disease Activity Index) activity categories, scored in five versus more than ninety seconds. Arthritis Care Res (Hoboken) 2010;62(2):181–9.
81. Meenan RF, Gertman PM, Mason JH. Measuring health status in arthritis. The arthritis impact measurement scales. Arthritis Rheum 1980;23(2):146–52.
82. Meenan RF, Mason JH, Anderson JJ, et al. AIMS2. The content and properties of a revised and expanded arthritis impact measurement scales health status questionnaire. Arthritis Rheum 1992;35(1):1–10.
83. Gignac MA, Cao X, McAlpine J, et al. Measures of disability: Arthritis Impact Measurement Scales 2 (AIMS2), Arthritis Impact Measurement Scales 2-Short Form (AIMS2-SF), The Organization for Economic Cooperation and Development (OECD) Long-Term Disability (LTD) Questionnaire, EQ-5D, World Health Organization Disability Assessment Schedule II (WHODASII), Late-Life Function and Disability Instrument (LLFDI), and Late-Life Function and Disability Instrument-Abbreviated Version (LLFDI-Abbreviated). Arthritis Care Res (Hoboken) 2011; 63(Suppl 11):S308–24.
84. Maska L, Anderson J, Michaud K. Measures of functional status and quality of life in rheumatoid arthritis: Health Assessment Questionnaire Disability Index (HAQ), Modified Health Assessment Questionnaire (MHAQ), Multidimensional Health Assessment Questionnaire (MDHAQ), Health Assessment Questionnaire II (HAQ-II), Improved Health Assessment Questionnaire (Improved HAQ), and Rheumatoid Arthritis Quality of Life (RAQoL). Arthritis Care Res (Hoboken) 2011;63(Suppl 11):S4–13.
85. Pincus T, Summey JA, Soraci SA Jr, et al. Assessment of patient satisfaction in activities of daily living using a modified Stanford Health Assessment Questionnaire. Arthritis Rheum 1983;26(11):1346–53.
86. Wolfe F. Which HAQ is best? A comparison of the HAQ, MHAQ and RA-HAQ, a difficult 8 item HAQ (DHAQ), and a rescored 20 item HAQ (HAQ20): analyses in 2,491 rheumatoid arthritis patients following leflunomide initiation. J Rheumatol 2001;28(5):982–9.
87. Pincus T, Sokka T, Kautiainen H. Further development of a physical function scale on a MDHAQ [corrected] for standard care of patients with rheumatic disease. J Rheumatol 2005;32(8):1432–9.
88. Wolfe F, Michaud K, Pincus T. Development and validation of the health assessment questionnaire II: a revised version of the health assessment questionnaire. Arthritis Rheum 2004;50(10):3296–305.

89. Anderson J, Sayles H, Curtis JR, et al. Converting modified Health Assessment Questionnaire (HAQ), multidimensional HAQ, and HAQII scores into original HAQ scores using models developed with a large cohort of rheumatoid arthritis patients. Arthritis Care Res 2010;62(10):1481–8.
90. Reeve BB, Hays RD, Bjorner JB, et al. Psychometric evaluation and calibration of health-related quality of life item banks: plans for the Patient-Reported Outcomes Measurement Information System (PROMIS). Med Care 2007;45(5 Suppl 1): S22–31.
91. Fries JF, Krishnan E, Rose M, et al. Improved responsiveness and reduced sample size requirements of PROMIS physical function scales with item response theory. Arthritis Res Ther 2011;13(5):R147.
92. Mularski RA, White-Chu F, Overbay D, et al. Measuring pain as the 5th vital sign does not improve quality of pain management. J Gen Intern Med 2006;21(6): 607–12.
93. Lorenz KA, Sherbourne CD, Shugarman LR, et al. How reliable is pain as the fifth vital sign? J Am Board Fam Med 2009;22(3):291–8.
94. Wolfe F, Michaud K. Assessment of pain in rheumatoid arthritis: minimal clinically significant difference, predictors, and the effect of anti-tumor necrosis factor therapy. J Rheumatol 2007;34(8):1674–83.
95. Tubach F, Ravaud P, Martin-Mola E, et al. Minimum clinically important improvement and patient acceptable symptom state in pain and function in rheumatoid arthritis, ankylosing spondylitis, chronic back pain, hand osteoarthritis, and hip and knee osteoarthritis: Results from a prospective multinational study. Arthritis Care Res (Hoboken) 2012;64(11):1699–707.
96. Farrar JT, Young JP Jr, LaMoreaux L, et al. Clinical importance of changes in chronic pain intensity measured on an 11-point numerical pain rating scale. Pain 2001;94(2):149–58.
97. Farrar JT, Pritchett YL, Robinson M, et al. The clinical importance of changes in the 0 to 10 numeric rating scale for worst, least, and average pain intensity: analyses of data from clinical trials of duloxetine in pain disorders. J Pain 2010;11(2):109–18.
98. Bradley LA. Pain measurement in arthritis. Arthritis Care Res 1993;6(4):178–86.
99. Williamson A, Hoggart B. Pain: a review of three commonly used pain rating scales. J Clin Nurs 2005;14(7):798–804.
100. Anderson DL. Development of an instrument to measure pain in rheumatoid arthritis: Rheumatoid Arthritis Pain Scale (RAPS). Arthritis Rheum 2001;45(4): 317–23.
101. Wolfe F. Pain extent and diagnosis: development and validation of the regional pain scale in 12,799 patients with rheumatic disease. J Rheumatol 2003;30(2): 369–78.
102. Sokka T. Assessment of pain in rheumatic diseases. Clin Exp Rheumatol 2005; 23(5 Suppl 39):S77–84.
103. Englbrecht M, Tarner IH, van der Heijde DM, et al. Measuring pain and efficacy of pain treatment in inflammatory arthritis: a systematic literature review. J Rheumatol 2012;90:3–10.
104. Bartlett SJ, Orbai AM, Duncan T, et al. Reliability and validity of selected PROMIS measures in people with rheumatoid arthritis. PLoS One 2015;10(9): e0138543.
105. Krause NM, Jay GM. What do global self-rated health items measure? Med Care 1994;32(9):930–42.

106. Fries JF, Ramey DR. "Arthritis specific" global health analog scales assess "generic" health related quality-of-life in patients with rheumatoid arthritis. J Rheumatol 1997;24(9):1697–702.
107. Khan NA, Spencer HJ, Abda EA, et al. Patient's global assessment of disease activity and patient's assessment of general health for rheumatoid arthritis activity assessment: are they equivalent? Ann Rheum Dis 2012;71(12):1942–9.
108. Rohekar G, Pope J. Test-retest reliability of patient global assessment and physician global assessment in rheumatoid arthritis. J Rheumatol 2009;36(10): 2178–82.
109. Barton JL, Imboden J, Graf J, et al. Patient-physician discordance in assessments of global disease severity in rheumatoid arthritis. Arthritis Care Res (Hoboken) 2010;62(6):857–64.
110. Kalyoncu U, Dougados M, Daures J, et al. Reporting of patient-reported outcomes in recent trials in rheumatoid arthritis: a systematic literature review. Ann Rheum Dis 2009;68(2):183–90.
111. Tack BB. Fatigue in rheumatoid arthritis. Conditions, strategies, and consequences. Arthritis Care Res 1990;3(2):65–70.
112. Wolfe F, Hawley DJ, Wilson K. The prevalence and meaning of fatigue in rheumatic disease. J Rheumatol 1996;23(8):1407–17.
113. Wolfe F. Fatigue assessments in rheumatoid arthritis: comparative performance of visual analog scales and longer fatigue questionnaires in 7760 patients. J Rheumatol 2004;31(10):1896–902.
114. Hewlett S, Hehir M, Kirwan JR. Measuring fatigue in rheumatoid arthritis: a systematic review of scales in use. Arthritis Rheum 2007;57(3):429–39.
115. Repping-Wuts H, van Riel P, van Achterberg T. Fatigue in patients with rheumatoid arthritis: what is known and what is needed. Rheumatology (Oxford) 2009; 48(3):207–9.
116. Khanna D, Pope JE, Khanna PP, et al. The minimally important difference for the fatigue visual analog scale in patients with rheumatoid arthritis followed in an academic clinical practice. J Rheumatol 2008;35(12):2339–43.
117. Wolfe F, Michaud K. Fatigue, rheumatoid arthritis, and anti-tumor necrosis factor therapy: an investigation in 24,831 patients. J Rheumatol 2004;31(11):2115–20.
118. Nikolaus S, Bode C, Taal E, et al. Fatigue and factors related to fatigue in rheumatoid arthritis: a systematic review. Arthritis Care Res (Hoboken) 2013;65(7): 1128–46.
119. Druce KL, Jones GT, Macfarlane GJ, et al. Determining pathways to improvements in fatigue in rheumatoid arthritis: results from the British Society for Rheumatology Biologics Register for Rheumatoid Arthritis. Arthritis Rheum 2015; 67(9):2303–10.
120. Hegarty RS, Conner TS, Stebbings S, et al. Feel the fatigue and be active anyway: physical activity on high-fatigue days protects adults with arthritis from decrements in same-day positive mood. Arthritis Care Res 2015;67(9): 1230–6.
121. Rongen-van Dartel SAA, Repping-Wuts H, Flendrie M, et al. Effect of aerobic exercise training on fatigue in rheumatoid arthritis: a meta-analysis. Arthritis Care Res 2015;67(8):1054–62.
122. Mahowald MW, Mahowald ML, Bundlie SR, et al. Sleep fragmentation in rheumatoid arthritis. Arthritis Rheum 1989;32(8):974–83.
123. Hirsch M, Carlander B, Vergé M, et al. Objective and subjective sleep disturbances in patients with rheumatoid arthritis. Arthritis Rheum 1994;37(1):41–9.

124. Drewes AM, Svendsen L, Taagholt SJ, et al. Sleep in rheumatoid arthritis: a comparison with healthy subjects and studies of sleep/wake interactions. Rheumatology (Oxford) 1998;37(1):71–81.
125. Abad VC, Sarinas PS, Guilleminault C. Sleep and rheumatologic disorders. Sleep Med Rev 2008;12(3):211–28.
126. Irwin MR, Olmstead R, Carrillo C, et al. Sleep loss exacerbates fatigue, depression, and pain in rheumatoid arthritis. Sleep 2012;35(4):537.
127. Westhovens R, Van der Elst K, Matthys A, et al. Sleep problems in patients with rheumatoid arthritis. J Rheumatol 2014;41(1):31–40.
128. Wells GA, Li T, Kirwan JR, et al. Assessing quality of sleep in patients with rheumatoid arthritis. J Rheumatol 2009;36(9):2077–86.
129. Wells G, Li T, Tugwell P. Investigation into the impact of abatacept on sleep quality in patients with rheumatoid arthritis, and the validity of the MOS-Sleep Questionnaire Sleep Disturbance Scale. Ann Rheum Dis 2010;69(10):1768–73.
130. Hawley DJ, Wolfe F. Depression is not more common in rheumatoid arthritis: a 10-year longitudinal study of 6,153 patients with rheumatic disease. J Rheumatol 1993;20(12):2025–31.
131. Dickens C, McGowan L, Clark-Carter D, et al. Depression in rheumatoid arthritis: a systematic review of the literature with meta-analysis. Psychosom Med 2002;64(1):52–60.
132. Matcham F, Rayner L, Steer S, et al. The prevalence of depression in rheumatoid arthritis: a systematic review and meta-analysis. Rheumatology (Oxford) 2013;52(12):2136–48.
133. Rathbun AM, Reed GW, Harrold LR. The temporal relationship between depression and rheumatoid arthritis disease activity, treatment persistence and response: a systematic review. Rheumatology (Oxford) 2013;52(10):1785–94.
134. Margaretten M, Yelin E, Imboden J, et al. Predictors of depression in a multiethnic cohort of patients with rheumatoid arthritis. Arthritis Rheum 2009;61(11):1586–91.
135. Wolfe F, Michaud K. Predicting depression in rheumatoid arthritis: the signal importance of pain extent and fatigue, and comorbidity. Arthritis Rheum 2009;61(5):667–73.
136. Margaretten M, Barton J, Julian L, et al. Socioeconomic determinants of disability and depression in patients with rheumatoid arthritis. Arthritis Care Res (Hoboken) 2011;63(2):240–6.
137. Rathbun AM, Harrold LR, Reed GW. Temporal effect of depressive symptoms on the longitudinal evolution of rheumatoid arthritis disease activity. Arthritis Care Res 2015;67(6):765–75.
138. Castrejón I, Gossec L, Carmona L. The EULAR outcome measures library: an evolutional database of validated patient-reported instruments. Ann Rheum Dis 2015;74(2):475–6.
139. Michaud K, Wolfe F, Inman CJ. Is there a difference in rheumatology patient reported outcomes when measured at home versus the clinic setting? Arthritis Rheum 2012;61(Suppl):S876.
140. Yazdany J, Myslinski R, Francisco M, et al. A National Electronic Health Record-Enabled Registry in rheumatology: the ACR's Rheumatology Informatics System for Effectiveness (RISE). Arthritis Rheum 2015;67(Suppl 10). Available at: http://acrabstracts.org/abstract/a-national-electronic-health-record-enabled-registry-in-rheumatology-the-acrs-rheumatology-informatics-system-for-effectiveness-rise/.

Patient-Reported Measures of Physical Function in Knee Osteoarthritis

Daniel K. White, PT, ScD, MSc*, Hiral Master, DPT, MPH

KEYWORDS

• Knee osteoarthritis • Patient-reported measures • WOMAC • KOOS • PROMIS

KEY POINTS

- The Western Ontario and McMaster Universities Osteoarthritis Index (WOMAC) physical function subscale is a well-validated and reliable patient-reported measure, although it is questionable if the constructs of physical function and pain are separately evaluated.
- The Knee Injury and Osteoarthritis Outcome Score (KOOS) Function in Sport and Recreation subscale is a well-validated measure of physical function, although floor effects are present for people with moderate to severe functional limitation.
- The Patient Reported Outcomes Measurement Information System (PROMIS) Physical Function measure is a newer measurement instrument, and preliminary studies show high test-retest reliability and no floor or ceiling effects among people with osteoarthritis (OA).

INTRODUCTION

Knee OA is a leading cause of functional limitation worldwide.[1,2] People with knee OA have pain, which limits commonly performed daily activities. Functional limitation is defined by Nagi as restriction in the performance of an individual, such as difficulty getting up out of bed, getting up from a chair, walking, and climbing stairs.[3] Functional limitation is a construct that is unique and separate from impairments (eg, knee pain) and disease (eg, knee OA).

Accurately assessing the type and severity of functional limitation is important for people with knee OA. From a societal perspective, proper measurement helps determine the burden of disease on function. From a research perspective, evaluating the efficacy and effectiveness of new treatment interventions requires measurement of physical function using appropriate measures. Lastly, from a clinical perspective,

The authors have no conflicts of interest.
Funding for the authors was provided by NIH U54 GM104941.
Department of Physical Therapy, University of Delaware, 540 South College Avenue, 210L, Newark, DE 19713, USA
* Corresponding author. 540 South College Avenue, 210L, Newark, DE 19713.
E-mail address: dkw@udel.edu

Rheum Dis Clin N Am 42 (2016) 239–252
http://dx.doi.org/10.1016/j.rdc.2016.01.005 rheumatic.theclinics.com
0889-857X/16/$ – see front matter

assessing functional limitation is important to demonstrate the efficacy of one-on-one intervention and describe worsening or improvement over time.[4] Measurement in knee OA is challenging because there is a wide spectrum of functional limitation types and severity.

Examples of commonly used fixed-length questionnaires of physical function in knee OA include the WOMAC, the KOOS, and the PROMIS Physical Function subscale. WOMAC is a disease-specific instrument that measures the domains of pain, stiffness, and physical function.[5] This article focuses on the physical function subscale. The KOOS is another disease-specific instrument that has similar items as the WOMAC physical function subscale with the addition of questions about sport and recreation and knee-related quality of life (QOL).[6,7] The PROMIS Physical Function instrument is a recently developed general measure of health.[8]

The purpose of this article is to review psychometric properties of commonly used patient-reported measures of physical function in knee OA and discuss the strengths and limitations of each measurement instrument.

THE IMPORTANCE OF MEASURING THE CONSTRUCT OF PHYSICAL FUNCTION

The disablement model is a useful tool to communicate the consequences of injury and disease. Jette[9] adopted Nagi's definition of disablement as "various impacts of chronic and acute conditions on the functioning of specific body systems, on basic human performance, and on people's functioning in necessary, usual, expected, and personally desired roles in society."[9] Physical function has a unique place in contemporary disablement frameworks. Functional limitation is a distinct phenomenon in the Nagi model that describes the construct of physical function, defined as restriction in the performance of an individual, such as difficulty getting up out of bed, getting up from a chair, walking, and climbing stairs.[3] In the more recent International Classification of Functioning, Disability and Health model from the World Health Organization, "activity" and "activity limitations" best describe physical function. Activity is "... the execution of a task or action by an individual. Activity limitations are defined as difficulties an individual may have in executing activities."[10,11]

From a measurement perspective, outcome instruments should measure specific underlying constructs and not mix 2 or more constructs together. For instance, although physical function is closely related to disease and pain, it is a unique construct of disablement. To best understand the prevalence and associated risk factors of functional limitation, an ideal measurement instrument should attempt to solely measure the construct of physical function.

PSYCHOMETRIC PROPERTIES

The authors reviewed the following psychometric properties of patient-reported measures: reliability, validity, and sensitivity to change and responsiveness (**Table 1**). The authors also investigated known group validity, which is the extent to which a measurement instrument can differentiate scores from groups that are known to be different. Lastly, sensitivity to change and responsiveness were evaluated. Sensitivity to change is the ability of measure to detect change that exceeds statistical error without regard to clinical relevance, whereas responsiveness refers to clinically relevant or meaningful change.[15] Responsiveness is determined using scores anchored to patient reported or provider-reported thresholds, such as the minimum clinical important difference (MCID).[15,16]

The greater number of psychometric properties studied and properly fulfilled, the better a measurement instrument assesses physical function. It is important for

Table 1
Definitions and implications of statistical values for psychometric testing of patient reported measures

Psychometric Property	Definition	Statistics
Reliability– internal consistency	Measure the relation of the items in a questionnaire to an underlying construct	Cronbach's alpha—items are considered to represent a similar construct when alpha is approximately ≥0.7.[12]
Reliability–test–retest or inter/intrarater	If the questionnaire measures a condition in a reproducible manner	Intraclass correlation coefficient ≥0.7 is considered acceptable for test-retest reliability.[13]
Validity: construct	Evaluation of the relationship of an instrument with other instruments	Correlation coefficient (Pearson r, Spearman ρ). Correlation coefficients of >0.50, 0.35–0.50, and <0.35 were considered strong, moderate, and weak, respectively.[14]
Validity: known groups	Measure of an instrument's ability to distinguish among different groups (eg, persons with functional limitation vs those without functional limitation)	*t* Test or analysis of variance, with post hoc analysis.
Sensitivity to change	Ability to detect change that exceeds statistical error without regard to clinical relevance	Effect size, standardized response mean, and MDC. Larger effect size and standardized response mean indicate more sensitivity to change.
Responsiveness	Ability to measure clinically relevant or meaningful change	MCID

clinicians and researchers to be familiar with the psychometric properties of commonly used measurement instruments to help guide clinical decision making and appropriately balance the implications of study findings.

WESTERN ONTARIO AND McMASTER UNIVERSITIES OSTEOARTHRITIS INDEXPHYSICAL FUNCTION SUBSCALE

The WOMAC physical function subscale is a widely used patient-reported measurement instrument for knee OA. The WOMAC was developed to fill the need for an outcome instrument that could be responsive to change in OA-related symptoms after a clinical trial.[5] Bellamy and Buchanan[17] interviewed 100 people with knee OA and identified 41 items in 5 dimensions that were important for people with knee OA, 1 being physical function. The WOMAC has been used in other patient populations, including hip OA,[18] rheumatoid arthritis (RA) and fibromyalgia,[19] and systemic lupus erythematosus,[18] among others.

The WOMAC physical function subscale begins with the question, "What degree of difficulty do you have due to pain, discomfort or arthritis…"; 17 items are evaluated, including going up and down stairs, sitting, standing, squatting to the floor, walking, getting in a car, shopping, putting on and taking off socks, getting out of bed, lying in bed, bathing, sitting, getting on and off the toilet, heavy domestic duties, and light domestic duties. There are 2 methods of scoring. The Likert method uses a 5-point scale with the choices of none, mild, moderate, severe, or extreme, and the physical function subscale ranges from 0 to 68. The Visual Analogue Scale (VAS) method uses a 100-mm horizontal line for each item and subjects mark a vertical line along the horizontal continuum for each item, which is measured and totaled with the other items on a 0 to 1700 scale.[20] For both scoring methods, higher scores represent more functional limitation.

Reliability

The WOMAC physical function subscale shows good reliability. Specifically, internal consistency of the WOMAC physical function subscale is high in English and other languages. High test-retest reliability over durations of time ranging from 6 days to 12 months has been shown as well (**Table 2**).

Validity

The WOMAC physical function subscale shows good construct validity with other known measures of physical function (see **Table 2**). The WOMAC physical function subscale also has been shown to have negligible flooring and ceiling effects.[24] The authors did not find studies that validated the WOMAC to known groups.

Sensitivity to Change and Responsiveness

Previous studies have shown the WOMAC physical function subscale as sensitive to change as other measures of physical function. Responsiveness thresholds have been established as well (**Table 3**).

Strengths and Weaknesses

The major strengths of the WOMAC physical function subscale are that this measurement instrument has been well validated, has good test-retest reliability, and has established MCID thresholds. Furthermore, because the instrument was developed as a disease-specific outcome, people with knee OA are likely to have difficulty with the items from the scale. Lastly, the instrument is easy to administer and has been translated into many different languages.

One potential major limitation of the WOMAC physical function subscale is its unclear delineation between the constructs of pain and function. This is because each item begins with the question, "What degree of difficulty do you have due to pain, discomfort or arthritis?" Hence, respondents technically only report the extent of functional limitation attributed to pain, discomfort, or arthritis, which may not reflect their total limitation. One previous study found the WOMAC physical function had a stronger association with measures of pain compared with performance measures of physical function.[39] Investigators should consider using an additional measure of physical function to accompany the WOMAC to fully measure the construct of physical function.

KNEE INJURY AND OSTEOARTHRITIS OUTCOME SCORE FUNCTION IN SPORT AND RECREATION SUBSCALE AND PHYSICAL FUNCTION SHORTFORM

Ewa Roos and colleagues[7] developed the KOOS using the WOMAC, a literature review, an expert panel of patients, orthopedic surgeons, physical therapists, and data from a pilot study of people with posttraumatic OA. An important innovation of the KOOS over the WOMAC is the addition of a high-functioning subscale, termed Function in Sport and Recreation. Respondents assess the degree of difficulty

Table 2
Reliability and validity of the Western Ontario and McMaster Universities Osteoarthritis Index physical function subscale

Study	N	Population Description	Internal Consistency: Cronbach's alpha	Test-Retest Reliability: Intraclass Correlation Coefficient	Comparator	Correlation
Bellamy et al,[5] 1988	57	People from Canada with knee or hip OA who were taking part in a randomized controlled trial of 2 nonsteroidal anti-inflammatory drugs	Likert Scale format = 0.95 VAS format = 0.89	—	Lequesne index physical function	r = 0.5
Xie et al,[21] 2008	131	People from Singapore with knee OA scheduled for total knee arthroplasty	>0.7	>0.8	SF-36 physical functioning and EQ-5D in Chinese and English	r >0.5
Nadrian et al,[22] 2012	116	People from Iran with physician diagnosis referred to a rheumatology clinic with knee or hip OA	0.95	>0.7	Lequesne index physical function	r >0.5
Thumboo et al,[23] 2001	66	English-speaking Chinese, Malay, or Indian people with knee or hip OA seen at a tertiary referral center	0.93	>0.8	SF-36 physical functioning	r = –0.4
Tüzün et al,[24] 2005	72	People from Turkey being seen in an outpatient physical therapy practice with knee OA	0.94	—	SF-36 physical functioning, Lequesne index physical function	r = –0.7, r = 0.7
Basaran et al,[25] 2010	117	People from Turkey with knee or hip OA	0.95	—	SF-36 physical functioning	r = –0.8
Williams et al,[26] 2012	168	People with knee OA participating in a rehabilitation program.	—	>0.8	—	—

Table 3
Sensitivity to change and responsiveness of the Western Ontario and McMaster Universities Osteoarthritis Index physical function subscale

Study	N	Effect Size and Standardized Response Mean of Western Ontario and McMaster Universities Osteoarthritis Index Physical Function vs Comparator	Minimal Detectable Change 90	Minimal Clinically Important Difference
Tubach et al,[27] 2005	1362	—	—	Minimally clinical important improvement = 26% change
Angst et al,[28] 2001	223	SRM = 0.63 vs SF-36 Physical function: SRM = 0.25	—	—
Williams et al,[26] 2012	116	—	Over 12 mo: MDC 90 change ≥11.8/100	Similar MCID as the lower extremity functional scale
Tüzün et al,[24] 2005	72	ES = 0.80 SRM = 0.94 vs Lequesne Physical function: ES = 0.83, SRM = 1.17	—	—

Abbreviations: ES, effect size; SRM, standardized response mean.

experienced during the past week due to their knee in 5 items: squatting, running, jumping, twisting/pivoting on the injured knee, and kneeling. Responses are on a Likert Scale, ranging from "None" to "Extreme."

KOOS–Physical Function Shortform (KOOS-PS) is a parsimonious measure of physical function derived from the KOOS. A working group tasked with constructing a composite measure of OA severity sponsored by the Osteoarthritis Research Society International and Outcome Measures in Rheumatology developed the KOOS-PS.[40] Respondents are asked to indicate the degree of difficulty experienced in the past week due to a knee problem in 7 tasks: rising from bed, putting on socks/stockings, rising from sitting, bending to the floor, twisting/pivoting on the injured knee, kneeling, and squatting. Responses are on a Likert Scale, ranging from "None" to "Extreme."

Reliability

The KOOS Function in Sport and Recreation subscale shows good internal consistency and test-retest reliability in multiple studies. The measurement instrument has good reported test-retest reliability measured over durations of time, ranging from 2 to 14 days (see **Table 4**). The KOOS-PS also has good internal consistency and high test-retest reliability, which was measured over durations of time, ranging from 2 to 14 days.

Validity

The Function in Sport and Recreation subscale was correlated with other known measures of physical function, namely the Short Form (SF)-36 physical functioning subscale. The authors did find several studies reporting floor effects.[29,30,32]

Table 4
Reliability and validity of the Knee Injury and Osteoarthritis Outcome Score Function in Sport and Recreation subscale and Knee Injury and Osteoarthritis Outcome Score Physical Function Shortform

Study	N	Population Description	Internal Consistency: Cronbach's Alpha	Test-Retest Reliability: Intraclass Correlation Coefficient	Comparator	Correlation
KOOS Function in Sport and Recreation subscale						
Xie et al,[29] 2006	127	People from Singapore with knee OA scheduled for total knee arthroplasty	>0.7	0.7	SF-36 physical functioning	r = 0.5
de Groot et al,[30] 2008	262	People from the Netherlands with knee OA or total knee arthroplasty	>0.9	>0.5	SF-36 physical functioning	r = 0.1–0.6
Ornetti et al,[31] 2008	67	People from France with knee OA or awaiting total knee replacement	0.8	0.8	Osteoarthritis knee and hip QOL questionnaire	r = 0.3
Goncalves et al,[32] 2009	223	People from Portugal with symptomatic knee OA	0.9	0.9	SF-36 physical functioning	r = 0.6
Paradowski et al,[33] 2015	68	People from Poland awaiting total knee replacement	0.9	0.9	SF-36 physical functioning	r = 0.4
KOOS-PS						
Ornetti et al,[34] 2009	87	People from France with knee OA	—	0.9	Osteoarthritis knee and hip QOL questionnaire	r = −0.4
Goncalves et al,[35] 2010	85	People from Portugal with symptomatic knee OA	0.9	0.9	—	—
Davis et al,[36] 2009	248	People from Canada 6 months after total knee replacement	0.9	—	WOMAC physical function	r = 0.9
Gul et al,[37] 2013	—	People from Turkey with symptomatic knee OA	0.9	0.8	WOMAC physical function	r = 0.8
Singh et al,[38] 2014	138	People from the US with knee OA	—	0.7	—	—

Abbreviations: ES, effect size; SRM, standardized response mean.

Statistically significant differences in scores were found for known groups, for example, severity of knee OA,[30] treatment approach,[31] and use of walking aids.[32] Several studies reported the KOOS Function in Sport and Recreation subscale to be sensitive to change,[31,32] although the authors found that less is known regarding responsiveness. For the KOOS-PS, the authors found high correlations with established measures of physical function and no reported floor or ceiling effects. One study reported differences in scores for people with symptomatic knee OA with and without assistive device use[35] (see **Table 6**).

Sensitivity to Change and Responsiveness

The Function in Sport and Recreation subscale was sensitive to change, although little is known about responsiveness. The KOOS-PS was also sensitive to change, and 1 study established an MCID (**Table 5**).

Strengths and Weaknesses

The KOOS Function in Sport and Recreation subscale and KOOS-PS have several strengths. First, both instruments are well studied from across the globe and are reliable, valid, and sensitive to change. Second, the KOOS is freely available by download, at http://www.koos.nu, in different languages. Third, the KOOS is disease specific to knee OA and builds on the strengths of the WOMAC. Lastly, the KOOS-PS is brief and takes minimal time to administer.

There are several limitations to the KOOS. First, the Function in Sport and Recreation subscale has reported floor effects with people with low functional status. This

Table 5
Sensitivity to change and responsiveness of the Knee Injury and Osteoarthritis Outcome Score Function in Sport and Recreation subscale and Knee Injury and Osteoarthritis Outcome Score Physical Function Shortform

Study	N	Effect Size and Standardized Response Mean of Knee Injury and Osteoarthritis Outcome Score	Minimal Detectable Change 95	Minimum Clinical Important Difference
KOOS Function in Sport and Recreation subscale				
Ornetti et al,[31] 2008	67	ES = 1.3 SRM = 0.9	—	—
Goncalves et al,[32] 2009	223	ES = 0.8 SRM = 0.8	—	—
Paradowski et al,[33] 2015	68	ES = 1.6 SRM = 0.9	In individuals: 24.3 In groups: 2.9	—
KOOS-PS				
Ornetti et al,[34] 2009	87	ES = 0.5 SRM = 0.8	—	—
Goncalves et al,[35] 2010	85	ES = 0.9 SRM = 1.2	—	—
Davis et al,[36] 2009	248	SRM = 1.5 vs WOMAC physical function SRM = 1.5	—	—
Singh et al,[38] 2014	138	—	—	MCID = 2.2 (0 to 100 scale)

may not be unexpected given this subscale was developed to measure higher level functional ability. Second, little is known about responsiveness of the KOOS. Although the KOOS is sensitive to change, few studies reported thresholds needed to reach meaningful change, whether by a distribution based (minimal detectable change [MDC]) or anchor-based methodology (MCID).

PATIENT REPORTED OUTCOMES MEASUREMENT INFORMATION SYSTEM PHYSICAL FUNCTION

PROMIS was created in response to the need to speed research discoveries by providing a national resource for accurate and efficient measurement of patient-reported outcomes. The initiative, funded under the National Institutes of Health Roadmap for Medical Research, sought to improve the reliability, validity, and precision of patient-reported outcomes and create new measurements that exceeded the psychometric performance of legacy measures.[41] Physical Function was included as a domain included within the PROMIS framework.

The authors summarize the steps used to develop the PROMIS Physical Function domain, which is described online at http://www.nihpromis.org/Documents/PROMIS_The_First_Four_Years.pdf. As a first step, an item bank was developed using both qualitative and quantitative methods. Items from established instruments were included in the item bank. Next, items were subjected to item-response theory analyses to better understand their dimensional structure. The number of items that were the most representative and informative were chosen through placing common items in a similar bin and then winnowing out items that were redundant or of less quality compared with alternative items in the same bin. The wording of remaining items was reviewed and revised by an expert panel. This was followed by focus groups to inform definitions of the domains and identify areas of future development and cognitive interviews to examine individual item comprehension.[42] Reviewed item banks were then field tested in the general population and in specific patient populations, including people with arthritis. The first wave of testing included 7000 people demographic that was similar to the US census in 2000.

Currently, PROMIS instruments are freely available online at http://www.assessmentcenter.net/. There are 5 physical function domain PROMIS instruments relevant to people with knee OA with the number of items ranging from 4 to 20. Response choices are in a Likert format. For items asking, "Does your health now limit you in ...? response choices range from "Not at all" to "Cannot do." For items asking, "Are you able to ...?" response choices range from "Without any difficulty" to "Unable to do." For each item, the item statistics are provided with the mean score and frequency of response choices using data from the first wave of testing.

Reliability

There were few studies to date that examined reliability among people with knee OA. The authors did find high internal consistency for people with RA and Spanish-speaking adults and also found 1 study that reported high test-retest reliability over 4 weeks among people with doctor-diagnosed OA (**Table 6**).

Validity

The authors found 1 study that showed high correlation of PROMIS Physical Function scores were found with SF-36 scores. PROMIS scores were also highly

Table 6
Reliability of Patient Reported Outcomes Measurement Information System Physical Function

Study	N	Population Description	Internal Consistency: Cronbach's Alpha	Test-Retest Reliability: Intraclass Correlation Coefficient
Bartlett et al,[43] 2015	177	People with RA at a routine clinic visit	0.99	—
Broderick et al,[44] 2013	98	People with doctor-diagnosed OA	—	0.95
Paz et al,[45] 2013	640	Adult Spanish-speaking Latinos	0.99	—

correlated with physical function measures in people with RA (**Table 7**). Among people with RA, the PROMIS Physical Function instrument covers a wider range of physical function levels than the Health Assessment Questionnaire Disability Index.[47] PROMIS also has worse scores with increased disease activity[43] and lower scores in those in remission compared with those with active RA disease.[47] Among 204 people with knee OA, almost none had floor or ceiling effects.[46]

Sensitivity to Change and Responsiveness

Little is known about sensitivity to change and responsiveness for PROMIS in knee OA. One study in RA reported the PROMIS Physical Function 20-item instrument as more sensitive to change than the PROMIS Physical Function 10-item instrument.[48]

Strengths and Weaknesses

A major strength of PROMIS Physical Function is the rigorous development of the item bank that yielded a conceptually clear and well-calibrated measurement instrument. This laid the groundwork for development of a computer adapted test format of the PROMIS Physical Function. Another strength is that all the PROMIS measures are freely available at http://www.assessmentcenter.net/.

Given the recent development of PROMIS Physical Function, literature demonstrating its reliability, validity, sensitivity to change, and responsiveness is a work in progress. To date, psychometric studies of PROMIS measures have shown positive results, although more work is needed.

Table 7
Construct validity of the Patient Reported Outcomes Measurement Information System Physical Function

Study	N	Comparator	Correlation
Bartlett et al,[43] 2015	177	Modified Health Assessment Questionnaire	r = −0.8
Driban et al,[46] 2015	204	SF-36 physical functioning	r = 0.8
Oude Voshaar et al,[47] 2015	690	Health Assessment Questionnaire Disability Index	r = −0.8

SUMMARY

Adequately assessing the burden of knee OA on physical function is challenging given the large number of functional limitations possible in this patient population. The WOMAC and KOOS are useful instruments that provide a valid and reliable measurement of functional limitation common in knee OA. PROMIS Physical Function is a newer measurement instrument that has a growing number of publications demonstrating its legitimacy in knee OA.

REFERENCES

1. Cross M, Smith E, Hoy D, et al. The global burden of hip and knee osteoarthritis: estimates from the global burden of disease 2010 study. Ann Rheum Dis 2014; 73(7):1323–30.
2. Guccione AA, Felson DT, Anderson JJ, et al. The effects of specific medical conditions on the functional limitations of elders in the Framingham Study. Am J Public Health 1994;84(3):351–8.
3. Jette AM. Toward a common language for function, disability, and health. Phys Ther 2006;86(5):726–34.
4. White D, Neogi T, Nguyen UD, et al. Trajectories of functional decline in knee osteoarthritis: the OAI. Rheumatology (Oxford) 2015. [Epub ahead of print].
5. Bellamy N, Buchanan WW, Goldsmith CH, et al. Validation study of WOMAC: a health status instrument for measuring clinically important patient relevant outcomes to antirheumatic drug therapy in patients with osteoarthritis of the hip or knee. J Rheumatol 1988;15(12):1833–40.
6. Roos EM, Roos HP, Ekdahl C, et al. Knee injury and osteoarthritis outcome score (KOOS)–validation of a Swedish version. Scand J Med Sci Sports 1998;8(6): 439–48.
7. Roos EM, Roos HP, Lohmander LS, et al. Knee injury and osteoarthritis outcome score (KOOS)–development of a self-administered outcome measure. J Orthop Sports Phys Ther 1998;28(2):88–96.
8. Rose M, Bjorner JB, Becker J, et al. Evaluation of a preliminary physical function item bank supported the expected advantages of the Patient-Reported Outcomes Measurement Information System (PROMIS). J Clin Epidemiol 2008; 61(1):17–33.
9. Jette AM. Physical disablement concepts for physical therapy research and practice. Phys Ther 1994;74(5):380–6.
10. International classification of functioning, disability, and health: ICF. Geneva (Switzerland): World Health Organization; 2001.
11. Furr RM, Bacharach VR. Psychometrics: an introduction. 2nd edition. Los Angeles (CA): SAGE; 2014.
12. Hays RD, Revicki D. Reliability and validity (including responsiveness). Oxford (NY): Oxford University Press; 1988.
13. Fayers PM, Machin D. Quality of life: assessment, analysis and interpretation. West Sussex (England): John Wiley & Sons; 2002.
14. Juniper EF, Guyatt GH, Jaeschke R. How to develop and validate a new health-related quality of life instrument. Philadelphia: LIpponcott-Raven Publishers; 1996.
15. Latham NK, Mehta V, Nguyen AM, et al. Performance-based or self-report measures of physical function: which should be used in clinical trials of hip fracture patients? Arch Phys Med Rehabil 2008;89(11):2146–55.

16. Beaton DE, Bombardier C, Katz JN, et al. Looking for important change/differences in studies of responsiveness. OMERACT MCID working group. Outcome measures in rheumatology. Minimal clinically important difference. J Rheumatol 2001;28(2): 400–5.
17. Bellamy N, Buchanan WW. A preliminary evaluation of the dimensionality and clinical importance of pain and disability in osteoarthritis of the hip and knee. Clin Rheumatol 1986;5(2):231–41.
18. Stucki G, Sangha O, Stucki S, et al. Comparison of the WOMAC (Western Ontario and McMaster Universities) osteoarthritis index and a self-report format of the self-administered Lequesne-Algofunctional index in patients with knee and hip osteoarthritis. Osteoarthritis Cartilage 1998;6(2):79–86.
19. Wolfe F, Kong SX. Rasch analysis of the Western Ontario MacMaster questionnaire (WOMAC) in 2205 patients with osteoarthritis, rheumatoid arthritis, and fibromyalgia. Ann Rheum Dis 1999;58(9):563–8.
20. Bruce B, Fries J. Longitudinal comparison of the health assessment questionnaire (HAQ) and the Western Ontario and McMaster Universities Osteoarthritis Index (WOMAC). Arthritis Rheum 2004;51(5):730–7.
21. Xie F, Li SC, Goeree R, et al. Validation of Chinese Western Ontario and McMaster Universities Osteoarthritis Index (WOMAC) in patients scheduled for total knee replacement. Qual Life Res 2008;17(4):595–601.
22. Nadrian H, Moghimi N, Nadrian E, et al. Validity and reliability of the Persian versions of WOMAC osteoarthritis index and lequesne algofunctional index. Clin Rheumatol 2012;31(7):1097–102.
23. Thumboo J, Chew LH, Soh CH. Validation of the Western Ontario and Mcmaster University osteoarthritis index in Asians with osteoarthritis in Singapore. Osteoarthritis Cartilage 2001;9(5):440–6.
24. Tüzün EH, Eker L, Aytar A, et al. Acceptability, reliability, validity and responsiveness of the Turkish version of WOMAC osteoarthritis index. Osteoarthritis Cartilage 2005;13(1):28–33.
25. Basaran S, Guzel R, Seydaoglu G, et al. Validity, reliability, and comparison of the WOMAC osteoarthritis index and Lequesne algofunctional index in Turkish patients with hip or knee osteoarthritis. Clin Rheumatol 2010;29(7):749–56.
26. Williams VJ, Piva SR, Irrgang JJ, et al. Comparison of reliability and responsiveness of patient-reported clinical outcome measures in knee osteoarthritis rehabilitation. J Orthop Sports Phys Ther 2012;42(8):716–23.
27. Tubach F, Ravaud P, Baron G, et al. Evaluation of clinically relevant changes in patient reported outcomes in knee and hip osteoarthritis: the minimal clinically important improvement. Ann Rheum Dis 2005;64(1):29–33.
28. Angst F, Aeschlimann A, Steiner W, et al. Responsiveness of the WOMAC osteoarthritis index as compared with the SF-36 in patients with osteoarthritis of the legs undergoing a comprehensive rehabilitation intervention. Ann Rheum Dis 2001;60(9):834–40.
29. Xie F, Li SC, Roos EM, et al. Cross-cultural adaptation and validation of Singapore English and Chinese versions of the Knee injury and Osteoarthritis Outcome Score (KOOS) in Asians with knee osteoarthritis in Singapore. Osteoarthritis Cartilage 2006;14(11):1098–103.
30. de Groot IB, Favejee MM, Reijman M, et al. The Dutch version of the knee injury and osteoarthritis outcome score: a validation study. Health Qual Life Outcomes 2008;6:16.

31. Ornetti P, Parratte S, Gossec L, et al. Cross-cultural adaptation and validation of the French version of the Knee injury and Osteoarthritis Outcome Score (KOOS) in knee osteoarthritis patients. Osteoarthritis Cartilage 2008;16(4):423–8.
32. Goncalves RS, Cabri J, Pinheiro JP, et al. Cross-cultural adaptation and validation of the Portuguese version of the Knee injury and Osteoarthritis Outcome Score (KOOS). Osteoarthritis Cartilage 2009;17(9):1156–62.
33. Paradowski PT, Keska R, Witonski D. Validation of the Polish version of the Knee injury and Osteoarthritis Outcome Score (KOOS) in patients with osteoarthritis undergoing total knee replacement. BMJ Open 2015;5(7):e006947.
34. Ornetti P, Perruccio AV, Roos EM, et al. Psychometric properties of the French translation of the reduced KOOS and HOOS (KOOS-PS and HOOS-PS). Osteoarthritis Cartilage 2009;17(12):1604–8.
35. Goncalves RS, Cabri J, Pinheiro JP, et al. Reliability, validity and responsiveness of the Portuguese version of the Knee injury and Osteoarthritis Outcome Score–Physical Function Short-form (KOOS-PS). Osteoarthritis Cartilage 2010;18(3):372–6.
36. Davis AM, Perruccio AV, Canizares M, et al. Comparative, validity and responsiveness of the HOOS-PS and KOOS-PS to the WOMAC physical function subscale in total joint replacement for osteoarthritis. Osteoarthritis Cartilage 2009;17(7):843–7.
37. Gul ED, Yilmaz O, Bodur H. Reliability and validity of the Turkish version of the knee injury and osteoarthritis outcome score-physical function short-form (KOOS-PS). J Back Musculoskelet Rehabil 2013;26(4):461–6.
38. Singh JA, Luo R, Landon GC, et al. Reliability and clinically important improvement thresholds for osteoarthritis pain and function scales: a multicenter study. J Rheumatol 2014;41(3):509–15.
39. Terwee CB, van der Slikke RM, van Lummel RC, et al. Self-reported physical functioning was more influenced by pain than performance-based physical functioning in knee-osteoarthritis patients. J Clin Epidemiol 2006;59(7):724–31.
40. Perruccio AV, Stefan Lohmander L, Canizares M, et al. The development of a short measure of physical function for knee OA KOOS-Physical Function Short-form (KOOS-PS) - an OARSI/OMERACT initiative. Osteoarthritis Cartilage 2008;16(5):542–50.
41. Fries JF, Bruce B, Cella D. The promise of PROMIS: using item response theory to improve assessment of patient-reported outcomes. Clin Exp Rheumatol 2005;23(5 Suppl 39):S53–7.
42. DeWalt DA, Rothrock N, Yount S, et al. Evaluation of item candidates: the PROMIS qualitative item review. Med Care 2007;45(5 Suppl 1):S12–21.
43. Bartlett SJ, Orbai AM, Duncan T, et al. Reliability and validity of selected PROMIS measures in people with rheumatoid arthritis. PLoS One 2015;10(9):e0138543.
44. Broderick JE, Schneider S, Junghaenel DU, et al. Validity and reliability of patient-reported outcomes measurement information system instruments in osteoarthritis. Arthritis Care Res (Hoboken) 2013;65(10):1625–33.
45. Paz SH, Spritzer KL, Morales LS, et al. Evaluation of the Patient-Reported Outcomes Information System (PROMIS(R)) Spanish-language physical functioning items. Qual Life Res 2013;22(7):1819–30.
46. Driban JB, Morgan N, Price LL, et al. Patient-Reported Outcomes Measurement Information System (PROMIS) instruments among individuals with symptomatic knee osteoarthritis: a cross-sectional study of floor/ceiling effects and construct validity. BMC Musculoskelet Disord 2015;16:253.

47. Oude Voshaar MA, Ten Klooster PM, Glas CA, et al. Validity and measurement precision of the PROMIS physical function item bank and a content validity-driven 20-item short form in rheumatoid arthritis compared with traditional measures. Rheumatology (Oxford) 2015;54(12):2221–9.
48. Fries JF, Krishnan E, Rose M, et al. Improved responsiveness and reduced sample size requirements of PROMIS physical function scales with item response theory. Arthritis Res Ther 2011;13(5):R147.

Patient-Reported Outcomes in Systemic Lupus Erythematosus

Mary Mahieu, MD[a,1], Susan Yount, PhD[b,1], Rosalind Ramsey-Goldman, MD, DrPH[a,*]

KEYWORDS

- Systemic lupus erythematosus (SLE, lupus) • Quality of life (QoL)
- Patient-reported outcomes (PROs)

KEY POINTS

- Successful management of complex conditions such as systemic lupus erythematosus (SLE) and comorbid conditions benefit significantly from patient-reported outcomes (PRO) instruments.
- Measuring health-related quality of life provides SLE patients with an opportunity to participate in their treatment and to facilitate better communication with the multidisciplinary team involved in care.
- Health outcomes research has produced a number of well-validated instruments that can be used across diseases; some have been specifically developed for SLE.
- The use of a generic or SLE-specific PRO depends on specific needs, including population monitoring, treatment decision making, clinical trials research, and for evaluating and comparing the effect of therapies.

INTRODUCTION

Systemic lupus erythematosus (SLE) is a chronic inflammatory autoimmune disorder with variable multi-system involvement. The survival of patients with SLE has significantly improved but like many chronic diseases, there is currently no cure, and morbidity and mortality remain high.[1] Treatment of more severe cases of SLE often involves a balance between managing the manifestations of the disease and minimizing the treatment-related side effects. The disease has a significant impact on many aspects of patients' lives and their overall well-being, or health-related quality of life

All authors have no conflicts of interest and have nothing to disclose.
[a] Division of Rheumatology, Department of Medicine, Northwestern University Feinberg School of Medicine, 240 East Huron Street, M-300, Chicago, IL 60611, USA; [b] Department of Medicine Social Sciences, Northwestern University Feinberg School of Medicine, 625 North Michigan Avenue, 27th Floor, Chicago, IL 60611, USA
[1] Contributed equally as first authors.
* Corresponding author. 240 East Huron Street, M-300, Chicago, IL 60611.
E-mail address: rgramsey@northwestern.edu

Rheum Dis Clin N Am 42 (2016) 253–263
http://dx.doi.org/10.1016/j.rdc.2016.01.001 rheumatic.theclinics.com
0889-857X/16/$ – see front matter

(HRQOL) because SLE affects a relatively younger age group and improved survival has translated into longer disease duration.[1–3] Therefore, patients with SLE must cope with a significant disease burden imposed by the numerous symptoms of the disease itself and its treatment, including fatigue, pain, sleep disturbance, renal and skin problems, and neurologic/psychiatric conditions (eg, anxiety, depression, headaches, motor/sensory deficits, seizures, cognitive impairment, neuropathy).[4–10] Increasing attention to comorbidities of patients with SLE, which themselves add to the burden of the disease, has a substantial impact on patient outcomes and HRQOL.[4,11]

Successful management of complex conditions such as SLE and comorbid conditions can benefit significantly from patient-reported outcomes (PRO) instruments that validly and precisely measure the relevant aspects of health status (eg, symptoms) and HRQOL. Physicians focus on disease activity and damage as their primary therapeutic goal[12]; however, there is a mixed literature with regard to the relationship between disease activity or organ damage and changes in HRQOL in patients with SLE.[13–20] Discordant perspectives between patient and provider when assessing disease burden and activity can result in treatment nonadherence, treatment interruptions, and misunderstandings in communication between patients and providers.[21–23] PROs can have a critical role in clinical trials and clinical care assessments because PROs provide relevant yet complementary information to disease activity and damage indices when it comes to prioritizing treatment decisions, managing symptoms, formulating interventions, providing a complete approach to the management of the disease, and possibly justifying the considerable costs of new therapies. HRQOL measures have been recommended for inclusion in core datasets for observational studies and clinical trials by Outcome Measures in Rheumatoid Arthritis Clinical Trials (OMERACT).[24,25] Further, measuring HRQOL and other aspects of health status (eg, symptoms, functioning) with PROs provides patients with an opportunity to participate more fully in their treatment and ultimately facilitate better communication with the multidisciplinary team of health professionals involved in their care.[13] We review both generic and SLE-specific PRO instruments and their use in patients with SLE herein.

GENERIC PATIENT-REPORTED OUTCOME INSTRUMENTS

Generic PRO tools have been used to assess HRQOL in SLE patients, including the Medical Outcomes Study Short Form 36 (SF-36)[26,27] and EuroQoL-5 Dimensions (EQ-5D).[28,29] Although these tools allow HRQOL comparisons between SLE patients and other patients with rheumatic and nonrheumatic diseases, some limitations in assessing SLE-specific outcomes exist.

The SF-36 is among the most widely used generic PRO tool in SLE studies. The 36-item questionnaire evaluates 8 separate HRQOL domains (physical functioning, general health, mental health, vitality, role physical, role emotional, bodily pain, and social functioning) and includes 2 summary scores (the physical component score and the mental component score).[26] Two versions of the SF-36 are available to evaluate health status in 1- or 4-week intervals. The questionnaire is scored from 0 (worse health) to 100 (better health). The SF-36 was originally validated in an SLE sample from the UK and found to have favorable psychometric properties including good internal consistency, criterion validity compared with the Medical Outcomes Study Short Form 20+ (SF20+), good discriminant validity compared with a British control population, and construct validity in comparisons with the British Isles Lupus Activity Group score,[27] but an inverse association with disease damage (using the Systemic Lupus International Collaborating Clinics/American College of Rheumatology Damage Index) was found only for the physical function domain. Responsiveness of SF-36 has since been shown in Canadian and French SLE samples.[30,31] Minimal clinically important differences (MCIDs) have been established in other rheumatic diseases, and range from 5 to 10 for individual domain scores and from 2.5 to 5 for physical component score and mental component score summary scores.[32]

The SF-36 has been used in both SLE clinical research studies (for example in[33–35]) and in clinical trials.[36–38] Further, the SF-36 is frequently used as a legacy HRQOL instrument to validate other tools, including SLE-specific PRO instruments.[39–42] One criticism of the SF-36 is that it does not assess all dimensions of health status that are important to SLE patients, such as body image and appearance, self-confidence, and social support.[43] Also, there have been concerns about the sensitivity of the SF-36 to capture the frequent changes in health status seen in SLE patients, especially over long periods of time. For example, little change in HRQOL was found in SLE patients who completed the SF-36 instrument over an 8-year period in one study,[44] whereas in another study change in SF-36 was seen only during the first 2 years after a diagnosis of SLE, and then remained stable for the subsequent 3 years of follow-up.[35] In contrast, certain components of the SF-36 have been sensitive to change over shorter periods of time in clinical drug trials.[36–38] These studies highlight the importance of critically evaluating the use of the SF-36 in certain clinical situations and suggest that use of the SF-36 to evaluate HRQOL may be most appropriate for SLE studies with short-term follow-up or SLE patients early in the disease course.

The EQ-5D has also been used in SLE studies, offering the advantage of allowing for economic evaluation in addition to measuring HRQOL.[28,29] The 6-item questionnaire assesses health on the day of completion, and assesses 5 dimensions of disability, such as mobility and self-care, with a single visual analog scale score for patient-reported overall health. The disability dimensions have a 3-item response scale and results are reported as a summary score from 0 (death or health worse than death) to 1.0 (best imaginable health). EQ-5D visual analog scale scores range from 0 (worst imaginable health) to 100 (best imaginable health) and can be used to calculate quality-adjusted life-years for economic analysis. When psychometric properties of the EQ-5D in patients with SLE were assessed in a US multiethnic population,[45] no floor or ceiling effects were found. Discriminant validity was detected among patients with high versus low SLE disease activity, but the EQ-5D did not differ among patients with a range of disease damage. Content validity and reliability of the EQ-5D were not assessed. The EQ-5D summary score was sensitive to changes over time when compared with EQ-5D visual analog scale and self-reported improvements, but the overall effect size was small. More recently, construct validity was established in a Chinese sample of SLE patients when compared with the Lupus Quality of Life Questionnaire (LupusQoL), and discriminant validity was seen with both SLE disease activity and damage scores.[46] Additionally, significant ceiling effects were detected in the EQ-5D, with almost one-half of participants reporting no problems in some disability domains including self-care. The EQ-5D has been used primarily in clinical SLE research studies.[47–51] For example, Strand and colleagues[50] found that SLE patients taking corticosteroids had lower HRQOL, measured by the EQ-5D, than those who were not taking corticosteroids, and concluded that medication side effects contribute to poorer HRQOL in these patients. EQ-5D was also included in the belimumab clinical trials, with changes in patient-reported pain/discomfort domain noted.[38]

The National Institutes of Health initiative Patient-Reported Outcomes Measurement Information System™ (PROMIS™) was established to develop self-report measures of adult and pediatric health status across a range of areas, or domains (eg, fatigue, pain) that are applicable to a broad array of health conditions.[52] PROMIS is domain specific but is not disease specific.

Computerized adaptive testing (CAT) enables precise and efficient estimation of a person's trait levels with only a subset of items from the item pool or "bank," and not all participants answer the same items. This efficiency and precision have been demonstrated with PROMIS CATs in Dutch patients with rheumatoid arthritis and in US patients with rheumatoid arthritis, osteoarthritis, and normal aging cohorts comparing PROMIS Physical Function short forms and CATs relative to existing "legacy" measures (eg, HAQ-DI, SF-36).[53,54]

The content relevance of PROMIS to SLE has been evaluated in a qualitative study of multiethnic Asian individuals with SLE, which confirmed that PROMIS domains (eg, physical function, pain, fatigue, sleep disturbance, sleep-related impairment, anger, anxiety, and depression) address the priority domains identified by these patients and could reasonably serve as a core set of HRQOL instruments, although some content gaps remain to be filled.[55]

The body of literature demonstrating the validity of PROMIS measures in specific clinical populations remains very much in a nascent stage, but has included several studies in patients with SLE, including one with juvenile-onset SLE[56] and several studies of adults with SLE described elsewhere in this paper. A cross-sectional study of SLE patients recruited through an Internet panel company used measures from PROMIS and another National Institutes of Health-funded initiative, the Quality of Life in Neurologic Disorders, to assess the PRO measures' associations with patient-reported SLE disease severity (Lai J-S, Jensen SE, Kaiser K, et al. An evaluation of health-related quality of life in patients with systemic lupus erythematosus using PROMIS, unpublished.). The PROMIS measures included the PROMIS-29 health profile, a measure composed of 4 items from each of 7 domains (depression, anxiety, physical function, pain interference, fatigue, sleep disturbance, and ability to participate in social roles and activities) and a 0 to 10 pain intensity item, and the psychosocial illness impact-negative short form. Compared with the general population norms, nearly all scores were at least one-half of a standard deviation worse (ie, 5 T-score units) with fatigue, pain interference, physical function, and psychosocial illness impact being the worst (ie, 1 standard deviation worse than the norms). Acceptable test–retest reliability (>0.7) was found on all instruments (range, 0.78–0.94).

The Activity in Lupus to Energize and Renew study was a cross-sectional study designed to test the relationship between subjective fatigue and objectively measured physical activity in patients with SLE.[57,58] The study included PROMIS measures (PROMIS Version 1.0; 8-item short forms for fatigue, pain interference, anxiety, depression, sleep disturbance, sleep-related impairment, and physical function), and accelerometer-based physical activity in patients with SLE. All PROMIS short forms demonstrated excellent internal consistency reliability (Cronbach alpha, all >0.90). Results demonstrated significant negative correlations between minutes of bouted moderate-to-vigorous physical activity and physical function, fatigue, and pain interference. Bouted moderate/vigorous physical activity minutes correlated with lower PROMIS-measured fatigue (r = -0.20; P = .03). Both light physical activity and moderate/vigorous physical activity minutes correlated with better physical function (r = 0.19 [P = .04] and r = 0.25 [P = .006], respectively). Mean PROMIS T-scores for fatigue, pain interference, anxiety, sleep disturbance, sleep-related impairment, and physical function were each one-half of a standard deviation worse than the general US population mean.

PROMIS allows for standardized comparison of health status across chronic disease populations in addition to comparing with population-normed data; PROMIS measures are disease agnostic. For example, comparisons of the PROMIS scores reported by SLE patients in this study to a large sample of individuals with arthritis (either rheumatoid arthritis or osteoarthritis) who completed the same PROMIS measures demonstrated that anxiety, depression, fatigue, and pain Interference scores were worse in this SLE sample, whereas physical function and satisfaction with social role scores were similar.[59] Studies of rheumatic disease patients incorporating PROMIS measures have also shown that, compared with patients with systemic sclerosis,[60] patients with SLE reported similar fatigue, more sleep disturbance, and better physical function. Compared with patients with osteoarthritis,[61] SLE patients had more fatigue but better physical function.[57,58]

PROMIS measures offer several advantages, including brevity and reduced burden; improved measurement with increased precision, allowing for increased power and reduced sample sizes; and flexible administration (established short forms of various lengths, custom short forms, CATs). They are domain specific rather than disease specific, and have a standardized scoring/metric, with a mean of 50 and standard deviation of 10, with most domains centered around the US general population, allowing for comparability across short forms and CATs and across studies and clinical conditions. Users of PROMIS measures have the ability to transform scores from other measures to the PROMIS score metric through PROsetta Stone linking methodology, and the measures are psychometrically sound, developed using state-of-the-science methods.

Although studies using PROMIS measures in people with SLE are only just emerging, these measurement tools seem to be appropriate for use in this population. The evidence to date suggests that PROMIS represents a system of valid and psychometric robust measurement tools that can provide brief yet precise scores for monitoring patients' HRQOL across relevant domains with minimal respondent burden. Additional research is needed to contribute to the evidence supporting the validity of the PROMIS measures in SLE. There is a need for studies to focus on the development of interpretive aids for PROMIS measures so researchers, clinicians, and patients can better understand what the scores and score changes mean in an informative, clinical context.

SYSTEMIC LUPUS ERYTHEMATOSUS-SPECIFIC PATIENT-REPORTED OUTCOME TOOLS

More recently, there has been an emphasis on developing SLE-specific PRO tools for use in clinical studies and clinical trials. Generic PRO tools may inadequately assess certain domains of the lupus experience, such as self-image or family planning, and SLE-specific PRO tools address these gaps. Further, generic instruments may not be sensitive enough to capture the frequent fluctuations in health status that are seen with SLE. Examples of SLE-specific PRO measures include LupusQoL,[39] Lupus Patient-Reported Outcome (LupusPRO),[40] SLE-specific Quality of Life Questionnaire (SLEQOL),[41] and SLE Quality of Life Questionnaire (L-QoL).[42]

The most widely studied SLE-specific PRO is the LupusQoL tool. Originally developed in the UK,[39] the instrument has since been validated in a US sample of patients with SLE.[62] Validity and other psychometric properties of non-English translations of LupusQoL have been published for Spanish,[63] Turkish,[64,65] Persian,[66] Italian,[67] French,[68] and Chinese[69] language cohorts. LupusQoL evaluates 8 domains including physical health, pain, planning, intimate relationships, burden to others, emotional health, body image, and fatigue. Questions pertain to the patient experience in the preceding 4 weeks and responses are given on a 5-item scale. A LupusQoL summary score is reported on 0 to 100 scale, with greater values indicating better HRQOL. LupusQoL has been shown to have favorable psychometric properties in the original UK version and in other language iterations of the tool. In the original UK sample, LupusQoL demonstrated good acceptability, reliability, and test–retest reliability. Concurrent validity was established by comparing with domains of SF-36 with good correlations. Patients with higher SLE disease activity, assessed with the British Isles Lupus Activity Group score, had poorer HRQOL in all domains except fatigue, establishing construct validity.[39] Responsiveness of Lupus QoL was assessed by comparison to the SF-36, with one study of Canadian patients with SLE reporting responsiveness equivalent to the SF-36[30] and another in a French sample finding that LupusQoL may be better than the SF-36 at capturing changes in respondents with improving health status.[31] In the French SLE sample, MCIDs ranged from 1.1 to 9.2 for respondents with global improvement in health status and from -0.5 to -6.4 for respondents with worsening health status.[31] Additional studies are needed to more firmly establish MCIDs. Finally, LupusQoL has been used in clinical research studies,[70–73] but not yet in clinical trials.

The LupusPRO tool was developed in a US SLE sample to allow improved generalizability to US patients.[40] The developers also sought to include issues pertinent to male patients with SLE and assess non-HRQOL domains. Cross-cultural validations of the English version of LupusPRO have been established in Canada[74] and the Philippines,[75] and the validity of translations into French Canadian,[76] Spanish,[77] Turkish,[78] and Chinese[79] have also been reported. The 43-item questionnaire includes 8 HRQOL domains such as lupus symptoms, physical health, and body image, as well as 4 non-HRQOL domains, including desires/goals and satisfaction with care. Respondents indicate their experience in the preceding 4 weeks on a 5-item response scale, and scores range from 0 (worst QOL) to 100 (best QOL). The initial validation cohort[40] demonstrated good internal consistency for all domains except lupus medication. Good test–retest reliability was noted for all HRQOL domains, but test–retest reliability was less for some of the non-HRQOL domains. Strong correlations with domains of the SF-36 were found, establishing concurrent validity. Criterion validity was suggested by strong correlations of LupusPRO domains with measures of disease activity, such as British Isles Lupus Activity Group, Safety of Estrogens in Lupus Erythematosus National Assessment-Systemic Lupus Erythematosus Disease Activity Index, and Lupus Foundation of America definition of disease flare, but correlations with disease damage were moderate. LupusPRO domains were compared with change in self-reported health status, physician global assessment, and Lupus Foundation of America flare status to evaluate responsiveness, but only weak to moderate correlations were found. MCIDs have also not been established for the Lupus PRO. Finally, beyond validation studies, LupusPRO has been used in one clinical research study[80] and no clinical trials to date.

Additional SLE-specific PRO tools include SLEQOL and L-QoL. SLEQOL was originally developed and validated in an English-speaking SLE sample in Singapore[41] but have not been assessed in a US cohort. Although the SLEQOL had acceptable internal consistency, test–retest reliability, construct validity, and responsiveness, it also demonstrated significant floor effects, such that respondents reported good QOL beyond what can be measured by the instrument, and concurrent validity of the tool was low when the summary score was compared with the SF-36.[41] Thus, coadministration of SLEQOL with a second validated HRQOL measure, such as the SF-36, may be required to address these limitations.

The L-QoL is the only SLE-specific PRO developed using a needs-based QOL model, and validation has only been assessed in a UK SLE sample thus far.[42] The L-QoL had excellent internal consistency, test–retest reliability and concurrent validity. Construct validity was assessed only against patient-reported disease activity and severity, and no validated physician assessments were used. The L-QoL has not been used in any clinical research studies or clinical trials to date, and further assessment of L-QoL construct validity and responsiveness will strengthen its use in future studies.

SUMMARY/DISCUSSION

Health outcomes research has produced a number of well-validated instruments that can be used across diseases and some have been specifically developed for SLE. Some of the most precise and comprehensive questionnaires are lengthy and complex, leading to a level of respondent burden that can hinder recruitment, limit the representativeness of the patient population being studied, and lead to problems of missing data.[24] Another approach has been to develop shorter questionnaires, which represent a compromise in measurement precision and range, but offer other desirable attributes in favor of practicality and the ability to compare with other chronic diseases as well as the general population. The use of either a generic or SLE-specific PRO is likely to depend on the variety of clinical applications including population monitoring, treatment decision making in clinical practice, clinical trials research, and for evaluation and comparison of the effect of therapies across conditions, therapies, trials, and patients in clinical research studies.[24]

REFERENCES

1. Cervera R, Khamashta MA, Font J, et al. Morbidity and mortality in systemic lupus erythematosus during a 10-year period: a comparison of early and late manifestations in a cohort of 1,000 patients. Medicine (Baltimore) 2003;82(5):299–308.
2. Siegel M, Lee SL. The epidemiology of systemic lupus erythematosus. Semin Arthritis Rheum 1973;3(1):1–54.
3. Trager J, Ward MM. Mortality and causes of death in systemic lupus erythematosus. Curr Opin Rheumatol 2001;13(5):345–51.
4. Bichile T, Petri M. Prevention and management of co-morbidities in SLE. Presse Med 2014;43(6 Pt 2):e187–95.
5. Tessier-Cloutier B, Clarke AE, Ramsey-Goldman R, et al. Systemic lupus erythematosus and malignancies: a review article. Rheum Dis Clin North Am 2014;40(3):497–506, viii.
6. Merrill JT. Treatment of systemic lupus erythematosus: a 2012 update. Bull NYU Hosp Jt Dis 2012;70(3):172–6.
7. Palagini L, Mosca M, Tani C, et al. Depression and systemic lupus erythematosus: a systematic review. Lupus 2013;22(5):409–16.
8. Palagini L, Tani C, Mauri M, et al. Sleep disorders and systemic lupus erythematosus. Lupus 2014;23(2):115–23.
9. Schoenfeld SR, Kasturi S, Costenbader KH. The epidemiology of atherosclerotic cardiovascular disease among patients with SLE: a systematic review. Semin Arthritis Rheum 2013;43(1):77–95.
10. Wekking EM. Psychiatric symptoms in systemic lupus erythematosus: an update. Psychosom Med 1993;55(2):219–28.
11. Bernatsky S, Boivin JF, Joseph L, et al. Mortality in systemic lupus erythematosus. Arthritis Rheum 2006;54(8):2550–7.

12. Schmeding A, Schneider M. Fatigue, health-related quality of life and other patient-reported outcomes in systemic lupus erythematosus. Best Pract Res Clin Rheumatol 2013;27(3):363–75.
13. McElhone K, Abbott J, Teh LS. A review of health related quality of life in systemic lupus erythematosus. Lupus 2006;15(10):633–43.
14. Feld J, Isenberg D. Why and how should we measure disease activity and damage in lupus? Presse Med 2014;43(6 Pt 2):e151–6.
15. Abu-Shakra M, Mader R, Langevitz P, et al. Quality of life in systemic lupus erythematosus: a controlled study. J Rheumatol 1999;26(2):306–9.
16. Fortin PR, Abrahamowicz M, Neville C, et al. Impact of disease activity and cumulative damage on the health of lupus patients. Lupus 1998;7(2):101–7.
17. Burckhardt CS, Archenholtz B, Bjelle A. Quality of life of women with systemic lupus erythematosus: a comparison with women with rheumatoid arthritis. J Rheumatol 1993;20(6):977–81.
18. Wang C, Mayo NE, Fortin PR. The relationship between health related quality of life and disease activity and damage in systemic lupus erythematosus. J Rheumatol 2001;28(3):525–32.
19. Hanly JG. Disease activity, cumulative damage and quality of life in systematic lupus erythematosus: results of a cross-sectional study. Lupus 1997;6(3):243–7.
20. Thumboo J, Fong KY, Chan SP, et al. A prospective study of factors affecting quality of life in systemic lupus erythematosus. J Rheumatol 2000;27(6):1414–20.
21. Pons-Estel GJ, Alarcón GS, Scofield L, et al. Understanding the epidemiology and progression of systemic lupus erythematosus. Semin Arthritis Rheum 2010; 39(4):257–68.
22. Neville C, Clarke AE, Joseph L, et al. Learning from discordance in patient and physician global assessments of systemic lupus erythematosus disease activity. J Rheumatol 2000;27(3):675–9.
23. Yen JC, Neville C, Fortin PR. Discordance between patients and their physicians in the assessment of lupus disease activity: relevance for clinical trials. Lupus 1999;8(8):660–70.
24. Strand V, Gladman D, Isenberg D, et al. Endpoints: consensus recommendations from OMERACT IV. Outcome measures in rheumatology. Lupus 2000;9(5):322–7.
25. Tugwell P, Chambers L, Torrance G, et al. The population health impact of arthritis. POHEM workshop group. J Rheumatol 1993;20(6):1048–51.
26. Ware JE Jr, Sherbourne CD. The MOS 36-item short-form health survey (SF-36). I. Conceptual framework and item selection. Med Care 1992;30(6):473–83.
27. Stoll T, Gordon C, Seifert B, et al. Consistency and validity of patient administered assessment of quality of life by the MOS SF-36; its association with disease activity and damage in patients with systemic lupus erythematosus. J Rheumatol 1997; 24(8):1608–14.
28. Hurst NP, Jobanputra P, Hunter M, et al. Validity of Euroqol–a generic health status instrument–in patients with rheumatoid arthritis. Economic and health outcomes research group. Br J Rheumatol 1994;33(7):655–62.
29. Hurst NP, Kind P, Ruta D, et al. Measuring health-related quality of life in rheumatoid arthritis: validity, responsiveness and reliability of EuroQol (EQ-5D). Br J Rheumatol 1997;36(5):551–9.
30. Touma Z, Gladman DD, Ibañez D, et al. Is there an advantage over SF-36 with a quality of life measure that is specific to systemic lupus erythematosus? J Rheumatol 2011;38(9):1898–905.

31. Devilliers H, Amoura Z, Besancenot JF, et al. Responsiveness of the 36-item short form health survey and the lupus quality of life questionnaire in SLE. Rheumatology (Oxford) 2015;54(5):940–9.
32. Strand V, Singh JA. Newer biological agents in rheumatoid arthritis: impact on health-related quality of life and productivity. Drugs 2010;70(2):121–45.
33. Kiani AN, Strand V, Fang H, et al. Predictors of self-reported health-related quality of life in systemic lupus erythematosus. Rheumatology (Oxford) 2013;52(9): 1651–7.
34. Mok CC, Ho LY, Cheung MY, et al. Effect of disease activity and damage on quality of life in patients with systemic lupus erythematosus: a 2-year prospective study. Scand J Rheumatol 2009;38(2):121–7.
35. Urowitz M, Gladman DD, Ibañez D, et al. Changes in quality of life in the first 5 years of disease in a multicenter cohort of patients with systemic lupus erythematosus. Arthritis Care Res (Hoboken) 2014;66(9):1374–9.
36. Strand V, Aranow C, Cardiel MH, et al. Improvement in health-related quality of life in systemic lupus erythematosus patients enrolled in a randomized clinical trial comparing LJP 394 treatment with placebo. Lupus 2003;12(9):677–86.
37. Wallace DJ, Stohl W, Furie RA, et al. A phase II, randomized, double-blind, placebo-controlled, dose-ranging study of belimumab in patients with active systemic lupus erythematosus. Arthritis Rheum 2009;61(9):1168–78.
38. Strand V, Levy RA, Cervera R, et al. Improvements in health-related quality of life with belimumab, a B-lymphocyte stimulator-specific inhibitor, in patients with autoantibody-positive systemic lupus erythematosus from the randomised controlled BLISS trials. Ann Rheum Dis 2014;73(5):838–44.
39. McElhone K, Abbott J, Shelmerdine J, et al. Development and validation of a disease-specific health-related quality of life measure, the LupusQol, for adults with systemic lupus erythematosus. Arthritis Rheum 2007;57(6):972–9.
40. Jolly M, Pickard AS, Block JA, et al. Disease-specific patient reported outcome tools for systemic lupus erythematosus. Semin Arthritis Rheum 2012;42(1):56–65.
41. Leong KP, Kong KO, Thong BY, et al. Development and preliminary validation of a systemic lupus erythematosus-specific quality-of-life instrument (SLEQOL). Rheumatology (Oxford) 2005;44(10):1267–76.
42. Doward LC, McKenna SP, Whalley D, et al. The development of the L-QoL: a quality-of-life instrument specific to systemic lupus erythematosus. Ann Rheum Dis 2009;68(2):196–200.
43. Stamm TA, Bauernfeind B, Coenen M, et al. Concepts important to persons with systemic lupus erythematosus and their coverage by standard measures of disease activity and health status. Arthritis Rheum 2007;57(7):1287–95.
44. Kuriya B, Gladman DD, Ibañez D, et al. Quality of life over time in patients with systemic lupus erythematosus. Arthritis Rheum 2008;59(2):181–5.
45. Aggarwal R, Wilke CT, Pickard AS, et al. Psychometric properties of the EuroQol-5D and short form-6D in patients with systemic lupus erythematosus. J Rheumatol 2009;36(6):1209–16.
46. Wang SL, Wu B, Zhu LA, et al. Construct and criterion validity of the Euro Qol-5D in patients with systemic lupus erythematosus. PLoS One 2014;9(6):e98883.
47. Wolfe F, Michaud K, Li T, et al. EQ-5D and SF-36 quality of life measures in systemic lupus erythematosus: comparisons with rheumatoid arthritis, noninflammatory rheumatic disorders, and fibromyalgia. J Rheumatol 2010;37(2):296–304.
48. Dua AB, Aggarwal R, Mikolaitis RA, et al. Rheumatologists' quality of care for lupus: comparison study between a university and county hospital. Arthritis Care Res (Hoboken) 2012;64(8):1261–4.

49. Bexelius C, Wachtmeister K, Skare P, et al. Drivers of cost and health-related quality of life in patients with systemic lupus erythematosus (SLE): a Swedish nationwide study based on patient reports. Lupus 2013;22(8):793–801.
50. Strand V, Galateanu C, Pushparajah DS, et al. Limitations of current treatments for systemic lupus erythematosus: a patient and physician survey. Lupus 2013;22(8): 819–26.
51. Bjork M, Dahlström Ö, Wetterö J, et al. Quality of life and acquired organ damage are intimately related to activity limitations in patients with systemic lupus erythematosus. BMC Musculoskelet Disord 2015;16:188.
52. Cella D, Riley W, Stone A, et al. The Patient Reported Outcomes Measurement Information System (PROMIS) developed and tested its first wave of adult self-reported health outcome item banks: 2005-2008. J Clin Epidemiol 2010;63(11): 1179–94.
53. Oude Voshaar MA, ten Klooster PM, Glas CA, et al. Calibration of the PROMIS physical function item bank in Dutch patients with rheumatoid arthritis. PLoS One 2014;9(3):e92367.
54. Fries JF, Cella D, Rose M, et al. Progress in assessing physical function in arthritis: PROMIS short forms and computerized adaptive testing. J Rheumatol 2009;36(9):2061–6.
55. Ow YL, Thumboo J, Cella D, et al. Domains of health-related quality of life important and relevant to multiethnic English-speaking Asian systemic lupus erythematosus patients: a focus group study. Arthritis Care Res (Hoboken) 2011;63(6): 899–908.
56. Jones JT, Nelson SL, Wootton J, et al. A134: validation of patient reported outcomes measurement information system modules for use in childhood-onset lupus. Arthritis Rheumatol 2014;66:S176–7.
57. Ahn G, Chmiel JS, Dunlop DD, et al. Accelerometer physical activity measurements, physical function, fatigue, anxiety, depression, pain, and sleep in adults with systemic lupus erythematosus (SLE): the Activity in Lupus to Energize and Renew (ALTER) study, in 10th International Congress on SLE. Buenos Aires, Argentina, April 18–21, 2013. p. P063.
58. Mahieu MA, Ahn GE, Chmiel JS, et al. Fatigue, patient reported outcomes, and objective measurement of physical activity in systemic lupus erythematosus. Lupus 2016; in press.
59. Rothrock NE, Hays RD, Spritzer K, et al. Relative to the general US population, chronic diseases are associated with poorer health-related quality of life as measured by the Patient-reported Outcomes Measurement Information System (PROMIS). J Clin Epidemiol 2010;63(11):1195–204.
60. Khanna D, Maranian P, Rothrock N, et al. Feasibility and construct validity of PROMIS and “legacy” instruments in an academic scleroderma clinic. Value Health 2012;15(1):128–34.
61. Broderick JE, Schneider S, Junghaenel DU, et al. Validity and reliability of Patient-reported Outcomes Measurement Information System instruments in osteoarthritis. Arthritis Care Res (Hoboken) 2013;65(10):1625–33.
62. Jolly M, Pickard AS, Wilke C, et al. Lupus-specific health outcome measure for US patients: the LupusQoL-US version. Ann Rheum Dis 2010;69(1):29–33.
63. Gonzalez-Rodriguez V, Peralta-Ramírez MI, Navarrete-Navarrete N, et al. Adaptation and validation of the Spanish version of a disease-specific quality of life measure in patients with systemic lupus erythematosus: the Lupus quality of life. Med Clin (Barc) 2010;134(1):13–6 [in Spanish].

64. Yilmaz-Oner S, Oner C, Dogukan FM, et al. Health-related quality of life assessed by LupusQoL questionnaire and SF-36 in Turkish patients with systemic lupus erythematosus. Clin Rheumatol 2015. [Epub ahead of print].
65. Pamuk ON, Onat AM, Donmez S, et al. Validity and reliability of the Lupus QoL index in Turkish systemic lupus erythematosus patients. Lupus 2015;24(8): 816–21.
66. Hosseini N, Bonakdar ZS, Gholamrezaei A, et al. Linguistic validation of the LupusQoL for the assessment of quality of life in Iranian patients with systemic lupus erythematosus. Int J Rheumatol 2014;2014:151530.
67. Conti F, Perricone C, Reboldi G, et al. Validation of a disease-specific health-related quality of life measure in adult Italian patients with systemic lupus erythematosus: LupusQoL-IT. Lupus 2014;23(8):743–51.
68. Devilliers H, Amoura Z, Besancenot JF, et al. LupusQoL-FR is valid to assess quality of life in patients with systemic lupus erythematosus. Rheumatology (Oxford) 2012;51(10):1906–15.
69. Wang SL, Wu B, Leng L, et al. Validity of LupusQoL-China for the assessment of health related quality of life in Chinese patients with systemic lupus erythematosus. PLoS One 2013;8(5):e63795.
70. Jolly M, Pickard SA, Mikolaitis RA, et al. LupusQoL-US benchmarks for US patients with systemic lupus erythematosus. J Rheumatol 2010;37(9):1828–33.
71. McElhone K, Castelino M, Abbott J, et al. The LupusQoL and associations with demographics and clinical measurements in patients with systemic lupus erythematosus. J Rheumatol 2010;37(11):2273–9.
72. Gordon C, Isenberg D, Lerstrøm K, et al. The substantial burden of systemic lupus erythematosus on the productivity and careers of patients: a European patient-driven online survey. Rheumatology (Oxford) 2013;52(12):2292–301.
73. Mirbagher L, Gholamrezaei A, Hosseini N, et al. Sleep quality in women with systemic lupus erythematosus: contributing factors and effects on health-related quality of life. Int J Rheum Dis 2014. [Epub ahead of print].
74. Bourre-Tessier J, Clarke AE, Mikolaitis-Preuss RA, et al. Cross-cultural validation of a disease-specific patient-reported outcome measure for systemic lupus erythematosus in Canada. J Rheumatol 2013;40(8):1327–33.
75. Navarra SV, Tanangunan RM, Mikolaitis-Preuss RA, et al. Cross-cultural validation of a disease-specific patient-reported outcome measure for lupus in Philippines. Lupus 2013;22(3):262–7.
76. Bourre-Tessier J, Clarke AE, Kosinski M, et al. The French-Canadian validation of a disease-specific, patient-reported outcome measure for lupus. Lupus 2014; 23(14):1452–9.
77. Jolly M, Toloza S, Block J, et al. Spanish LupusPRO: cross-cultural validation study for lupus. Lupus 2013;22(5):431–6.
78. Kaya A, Goker B, Cura ES, et al. Turkish lupusPRO: cross-cultural validation study for lupus. Clin Rheumatol 2014;33(8):1079–84.
79. Mok CC, Kosinski M, Ho LY, et al. Validation of the LupusPRO in Chinese patients from Hong Kong with systemic lupus erythematosus. Arthritis Care Res (Hoboken) 2015;67(2):297–304.
80. Jolly M, Peters KF, Mikolaitis R, et al. Body image intervention to improve health outcomes in lupus: a pilot study. J Clin Rheumatol 2014;20(8):403–10.

Patient-Reported Outcomes in Psoriatic Arthritis

Ana-Maria Orbai, MD, MHS[a,*], Alexis Ogdie, MD, MSCE[b]

KEYWORDS

- Psoriatic arthritis • Patient reported outcome • Outcome measure
- Composite measures

KEY POINTS

- Psoriatic arthritis is a chronic and heterogeneous inflammatory arthritis associated with psoriasis.
- Patient-reported outcomes are essential in assessing health status and treatment effects in psoriatic arthritis.
- Additional studies are needed to understand what patients think is important in defining the activity of their disease.

INTRODUCTION

Psoriatic arthritis (PsA) is a chronic inflammatory arthritis associated with psoriasis. It affects people heterogeneously with a range of clinical manifestations (eg, inflammatory arthritis, dactylitis, enthesitis, spondylitis, skin psoriasis, nail disease). The disease has a significant impact on patients' physical function, energy level, social participation, mood, and quality of life.[1] Physician-based outcome measures do not capture the patient's experience of the disease. Patient input in assessing disease status and the effectiveness of their treatments is an important aspect of the management of PsA. Patient-reported outcomes (PROs) give us the ability to integrate patient input in a way that is complementary to physician assessments and laboratory measures. PROs are measures of self-reported health status used to evaluate the

Disclosure Statement: The authors have nothing to disclose.
Dr A.M. Orbai's work is supported by the Rheumatology Research Foundation Scientist Development Award and by the Johns Hopkins Arthritis Discovery Fund. Dr A. Ogdie is supported by National Institute of Arthritis and Musculoskeletal and Skin Diseases (K23 AR063764).
[a] Division of Rheumatology, Johns Hopkins University, Asthma and Allergy Building, Room 1B19, 5501 Hopkins Bayview Circle, Baltimore, MD 21224, USA; [b] Division of Rheumatology, Center for Clinical Epidemiology and Biostatistics, Perelman School of Medicine, University of Pennsylvania, White Building, Room 5024, 3400 Spruce Street, Philadelphia, PA 19104, USA
* Corresponding author.
E-mail address: aorbai1@jhmi.edu

Rheum Dis Clin N Am 42 (2016) 265–283
http://dx.doi.org/10.1016/j.rdc.2016.01.002 rheumatic.theclinics.com
0889-857X/16/$ – see front matter

patient's perception of symptoms, function, and other aspects of his or her life potentially impacted by disease.

In PsA, PROs are used in clinical trials and clinical practice. PROs are key components of efficacy endpoints in clinical trials and are incorporated with physician-based measures in composite disease activity indices, including the primary outcome in PsA randomized controlled trials (RCTs), the American College of Rheumatology 20% improvement response criteria (ACR20). As a part of the OMERACT (Outcome Measures in Rheumatology Clinical Trials) PsA Core Domain Set,[2] PROs representing patient global assessment, pain, physical function, and health-related quality of life are expected to be measured in all PsA RCTs in addition to physician assessments of joints and skin. Beyond these domains, PROs are used to capture work productivity, fatigue, psychological endpoints, and other symptoms. A wide range of PROs exist and few have been developed specifically for PsA. Most measures used in PsA have been developed for other diseases (eg, Health Assessment Questionnaire Disability index for rheumatoid arthritis, Functional Assessment of Chronic Illness Therapy-Fatigue for cancer-related anemia) or are generic and meant to assess population health (eg, Medical Outcomes Study Short Form-36 [SF-36], European Quality of Life Index-5 Dimensions [EQ-5D]). Furthermore, even fewer PROs have been developed with input from patients with PsA. Patient input into PsA outcome measures has previously been reviewed, and for most measures there has been no patient input.[3] For a few measures, patient input has been incorporated by developing items from qualitative research among patients with PsA (Psoriatic Arthritis Quality of Life index, Psoriasis Symptom Inventory, Worst Itch-Numerical Rating Scale) or using patient research partner opinions of the relative importance of domains (Psoriatic Arthritis Impact of Disease).[4] Measures of PsA have been reviewed previously.[5]

In this review, we discuss PROs used in observational and interventional studies of PsA. We have organized the PROs into categories based on the domains they address.

METHODS

We performed a systematic literature search on July 22, 2015, in PubMed. We included the following search terms for PsA: ("Arthritis, Psoriatic"[Mesh] OR "Psoriatic arthritis" OR "psoriatic arthropathy" OR "arthritis psoriatica" OR "arthropathic psoriasis" OR "psoriasis arthropathica" OR "psoriatic arthropathy" OR "psoriatic polyarthritis" OR "psoriatic rheumatism") and the Oxford Patient-Reported Outcome Measurement filter (source: Oxford Department of Public Health PROM Group). We obtained 1422 entries, which were reviewed by title and abstract for inclusion. We excluded duplicates and studies specifically for children. After this review, 247 articles were retained. We performed additional searches for individual outcome measures. For each measure, we synthesized the available data on the use of the outcome measure in PsA.

PATIENT-REPORTED OUTCOMES IN PSORIATIC ARTHRITIS STUDIES

PROs may be disease specific or generic and may address one or more health dimensions or domains. Domains assessed by PROs used in PsA are shown in **Table 1** and the most frequently used are discussed as follows. Studied measurement characteristics of PRO measurement instruments are summarized in **Table 2**.

Pain

Pain is a prevalent and debilitating symptom in arthritis. Pain assessment is part of the Outcome Measures in Rheumatology Clinical Trials core domain set and 1 of the 3 PROs in the ACR response indices. It is an outcome measure that is, uniformly

Table 1
Domains and patient-reported outcomes in psoriatic arthritis studies

Domain	Patient-Reported Outcome
Pain	Pain visual analog scale
Patient global	Patient global Skin Joints Skin and Joints
Health-related quality of life	Medical Outcomes Study Short Form-36 Euro-Qol 5 Dimensions PsA Quality of Life Index Dermatologic Life Quality Index Ankylosing Spondylitis Quality of Life Index
Impact of disease	Arthritis Impact Measurement Scales Psoriatic Arthritis Impact of Disease
Disease activity	Routine Assessment of Patient Index Data Rheumatoid Arthritis Disease Activity Index Bath Ankylosing Spondylitis Disease Activity Index
Disability and physical function	Health Assessment Questionnaire Disability Index Bath Ankylosing Spondylitis Functional Index Disabilities of Arm, Shoulder, and Hand Questionnaire
Skin	Psoriasis Symptom Inventory Worst Itch Numerical Rating Scale
Fatigue	Functional Assessment Chronic Illness Therapy-Fatigue Fatigue Visual Analog Scale/Numerical Rating Scale
Productivity	Work Productivity Survey (arthritis specific)

collected in PsA RCTs and longitudinal studies. Pain is generally measured using a 100-mm visual analog scale (VAS) or an 11-point numerical rating scale (NRS) (range 0–10) with anchors "no pain" (left, 0) to "pain as bad as it could be" (right, 100 or 10 respectively) and a recall period of 7 days.

Psoriatic Arthritis Global Assessment Scales

As noted previously, global assessment scales are a part of the 2006 OMERACT PsA Core Domain Set and are captured in most clinical trials and as part of many composite measures. Global assessment scales are meant to measure the impact of a patient's disease on his or her life. These questions may be phrased in slightly different ways and generally specify a time period over which to rate the effect of their disease. The Group for Research and Assessment of Psoriasis and Psoriatic Arthritis (GRAPPA) has advocated for measuring 3 distinct global assessments that include separate skin and joint global assessments and a dual skin and joint global assessment.[6] The skin and joint global item is formulated as follows: "In all the ways in which your PSORIASIS and ARTHRITIS, as a whole, affects you, how would you rate the way you felt over the past week?" and responses are recorded on a 100-mm VAS with anchors "Excellent" (left) and "Poor" (right). VASs are most often used in measuring a global assessment, although some have used NRS or Likert-type scales, such as the Multi-Dimensional Health Assessment Questionnaire (MDHAQ).[7]

Health-Related Quality of Life

Although the term "health-related quality of life" (HRQL)[8] has not been precisely defined, measures of HRQL are generally felt to measure the impact of chronic

Table 2
Studied measurement characteristics of patient-reported outcomes in psoriatic arthritis

Patient-Reported Outcome	Population	Reliability Internal Consistency	Reliability, for Example Test-Retest	Measurement Error	Content Validity	Construct Validity	Criterion Validity	Responsiveness	Interpretability (Existence of Cutoffs)
Medical Outcomes Study Short Form-36 (SF-36)	General	Cronbach alpha >0.8 for all 8 scales[30]	NR	NR	NR	Hypothesis testing based on convergent/ divergent validity[30] Structural validity of PCS and MCS dimensions with confirmatory factor analysis[73]	NR	Area under receiver operator curve[74]	PsA MID calculated[13]
Euro-Qol 5 Dimensions (EQ-5D)	General	NR	NR	NR	NR	NR	NR	NR	NR
PsA Quality of Life Index (PsAQoL)	Psoriatic arthritis	Internal consistency 0.91 Rasch analysis: person separation index 0.93[23]	Test-retest reliability 0.89[23]	NR	Qualitative research	Hypothesis testing convergent validity[23]	NR	NR	NR
Dermatologic Life Quality Index (DLQI)	Dermatologic conditions	NR	NR	NR	NR	NR	NR	NR	NR
Psoriatic Arthritis Impact of Disease (9 and 12 item)	Psoriatic arthritis	Cronbach alpha = 0.93–0.94[4]	Test-retest reliability at 2–10 d ICC 0.95 and 0.94[4]	NR	Patient prioritized domains[4]	Hypothesis testing convergent validity[4]	NR	Provided SRM[4]	Preliminary values PASS = 4 MCII = 3[4]

Bath Ankylosing Spondylitis Disease Activity Index (BASDAI)	Ankylosing spondylitis	NR	NR	NR	NR	Hypothesis testing correlation with disease activity[44,45]	NR	Area under receiver operator curve calculated for predicting high disease activity/ change in treatment[45]	NR
Health Assessment Questionnaire Disability Index (HAQ-DI)	RA	NR	NR	NR	NR	NR	NR	Area under receiver operator curve calculated[74]	PsA MID 0.131[75] PsA MCII 0.35[50]
Disabilities of Arm, Shoulder, and Hand Questionnaire (DASH)	RA	NR	NR	NR	NR	Hypothesis testing, correlations with disease activity measures[55]	NR	NR	NR
Psoriasis Symptom Inventory (PSI)	Psoriasis	Cronbach alpha = 0.95–0.97[63]	Test- retest (0–2 wk and 2–4 wk) ICC = 0.7 and 0.87[63]	(psoriasis) Limits of agreement[62]	Qualitative research	Structural validity using confirmatory factor analysis and Rasch analysis: unidimensionality Hypothesis testing correlations with BSA, SF-36[63]	NR	Comparison of PSI change scores w change in patient global[63]	NR
Functional Assessment Chronic Illness Therapy-Fatigue (FACIT-F)	Cancer	Cronbach alpha = 0.96[66]	Test-retest ICC = 0.95[66]	NR	NR	Hypothesis testing[66]	Correlation with Fatigue Severity Scale = –0.79	NR	No PsA MID RA MID is 4
Work Productivity Survey (WPS)	RA	NR	NR	NR	Literature review	Hypothesis testing[72]	NR	Report SRM[72]	NR

Abbreviations: BSA, body surface area; ICC, intraclass correlation coefficient; MCII, minimal clinically important improvement; MID, minimally important difference; NR, not reported; PASS, patient acceptable symptoms state; PsA, psoriatic arthritis; RA, rheumatoid arthritis; SRM, standardized response mean.

disease or therapeutic interventions on a patient's quality of life. Self-rated health has long been shown to predict short-term and long-term mortality in the elderly after adjustment for physician assessment, comorbidities, health-service utilization, demographics, income, and life satisfaction.[9] HRQL represents a broad concept and draws from different domains of health (such as fatigue, physical function, and emotional function) to derive a final score. The most commonly used HRQL outcome measures are generic (eg, SF-36 and EQ-5D), although some HRQL measures have been developed specifically for PsA (Psoriatic Arthritis Quality of Life [PsAQoL]). HRQL measures are often secondary efficacy endpoints in RCTs and can be incorporated into composite measures assessing the cost-effectiveness of interventions in PsA. We discuss those measures most frequently used in PsA in the following paragraphs. Other measures that are less commonly used in PsA include the Arthritis Impact Measurement Scales (AIMS and AIMS2), Ankylosing Spondylitis Quality of Life index (ASQoL), Routine Assessment of Patient Index Data (RAPID3), and the Rheumatoid Arthritis Disease Activity Index (RADAI).

The Medical Outcomes Study Short Form-36

The SF-36 was developed for use in the general population for clinical care, economic evaluations, and health surveys.[10,11] It can be administered as a PRO, but also has been administered by trained individuals via telephone. Although a free version of the questionnaire (RAND-36) is available,[12] the SF-36 is proprietary and the scoring is complex. The SF-36 questionnaire assesses the following 8 health domains on a scale of 0 to 100, with 100 being the best score: (1) limitations in physical activities (due to health problems); (2) limitations in social activities (due to physical or emotional problems); (3) limitations in usual role activities (due to physical health problems); (4) bodily pain; (5) general mental health (psychological distress and well-being); (6) limitations in usual role activities (due to emotional problems); (7) vitality (energy and fatigue); and (8) general health perceptions. Scores can also be summarized on 2 components using a population-normed T-score metric with a mean of 50 and SD of 10. These subscores are termed the Physical Component Score (PCS) and Mental Component Score (MCS). Minimal important differences for improvement in PsA were examined using Rasch analysis in one[13] small study (20 patients with PsA starting biologic) and are estimated at 3.74 for PCS and 1.7 for MCS. Corresponding changes in a population with rheumatoid arthritis (RA) are 4.4 for PCS and 3.1 for MCS.[14] The SF-36 is widely used in PsA RCTs as the preferred measure for HRQL due to its responsiveness with treatment.[13,15,16]

The European Quality of Life Index-5 Dimensions

The EQ-5D is a commonly used generic quality-of-life instrument developed in Europe. It assesses mobility, self-care, usual activities, pain and anxiety/depression. The final score is calculated using a derived formula. The score ranges from −0.594 to 1, where zero is equivalent to death (and therefore patients can rate their health status as being worse than death). EQ-5D has been measured in many PsA RCTs, particularly those conducted in Europe. However, it is widely used among many different diseases and has been validated in a variety of disease states. It is frequently used in economic analyses. An advantage and disadvantage of the EQ-5D is its brevity: it is easily and rapidly completed; however, there are only 3 possible answers for each question, which contributes to a ceiling effect.[17–22]

Psoriatic Arthritis Quality of Life Index

The PsAQoL is a PsA disease-specific measure of quality of life composed of 20 yes/no questions, making this a relatively easy and rapid questionnaire for completion. The items address domains including social participation, fatigue, mood, and daily activities. This instrument was developed using results from focus groups conducted among patients with PsA and subsequent item surveys with patients. The PsAQoL had excellent test-retest reliability and 2 studies have demonstrated correlation of PsAQoL with other instruments, suggesting construct validity.[23,24] Additionally, the PsAQoL is sensitive to change. The PsAQoL has been adapted in additional languages for Sweden and the Netherlands.[25–28] Similar to the SF-36, the PsAQoL is proprietary. Although not frequently used in clinical trials, the PsAQoL was used in the recent Tight Control in Psoriatic Arthritis (TiCOPA) trial and it is part of several candidate PsA disease activity indices (see **Table 3**).[29–31]

Psoriatic Arthritis Impact of Disease

The Psoriatic Arthritis Impact of Disease (PsAID) is a measure developed by the European League Against Rheumatism (EULAR) and is composed of domains selected by an international group of patients with PsA. The PsAID is not specifically an HRQL PRO. It is instead intended for use as a patient-reported measure of disease impact on life in general. The PsAID has 2 versions: 1 with 9 domains for RCTs and 1 with 12 domains for clinical care. PsAID domains include the following: (1) pain (pain in joints, spine, and skin); (2) skin problems (including itching); (3) fatigue (being physically tired, but also mental fatigue, lack of energy); (4) ability to work/leisure; (5) functional capacity; (6) feeling of discomfort; (7) sleep disturbance; (8) anxiety, fear, and uncertainty (about the future, treatments, fear of loneliness); (9) coping (adjustment to the disease, managing, being in charge, making do with the disease); (10) embarrassment and/or shame due to appearance; (11) social participation; and (12) depression (numbers 10–12 are added to the 9-item questionnaire). The questionnaire uses a weighted scoring system (weights were derived by patient impression of importance) and has a range of 0 to 10 (higher scores are worse) with 4 being considered a patient-acceptable symptom state.[4] The proposed Minimal Clinically Important Difference (MCID) is 3. Given that this is a relatively new measure, few studies have included the PsAID, but studies are under way to determine sensitivity to change and convergent validity.

Patient-Reported Disease Activity, Disability, and Physical Function

Patient-reported disease activity measures have been developed for RA (eg, RAPID3) and ankylosing spondylitis (AS) (eg, Bath Ankylosing Spondylitis Disease Activity Index [BASDAI]), and these measures have been extended to other rheumatologic diseases including PsA. One issue with patient-reported disease activity measures is the lack of correlation between self-reported joint counts with physician assessments in PsA.[32] In one study, there was weak correlation for tender joints, no correlation for swollen joints, and weak to moderate correlation for damaged joints. A study in the same cohort showed discrepancies between patient and physician global assessments[33]; these patient-physician discrepancies were significantly associated in a multivariable regression model with scores for fatigue, pain, tender and swollen joints, and HRQL. Nevertheless, these measures may provide different and complimentary information to physician-reported measures. We discuss the most commonly used patient-reported disease activity measures in PsA trials and in the clinical management of PsA in the following sections. Additionally, we discuss PRO measures for disability and physical function, which have different meanings from disease activity. Although physical function may correlate with disease activity, disability may not.[34–41]

Bath Ankylosing Spondylitis Disease Activity Index

The BASDAI was developed in patients with AS and exclusively axial disease.[42] BASDAI is a questionnaire consisting of 6 VAS items assessing fatigue, axial joint pain, peripheral joint pan, soft tissue tenderness to touch, and severity and duration of morning stiffness. Responses are recorded on unlabeled 10-cm VAS with left and right anchor "None" and "Very severe," except for the morning stiffness duration item, from "0" to "2 or more hours" with additional labels for 0.5, 1.0, and 1.5 hours. Score range is 0 to 10, calculated as the mean of the 6 items. BASDAI has been used in PsA with and without axial disease and scores were generally higher in the axial versus peripheral PsA phenotype.[43,44] In axial PsA (grade 2 or more unilateral sacroiliitis, inflammatory back pain, and stiffness), BASDAI did not differentiate between levels of disease activity defined by change in treatment in either axial or peripheral PsA.[44] In the Toronto PsA cohort, BASDAI showed good discriminative ability for high and low disease activity in axial PsA (similarly defined as grade 2 or more sacroiliitis, inflammatory back pain, or spinal mobility limitation). Three definitions were used for high disease activity: patient global greater than 6, physician global greater than 6, and change in treatment. BASDAI discriminative ability for high disease activity using the 3 definitions was calculated as area under the curve (AUC) (95% confidence interval): 0.92 (0.88–0.95), 0.78 (0.67–0.88), and 0.69 (0.63–0.76) respectively.[45]

Health Assessment Questionnaire Disability Index

Health Assessment Questionnaire Disability Index (HAQ-DI) is a widely used outcome measurement instrument for disability, developed in patients with RA.[46] HAQ-DI scores have been shown to predict future function, survival, and resource utilization in RA,[47] and correlate with radiographic scores in RA.[48] Total HAQ-DI score range is 0 to 3 and normal scores are 0.5 or lower. Minimal clinically important improvement (MCII) in RA has been determined to be a decrease of 0.375 in the total score[49] (equivalent to 3 points improvement in the raw score), and very similar, a decrease of 0.35 in PsA.[50] The HAQ-DI has been measured in every PsA RCT, as it is part of the ACR responder indices and is usually also reported as a separate endpoint. HAQ-DI has been shown to be limited by floor effect much more in PsA (30%) than RA (8%),[51–53] a fact supported by a comparative review of RA versus PsA RCTs in which mean HAQ-DI scores are systematically higher in RA versus PsA.[54] Although this may be interpreted as a lower level of disability, it may in fact be a reflection of common oligoarticular involvement with PsA.

Disabilities of Arm, Shoulder, and Hand Questionnaire

The Disabilities of Arm, Shoulder, and Hand Questionnaire (DASH) was studied in one longitudinal PsA cohort. Correlations with clinical measures of disease/joint activity were lower for the total joint core compared with upper extremity score as expected because DASH measures upper limb function.[55] Due to common lower extremity involvement in PsA, the measure is not sufficient for assessing the construct of disability in most patients with PsA.

Skin Symptoms and Related Impact

Although a complete review of the quality-of-life and disease activity indices for skin are beyond the scope of this review, we briefly discuss those commonly included in clinical trials of PsA.

Dermatology Life Quality Index

The Dermatology Life Quality Index (DLQI) is a quality-of-life index designed for patients with skin disease. This 10-item questionnaire (with one additional item that branches) ascertains the impact of skin disease on work and leisure activities, social participation/relationships, and symptoms related to skin disease, such as itch and pain.[56,57] The DLQI is widely used in clinical trials for psoriasis and PsA and correlates well with the Psoriasis Area and Severity Index.[58] This questionnaire is easy to complete, sensitive to change, and has been validated in multiple populations, in particular psoriasis.[59]

Psoriasis Symptom Inventory

The Psoriasis Symptom Inventory (PSI) is a recently developed PRO assessing psoriasis symptoms that can be administered on paper or electronically.[60] Rather than an HRQL index, this can be used more as a disease activity index. The PSI was developed in people with psoriasis in the United States who participated in focus groups and interviews to generate and subsequently clarify concepts and patient-preferred terms. The PSI has 8 items assessing the severity of each of these symptoms: (1) itch, (2) redness, (3) scaling, (4) burning, (5) stinging, (6) cracking, (7) flaking, and (8) pain due to psoriasis.[61] Item response options are a 5-point Likert type (score 0: not at all severe; 1: mild; 2: moderate; 3: severe; 4: very severe), and 2 versions exist, differing only in the recall period (24 hours and 7 days). The PSI score range is 0 to 32 with higher score representing worse symptoms. The test-retest reliability of PSI items has been studied in 139 patients with psoriasis and it was good (individual items intraclass correlation coefficients [ICCs] >0.7) as well as correlations with DLQI and SF-36 items. As expected, the highest correlations were observed with corresponding skin symptom items.[62] The PSI was tested in 154 people, with PsA showing good test-retest reliability (total score ICC 0.7), moderate correlation with body surface area and patient global (–0.5 and 0.4, respectively) and low correlations with SF-36 concepts and physician global.[63]

Worst Itch Numerical Rating Scale

The Worst Itch NRS was developed in patients with psoriasis (n = 22) and PsA (n = 12) and consists of a single NRS (0–10, “no itch” to “worst imaginable itch”) for itch with an assessment over the past 24 hours. The item was developed using qualitative research with patients with psoriasis and PsA followed by item cognitive debriefing.[64]

Fatigue

Functional Assessment Chronic Illness Therapy-Fatigue

The Functional Assessment Chronic Illness Therapy-Fatigue (FACIT-F) is a 13-item PRO initially developed in patients with cancer as the Functional Assessment of Cancer Therapy[65] and adapted for use in other chronic conditions. Score range is 0 to 52 with higher scores reflecting less fatigue. FACIT-F reliability and validity was examined in a longitudinal PsA study.[66] Minimal important change in RA is 4 points[67] and it has not been specifically studied in PsA.

Fatigue Visual Analog Scale

Fatigue VAS use is common especially in clinical care (including an 11-point NRS scale as a part of the MDHAQ) and longitudinal studies. Fatigue VAS has been criticized for lack of standardization because this causes great difficulty with comparisons across studies.[68]

Work Productivity

Work productivity and work disability are related concepts. PsA is associated with increased work disability[69] that can be reversed with treatment.[70]

The arthritis-specific Work Productivity Survey (WPS) was developed in RA on the basis of a literature review[71] and has data supporting its validity in PsA from one RCT.[72] The WPS is an interviewer-administered 10-item questionnaire assessing employment status, missed workdays, productivity, and arthritis interference both in the work place and at home, with a recall period of 1 month. Two of the items are VASs with anchors "no interference" (left) and "complete interference" (right) and additional items are reports of numbers of days missed or not as productive.

Sleep Disturbance

There is evidence that PsA is associated with sleep disturbance[76] and patients prioritized this impact in the EULAR PsAID measure, yet sleep is rarely assessed in PsA research or clinical care. The Medical Outcomes Study Sleep Scale has been used in a study of psoriasis and fibromyalgia but not specifically in PsA.[77,78] The PsAID questionnaire is the only PsA-specific PRO assessing sleep disturbance as one of its domains. Further studies are needed to address optimal PROs for sleep in PsA.

INCLUSION OF PATIENT-REPORTED OUTCOMES IN COMPOSITE MEASURES FOR PSORIATIC ARTHRITIS

Composite outcome measures have been developed to attempt to integrate patient and clinician measures (**Table 3**) and to address several domains in a single measure. In composite indices, patient and physician measures are aggregated into a single score. There are 2 types of composite measures: those that are response indices and have a dichotomous cutoff (eg, ACR20) and those that calculate a score for disease activity (eg, Disease Activity for Psoriatic Arthritis [DAPSA]) that is sensitive to change and a cutoff is derived to serve as a threshold for "response." This second type of measure can be a static or dynamic measure of disease activity and often has defined categories of disease activity (eg, remission; low, moderate, and high disease activity). Patient measures most often included are the HAQ (or a functional assessment), pain, and global assessments. A few of the composite measures include quality of life (via the SF-36, PsAQoL, DLQI, and/or ASQoL). In the following sections we address the PROs in each composite index and how these were selected. The domains assessed by each composite measure are shown in **Table 3**. The Psoriatic Arthritis Joint Activity Index (PsAJAI) was previous developed but has not yet been used in additional studies since development and thus is not included below.[79]

American College of Rheumatology 20%, 50%, and 70% Response Criteria

The ACR20 is the most commonly used response index and is the primary outcome for trials in PsA. The ACR criteria define response as a binary outcome. These criteria were initially developed for RA and use a 28-joint count. This has been modified in PsA to include a 66/68 joint count. The ACR criteria were developed using physician surveys and analysis of RA clinical trial data. These criteria define response at the 20%, 50%, and 70% thresholds based on the reduction in tender and swollen joint counts, physician's global assessment, acute phase reactant, and 3 PROs, HAQ-DI, patient pain assessment, and patient global assessment.[80]

Disease Activity Score

Disease Activity Score (DAS) of 28 or 66/68 joints, the Clinical Disease Activity Index (CDAI), and the Simplified Disease Activity Index (SDAI). Similar to the ACR outcomes, these measures were developed initially in RA. The DAS has been modified for PsA to include the 66/68 joint counts. These disease activity measures include only one

Table 3
Composite outcome measures in psoriatic arthritis

	ACR20[a]	DAS28[a]	CDAI	SDAI	PsARC	DAPSA	CPDAI	PASDAS	AMDF
Peripheral arthritis[a]	■	■	■	■	■	■	■	■	■
Psoriasis skin disease							■		
Enthesitis							■	■	
Dactylitis							■	■	
Spinal disease							■		
Health-related quality of life							■	■	■
Physical function assessment (HAQ)	■						■		■
Patient global: arthritis activity									■
Patient global: skin disease activity									■
Patient global: disease activity	■	■	■	■	■	■		■	■
Patient pain assessment	■					■			■
Physician global assessment	■		■	■	■			■	
Acute-phase response	■	■		■		■		■	

Patient-reported outcomes are shown within the dark lines.

Abbreviations: ACR20, American College of Rheumatology 20% Response; AMDF, arithmetical mean of desirability functions; CDAI, clinical disease activity index; CPDAI, composite psoriatic disease activity index; DAPSA, disease activity in psoriatic arthritis; DAS28, Disease Activity Score 28 Joints; PASDAS, psoriatic arthritis disease activity score; PsAJAI, psoriatic arthritis joint activity index; SDAI, simplified disease activity index.

[a] Peripheral arthritis is captured through the number of swollen and tender joints. The ACR20 is defined as 20% improvement in tender and swollen joint counts as well as 20% improvement in 3 of the other 5 measures. The ACR20 and DAS28 assess the proximal interphalangeal and metacarpophalangeal joints, wrists, elbows, shoulders, and knees. DAPSA, CPDAI, PASDAS, and AMDF use the 66/68 joint counts. The DAS66/68 adds the hips, distal interphalangeal joints, sternoclavicular, temporomandibular, acromioclavicular, talotibial, midtarsal, metatarsophalangeal, and interphalangeal joints of the toes.

Adapted from Coates LC, FitzGerald O, Mease PJ, et al. Development of a disease activity and responder index for psoriatic arthritis–report of the Psoriatic Arthritis Module at OMERACT 11. J Rheumatol 2014;41(4):784; with permission.

PRO: the patient global assessment of health in the case of DAS, and the patient global assessment of arthritis for CDAI and SDAI. In addition, these measures include the swollen and tender joint counts and one or both of the C-reactive protein or sedimentation rate and physician (or evaluator) global assessment.[81]

Disease Activity Index for Psoriatic Arthritis

Development of the DAPSA was based on a principal component analysis that revealed 3 significant components: 2 PROs (patient pain and global assessments), joint involvement (66/68 swollen joint counts), and acute phase response (C-reactive protein).[82] The Disease Activity Index for Reactive Arthritis (DAREA) had previously been derived for reactive arthritis and contained these same elements. It was thus tested in PsA and found to have good discrimination (AUC 0.74–0.80)[83]; however, subsequent studies have suggested that other composite indices may have larger effect sizes.[84] Recently, DAPSA cutoffs for disease activity states and treatment response have been derived using patient-level data from 3 PsA RCTs[85] therefore this index is now usable and interpretable.

Composite Psoriatic Disease Activity Index

The domains of the Composite Psoriatic Disease Activity Index (CPDAI) were derived from consensus among GRAPPA members and include joint disease, skin involvement, enthesitis, dactylitis, and spinal disease. Instruments to measure each domain were similarly chosen by consensus. For each domain, activity is defined as none, mild, moderate, or severe, and these categories can be defined by more than one instrument. Each domain is assigned a point value depending on the severity (0–3 respectively), and these individual scores are then summed to a final score (range 0–15). PROs included in the CPDAI include the HAQ for peripheral arthritis, DLQI for skin disease, and BASDAI or ASQoL for spine disease.[86]

The Psoriatic Arthritis Disease Activity Score and the Arithmetical Mean of Desirability Functions

Both the Psoriatic Arthritis Disease Activity Score (PASDAS) and Arithmetical Mean of Desirability Functions (AMDF) were developed as a part of the GRAppa Composite Exercise (GRACE) project and were derived (although in different ways) from the same datasets. In this dataset (GRACE study), PROs included patient global assessments (overall global, skin, and joints), the DLQI, ASQoL index, PsAQoL index, SF-36 and the individual components, and the HAQ. The PASDAS was derived using a principal component analysis, and the AMDF was derived using desirability functions (desirability was derived using physician surveys). Both have somewhat complex formulas. The PASDAS includes the physician and patient global assessments, the SF-36 physical component scale, the tender and swollen joint counts, the Leeds enthesitis count, tender dactylitis count, and the C-reactive protein. The AMDF includes the same elements (different formula) but adds the mental component scale of the SF-36.[87] These measures have not yet been used in PsA clinical trials but have shown large effect sizes in a clinical trial dataset.[88]

Minimal Disease Activity

Minimal Disease Activity (MDA) is a set of criteria that define the “state of disease activity deemed a useful target of treatment by both the patient and physician, given current treatment possibilities and limitations.” Each domain is assessed as active or not active based on suggested thresholds. The OMERACT PsA Core Domains, agreed on in 2006, were used to define MDA. However, HRQL was excluded because of lack of correlation between HRQL and other measures of disease activity to be included. Rheumatologists and dermatologists were then asked to decide whether patient profiles were in a state of MDA. Thresholds for each of the domains were maintained when greater than 70% consensus was achieved. The final version of the MDA includes the following components: (threshold) patient pain and global VAS assessments (less than or equal to 15 and 20 respectively), the HAQ (less than or equal to 0.5), tender and swollen joint counts (less than or equal to 1), enthesitis count (less than or equal to 1), and psoriasis severity characterized by either Psoriasis Area and Severity Index (PASI) or body surface area (less than or equal to 1, and 3% respectively).[89] MDA state is defined as achieving the threshold for 5 of the 7 components.

Psoriatic Arthritis Response Criteria

The Psoriatic Arthritis Response Criteria (PsARC) is a composite responder index that includes tender[68] and swollen[66] joint counts and physician and patient global assessments (measured on 5-point Likert scales).[90] It was the first composite measure derived specifically for PsA. Similar to the ACR response criteria, this is a binary score in which patients can meet the definition of response if they have either a 30% reduction in tender joints or swollen joints or a 1-point improvement in either the physician or patient global assessment scale and the other items must not worsen.[91] The PsARC is generally not used as the primary outcome measure in RCTs but rather as a secondary outcome.[92–95]

SUMMARY

PsA is a complex disease. Patients with PsA have highly varied manifestations of PsA (eg, peripheral arthritis, spondylitis, enthesitis, dactylitis) and are likewise varied in terms of how they experience their disease and the level of impact it has on their lives. From these perspectives, PsA can be difficult to measure. The patients' perspective of their illness and their response to therapy can be captured using PROs. Although numerous PROs exist in general, only a few addressing each domain have been validated in PsA and even fewer have been developed specifically for PsA; however, some existing PROs do perform relatively well in PsA RCTs. Additional studies are needed to understand what patients think is important in defining the activity of their disease. With such knowledge, we can more precisely define the unidimensional concepts that need to be assessed in PsA such that a set of PROs with optimized measurement properties for PsA can be selected and standardized for PsA assessment in clinical trials and clinical practice.

REFERENCES

1. Taylor WJ, Mease PJ, Adebajo A, et al. Effect of psoriatic arthritis according to the affected categories of the international classification of functioning, disability and health. J Rheumatol 2010;37(9):1885–91.
2. Gladman DD, Mease PJ, Strand V, et al. Consensus on a core set of domains for psoriatic arthritis. J Rheumatol 2007;34(5):1167–70.
3. Tillett W, Adebajo A, Brooke M, et al. Patient involvement in outcome measures for psoriatic arthritis. Curr Rheumatol Rep 2014;16(5):418.
4. Gossec L, de Wit M, Kiltz U, et al. A patient-derived and patient-reported outcome measure for assessing psoriatic arthritis: elaboration and preliminary validation of the Psoriatic Arthritis Impact of Disease (PsAID) questionnaire, a 13-country EULAR initiative. Ann Rheum Dis 2014;73(6):1012–9.
5. Mease PJ. Measures of psoriatic arthritis: Tender and Swollen Joint Assessment, Psoriasis Area and Severity Index (PASI), Nail Psoriasis Severity Index (NAPSI), Modified Nail Psoriasis Severity Index (mNAPSI), Mander/Newcastle Enthesitis Index (MEI), Leeds Enthesitis Index (LEI), Spondyloarthritis Research Consortium of Canada (SPARCC), Maastricht Ankylosing Spondylitis Enthesis Score (MASES), Leeds Dactylitis Index (LDI), Patient Global for Psoriatic Arthritis, Dermatology Life Quality Index (DLQI), Psoriatic Arthritis Quality of Life (PsAQOL), Functional Assessment of Chronic Illness Therapy-Fatigue (FACIT-F), Psoriatic Arthritis Response Criteria (PsARC), Psoriatic Arthritis Joint Activity Index (PsAJAI), Disease Activity in Psoriatic Arthritis (DAPSA), and Composite Psoriatic Disease Activity Index (CPDAI). Arthritis Care Res (Hoboken) 2011;63(Suppl 11): S64–85.
6. Cauli A, Gladman DD, Mathieu A, et al. Patient global assessment in psoriatic arthritis: a multicenter GRAPPA and OMERACT study. J Rheumatol 2011;38(5): 898–903.

7. Pincus T, Skummer PT, Grisanti MT, et al. MDHAQ/RAPID3 can provide a roadmap or agenda for all rheumatology visits when the entire MDHAQ is completed at all patient visits and reviewed by the doctor before the encounter. Bull NYU Hosp Jt Dis 2012;70(3):177–86.
8. Guyatt GH, Feeny DH, Patrick DL. Measuring health-related quality of life. Ann Intern Med 1993;118(8):622–9.
9. Mossey JM, Shapiro E. Self-rated health: a predictor of mortality among the elderly. Am J Public Health 1982;72(8):800–8.
10. McHorney CA, Ware JE Jr, Raczek AE. The MOS 36-Item Short-Form Health Survey (SF-36): II. Psychometric and clinical tests of validity in measuring physical and mental health constructs. Med Care 1993;31(3):247–63.
11. Ware JE Jr, Sherbourne CD. The MOS 36-item short-form health survey (SF-36). I. Conceptual framework and item selection. Med Care 1992;30(6):473–83.
12. Hays RD, Morales LS. The RAND-36 measure of health-related quality of life. Ann Med 2001;33(5):350–7.
13. Leung YY, Zhu TY, Tam LS, et al. Minimal important difference and responsiveness to change of the SF-36 in patients with psoriatic arthritis receiving tumor necrosis factor-alpha blockers. J Rheumatol 2011;38(9):2077–9.
14. Kosinski M, Zhao SZ, Dedhiya S, et al. Determining minimally important changes in generic and disease-specific health-related quality of life questionnaires in clinical trials of rheumatoid arthritis. Arthritis Rheum 2000;43(7):1478–87.
15. Saad AA, Ashcroft DM, Watson KD, et al. Improvements in quality of life and functional status in patients with psoriatic arthritis receiving anti-tumor necrosis factor therapies. Arthritis Care Res (Hoboken) 2010;62(3):345–53.
16. Strand V, Sharp V, Koenig AS, et al. Comparison of health-related quality of life in rheumatoid arthritis, psoriatic arthritis and psoriasis and effects of etanercept treatment. Ann Rheum Dis 2012;71(7):1143–50.
17. Ahmad MA, Xypnitos FN, Giannoudis PV. Measuring hip outcomes: common scales and checklists. Injury 2011;42(3):259–64.
18. Leung YY, Png ME, Wee HL, et al. Comparison of EuroQol-5D and short form-6D utility scores in multiethnic Asian patients with psoriatic arthritis: a cross-sectional study. J Rheumatol 2013;40(6):859–65.
19. Gignac MA, Cao X, McAlpine J, et al. Measures of disability: arthritis impact measurement scales 2 (AIMS2), Arthritis Impact Measurement Scales 2-Short Form (AIMS2-SF), The Organization for Economic Cooperation and Development (OECD) Long-Term Disability (LTD) Questionnaire, EQ-5D, World Health Organization Disability Assessment Schedule II (WHODASII), Late-Life Function and Disability Instrument (LLFDI), and Late-Life Function and Disability Instrument-Abbreviated Version (LLFDI-Abbreviated). Arthritis Care Res 2011;63(Suppl 11):S308–24.
20. Husted J, Gladman DD, Farewell VT, et al. Validation of the revised and expanded version of the Arthritis Impact Measurement Scales for patients with psoriatic arthritis. J Rheumatol 1996;23(6):1015–9.
21. Husted J, Gladman DD, Long JA, et al. Relationship of the Arthritis Impact Measurement Scales to changes in articular status and functional performance in patients with psoriatic arthritis. J Rheumatol 1996;23(11):1932–7.
22. Long JA, Husted JA, Gladman DD, et al. The relationship between patient satisfaction with health and clinical measures of function and disease status in patients with psoriatic arthritis. J Rheumatol 2000;27(4):958–66.
23. McKenna SP, Doward LC, Whalley D, et al. Development of the PsAQoL: a quality of life instrument specific to psoriatic arthritis. Ann Rheum Dis 2004;63(2):162–9.

24. Brodszky V, Pentek M, Balint PV, et al. Comparison of the Psoriatic Arthritis Quality of Life (PsAQoL) questionnaire, the functional status (HAQ) and utility (EQ-5D) measures in psoriatic arthritis: results from a cross-sectional survey. Scand J Rheumatol 2010;39(4):303–9.
25. Billing E, McKenna SP, Staun M, et al. Adaptation of the Psoriatic Arthritis Quality of Life (PsAQoL) instrument for Sweden. Scand J Rheumatol 2010;39(3):223–8.
26. Wink F, Arends S, McKenna SP, et al. Validity and reliability of the Dutch adaptation of the Psoriatic Arthritis Quality of Life (PsAQoL) Questionnaire. PLoS One 2013;8(2):e55912.
27. Doward LC, Spoorenberg A, Cook SA, et al. Development of the ASQoL: a quality of life instrument specific to ankylosing spondylitis. Ann Rheum Dis 2003;62(1): 20–6.
28. Leung YY, Tam LS, Kun EW, et al. Comparison of 4 functional indexes in psoriatic arthritis with axial or peripheral disease subgroups using Rasch analyses. J Rheumatol 2008;35(8):1613–21.
29. Husted JA, Gladman DD, Cook RJ, et al. Responsiveness of health status instruments to changes in articular status and perceived health in patients with psoriatic arthritis. J Rheumatol 1998;25(11):2146–55.
30. Husted JA, Gladman DD, Farewell VT, et al. Validating the SF-36 health survey questionnaire in patients with psoriatic arthritis. J Rheumatol 1997;24(3):511–7.
31. Taal E, Rasker JJ, Riemsma RP. Sensitivity to change of AIMS2 and AIMS2-SF components in comparison to M-HAQ and VAS-pain. Ann Rheum Dis 2004; 63(12):1655–8.
32. Chaudhry SR, Thavaneswaran A, Chandran V, et al. Physician scores vs patient self-report of joint and skin manifestations in psoriatic arthritis. Rheumatology (Oxford) 2013;52(4):705–11.
33. Eder L, Thavaneswaran A, Chandran V, et al. Factors explaining the discrepancy between physician and patient global assessment of joint and skin disease activity in psoriatic arthritis patients. Arthritis Care Res (Hoboken) 2015;67(2):264–72.
34. Husted JA, Tom BD, Farewell VT, et al. A longitudinal study of the effect of disease activity and clinical damage on physical function over the course of psoriatic arthritis: does the effect change over time? Arthritis Rheum 2007;56(3):840–9.
35. Castrejon I, Bergman MJ, Pincus T. MDHAQ/RAPID3 to recognize improvement over 2 months in usual care of patients with osteoarthritis, systemic lupus erythematosus, spondyloarthropathy, and gout, as well as rheumatoid arthritis. J Clin Rheumatol 2013;19(4):169–74.
36. Pincus T, Swearingen CJ, Bergman M, et al. RAPID3 (Routine Assessment of Patient Index Data 3), a rheumatoid arthritis index without formal joint counts for routine care: proposed severity categories compared to disease activity score and clinical disease activity index categories. J Rheumatol 2008;35(11):2136–47.
37. Pincus T, Furer V, Keystone E, et al. RAPID3 (Routine Assessment of Patient Index Data 3) severity categories and response criteria: similar results to DAS28 (Disease Activity Score) and CDAI (Clinical Disease Activity Index) in the RAPID 1 (Rheumatoid Arthritis Prevention of Structural Damage) clinical trial of certolizumab pegol. Arthritis Care Res 2011;63(8):1142–9.
38. Castrejon I, Dougados M, Combe B, et al. Can remission in rheumatoid arthritis be assessed without laboratory tests or a formal joint count? possible remission criteria based on a self-report RAPID3 score and careful joint examination in the ESPOIR cohort. J Rheumatol 2013;40(4):386–93.
39. Danve A, Reddy A, Vakil-Gilani K, et al. Routine Assessment of Patient Index Data 3 score (RAPID3) correlates well with Bath Ankylosing Spondylitis Disease

Activity index (BASDAI) in the assessment of disease activity and monitoring progression of axial spondyloarthritis. Clin Rheumatol 2015;34(1):117–24.
40. Castrejon I, Yazici Y, Pincus T. Patient self-report RADAI (Rheumatoid Arthritis Disease Activity Index) joint counts on an MDHAQ (Multidimensional Health Assessment Questionnaire) in usual care of consecutive patients with rheumatic diseases other than rheumatoid arthritis. Arthritis Care Res 2013;65(2):288–93.
41. Leeb BF, Haindl PM, Brezinschek HP, et al. Patient-centered psoriatic arthritis (PsA) activity assessment by Stockerau Activity Score for Psoriatic Arthritis (SASPA). BMC Musculoskelet Disord 2015;16:73.
42. Garrett S, Jenkinson T, Kennedy LG, et al. A new approach to defining disease status in ankylosing spondylitis: the Bath ankylosing spondylitis disease activity index. J Rheumatol 1994;21(12):2286–91.
43. Taylor WJ, Harrison AA. Could the Bath Ankylosing Spondylitis Disease Activity Index (BASDAI) be a valid measure of disease activity in patients with psoriatic arthritis? Arthritis Rheum 2004;51(3):311–5.
44. Fernandez-Sueiro JL, Willisch A, Pertega-Diaz S, et al. Validity of the bath ankylosing spondylitis disease activity index for the evaluation of disease activity in axial psoriatic arthritis. Arthritis Care Res (Hoboken) 2010;62(1):78–85.
45. Eder L, Chandran V, Shen H, et al. Is ASDAS better than BASDAI as a measure of disease activity in axial psoriatic arthritis? Ann Rheum Dis 2010;69(12):2160–4.
46. Fries JF, Spitz P, Kraines RG, et al. Measurement of patient outcome in arthritis. Arthritis Rheum 1980;23(2):137–45.
47. Wolfe F, Kleinheksel SM, Cathey MA, et al. The clinical value of the Stanford Health Assessment Questionnaire Functional Disability Index in patients with rheumatoid arthritis. J Rheumatol 1988;15(10):1480–8.
48. Navarro-Compan V, Landewe R, Provan SA, et al. Relationship between types of radiographic damage and disability in patients with rheumatoid arthritis in the EURIDISS cohort: a longitudinal study. Rheumatology (Oxford) 2015;54(1):83–90.
49. Ward MM, Guthrie LC, Alba MI. Clinically important changes in individual and composite measures of rheumatoid arthritis activity: thresholds applicable in clinical trials. Ann Rheum Dis 2015;74(9):1691–6.
50. Mease PJ, Woolley JM, Bitman B, et al. Minimally important difference of Health Assessment Questionnaire in psoriatic arthritis: relating thresholds of improvement in functional ability to patient-rated importance and satisfaction. J Rheumatol 2011;38(11):2461–5.
51. Taylor WJ, McPherson KM. Using Rasch analysis to compare the psychometric properties of the Short Form 36 physical function score and the Health Assessment Questionnaire disability index in patients with psoriatic arthritis and rheumatoid arthritis. Arthritis Rheum 2007;57(5):723–9.
52. Fries JF, Bruce B, Rose M. Comparison of the health assessment questionnaire disability index and the short form 36 physical functioning subscale using Rasch analysis: comment on the article by Taylor and McPherson. Arthritis Rheum 2008; 59(4):598–9 [author reply: 9].
53. Calin A, Garrett S, Whitelock H, et al. A new approach to defining functional ability in ankylosing spondylitis: the development of the bath ankylosing spondylitis functional index. J Rheumatol 1994;21(12):2281–5.
54. Lee S, Mendelsohn A, Sarnes E. The burden of psoriatic arthritis: a literature review from a global health systems perspective. P T 2010;35(12):680–9.
55. Navsarikar A, Gladman DD, Husted JA, et al. Validity assessment of the disabilities of arm, shoulder, and hand questionnaire (DASH) for patients with psoriatic arthritis. J Rheumatol 1999;26(10):2191–4.

56. Finlay AY, Khan GK. Dermatology Life Quality Index (DLQI)–a simple practical measure for routine clinical use. Clin Exp Dermatol 1994;19(3):210–6.
57. Nichol MB, Margolies JE, Lippa E, et al. The application of multiple quality-of-life instruments in individuals with mild-to-moderate psoriasis. Pharmacoeconomics 1996;10(6):644–53.
58. Mattei PL, Corey KC, Kimball AB. Psoriasis Area Severity Index (PASI) and the Dermatology Life Quality Index (DLQI): the correlation between disease severity and psychological burden in patients treated with biological therapies. J Eur Acad Dermatol Venereol 2014;28(3):333–7.
59. Lundberg L, Johannesson M, Silverdahl M, et al. Health-related quality of life in patients with psoriasis and atopic dermatitis measured with SF-36, DLQI and a subjective measure of disease activity. Acta Derm Venereol 2000;80(6):430–4.
60. Bushnell DM, Martin ML, Scanlon M, et al. Equivalence and measurement properties of an electronic version of the Psoriasis Symptom Inventory. Qual Life Res 2014;23(3):897–906.
61. Martin ML, McCarrier KP, Chiou CF, et al. Early development and qualitative evidence of content validity for the Psoriasis Symptom Inventory (PSI), a patient-reported outcome measure of psoriasis symptom severity. J Dermatolog Treat 2013;24(4):255–60.
62. Bushnell DM, Martin ML, McCarrier K, et al. Validation of the Psoriasis Symptom Inventory (PSI), a patient-reported outcome measure to assess psoriasis symptom severity. J Dermatolog Treat 2013;24(5):356–60.
63. Wilson HD, Mutebi A, Revicki DA, et al. Reliability and validity of the psoriasis symptom inventory in patients with psoriatic arthritis. Arthritis Care Res (Hoboken) 2015;67(12):1750–6.
64. Naegeli AN, Flood E, Tucker J, et al. The Worst Itch Numeric Rating Scale for patients with moderate to severe plaque psoriasis or psoriatic arthritis. Int J Dermatol 2015;54(6):715–22.
65. Yellen SB, Cella DF, Webster K, et al. Measuring fatigue and other anemia-related symptoms with the Functional Assessment of Cancer Therapy (FACT) measurement system. J Pain Symptom Manage 1997;13(2):63–74.
66. Chandran V, Bhella S, Schentag C, et al. Functional assessment of chronic illness therapy-fatigue scale is valid in patients with psoriatic arthritis. Ann Rheum Dis 2007;66(7):936–9.
67. Cella D, Yount S, Sorensen M, et al. Validation of the functional assessment of chronic illness therapy fatigue scale relative to other instrumentation in patients with rheumatoid arthritis. J Rheumatol 2005;32(5):811–9.
68. Hewlett S, Dures E, Almeida C. Measures of fatigue: Bristol Rheumatoid Arthritis Fatigue Multi-Dimensional Questionnaire (BRAF MDQ), Bristol Rheumatoid Arthritis Fatigue Numerical Rating Scales (BRAF NRS) for severity, effect, and coping, Chalder Fatigue Questionnaire (CFQ), Checklist Individual Strength (CIS20R and CIS8R), Fatigue Severity Scale (FSS), Functional Assessment Chronic Illness Therapy (Fatigue) (FACIT-F), Multi-Dimensional Assessment of Fatigue (MAF), Multi-Dimensional Fatigue Inventory (MFI), Pediatric Quality of Life (PedsQL) Multi-Dimensional Fatigue Scale, Profile of Fatigue (ProF), Short Form 36 Vitality Subscale (SF-36 VT), and Visual Analog Scales (VAS). Arthritis Care Res 2011;63(Suppl 11):S263–86.
69. Tillett W, de-Vries C, McHugh NJ. Work disability in psoriatic arthritis: a systematic review. Rheumatology (Oxford) 2012;51(2):275–83.

70. Kristensen LE, Englund M, Neovius M, et al. Long-term work disability in patients with psoriatic arthritis treated with anti-tumour necrosis factor: a population-based regional Swedish cohort study. Ann Rheum Dis 2013;72(10):1675–9.
71. Osterhaus JT, Purcaru O, Richard L. Discriminant validity, responsiveness and reliability of the rheumatoid arthritis-specific Work Productivity Survey (WPS-RA). Arthritis Res Ther 2009;11(3):R73.
72. Osterhaus JT, Purcaru O. Discriminant validity, responsiveness and reliability of the arthritis-specific Work Productivity Survey assessing workplace and household productivity in patients with psoriatic arthritis. Arthritis Res Ther 2014; 16(4):R140.
73. Leung YY, Ho KW, Zhu TY, et al. Testing scaling assumptions, reliability and validity of medical outcomes study short-form 36 health survey in psoriatic arthritis. Rheumatology (Oxford) 2010;49(8):1495–501.
74. Husted JA, Cook RJ, Farewell VT, et al. Methods for assessing responsiveness: a critical review and recommendations. J Clin Epidemiol 2000;53(5):459–68.
75. Kwok T, Pope JE. Minimally important difference for patient-reported outcomes in psoriatic arthritis: health assessment questionnaire and pain, fatigue, and global visual analog scales. J Rheumatol 2010;37(5):1024–8.
76. Callis Duffin K, Wong B, Horn EJ, et al. Psoriatic arthritis is a strong predictor of sleep interference in patients with psoriasis. J Am Acad Dermatol 2009;60(4): 604–8.
77. Strober BE, Sobell JM, Duffin KC, et al. Sleep quality and other patient-reported outcomes improve after patients with psoriasis with suboptimal response to other systemic therapies are switched to adalimumab: results from PROGRESS, an open-label Phase IIIB trial. Br J Dermatol 2012;167(6):1374–81.
78. Williams DA, Arnold LM. Measures of fibromyalgia: fibromyalgia impact questionnaire (FIQ), Brief Pain Inventory (BPI), Multidimensional Fatigue Inventory (MFI-20), Medical Outcomes Study (MOS) Sleep Scale, and Multiple Ability Self-Report Questionnaire (MASQ). Arthritis Care Res 2011;63(Suppl 11):S86–97.
79. Gladman DD, Tom BD, Mease PJ, et al. Informing response criteria for psoriatic arthritis (PsA). II: further considerations and a proposal–the PsA joint activity index. J Rheumatol 2010;37(12):2559–65.
80. Felson DT, Anderson JJ, Boers M, et al. American College of Rheumatology preliminary definition of improvement in rheumatoid arthritis. Arthritis Rheum 1995; 38(6):727–35.
81. Prevoo ML, van 't Hof MA, Kuper HH, et al. Modified disease activity scores that include twenty-eight-joint counts. Development and validation in a prospective longitudinal study of patients with rheumatoid arthritis. Arthritis Rheum 1995; 38(1):44–8.
82. Nell-Duxneuner VP, Stamm TA, Machold KP, et al. Evaluation of the appropriateness of composite disease activity measures for assessment of psoriatic arthritis. Ann Rheum Dis 2010;69(3):546–9.
83. Schoels M, Aletaha D, Funovits J, et al. Application of the DAREA/DAPSA score for assessment of disease activity in psoriatic arthritis. Ann Rheum Dis 2010; 69(8):1441–7.
84. Helliwell PS, FitzGerald O, Fransen J. Composite disease activity and responder indices for psoriatic arthritis: a report from the GRAPPA 2013 meeting on development of cutoffs for both disease activity states and response. J Rheumatol 2014;41(6):1212–7.

85. Schoels MM, Aletaha D, Alasti F, et al. Disease activity in psoriatic arthritis (PsA): defining remission and treatment success using the DAPSA score. Ann Rheum Dis 2015. [Epub ahead of print].
86. Mumtaz A, Gallagher P, Kirby B, et al. Development of a preliminary composite disease activity index in psoriatic arthritis. Ann Rheum Dis 2011;70(2):272–7.
87. Helliwell PS, FitzGerald O, Fransen J, et al. The development of candidate composite disease activity and responder indices for psoriatic arthritis (GRACE project). Ann Rheum Dis 2013;72(6):986–91.
88. Helliwell PS, Kavanaugh A. Comparison of composite measures of disease activity in psoriatic arthritis using data from an interventional study with golimumab. Arthritis Care Res 2014;66(5):749–56.
89. Coates LC, Fransen J, Helliwell PS. Defining minimal disease activity in psoriatic arthritis: a proposed objective target for treatment. Ann Rheum Dis 2010;69(1): 48–53.
90. Clegg DO, Reda DJ, Mejias E, et al. Comparison of sulfasalazine and placebo in the treatment of psoriatic arthritis. A Department of Veterans Affairs cooperative study. Arthritis Rheum 1996;39(12):2013–20.
91. Fransen J, Antoni C, Mease PJ, et al. Performance of response criteria for assessing peripheral arthritis in patients with psoriatic arthritis: analysis of data from randomised controlled trials of two tumour necrosis factor inhibitors. Ann Rheum Dis 2006;65(10):1373–8.
92. Mease PJ, Fleischmann R, Deodhar AA, et al. Effect of certolizumab pegol on signs and symptoms in patients with psoriatic arthritis: 24-week results of a phase 3 double-blind randomised placebo-controlled study (RAPID-PsA). Ann Rheum Dis 2014;73(1):48–55.
93. Mease PJ, Goffe BS, Metz J, et al. Etanercept in the treatment of psoriatic arthritis and psoriasis: a randomised trial. Lancet 2000;356(9227):385–90.
94. Gladman DD, Tom BD, Mease PJ, et al. Informing response criteria for psoriatic arthritis. I: discrimination models based on data from 3 anti-tumor necrosis factor randomized studies. J Rheumatol 2010;37(9):1892–7.
95. Gladman DD1; ACCLAIM Study Investigators, Sampalis JS, et al. Responses to adalimumab in patients with active psoriatic arthritis who have not adequately responded to prior therapy: effectiveness and safety results from an open-label study. J Rheumatol 2010;37(9):1898–906.

35. Schoels MM, Aletaha D, Alasti F, et al. Disease activity in psoriatic arthritis (PsA): defining remission and treatment success using the DAPSA score. Ann Rheum Dis 2016. [Epub ahead of print].
36. Mumtaz A, Gallagher P, Kirby B, et al. Development of a preliminary composite disease activity index in psoriatic arthritis. Ann Rheum Dis 2011;70(2):272–7.
37. Helliwell PS, FitzGerald O, Fransen J, et al. The development of candidate composite disease activity and responder indices for psoriatic arthritis (GRACE project). Ann Rheum Dis 2013;72(6):986–91.
38. [illegible]

Patient-Reported Outcomes in Axial Spondyloarthritis

Derek T. Nhan, BS, BA[a,b], Liron Caplan, MD, PhD[a,b,*]

KEYWORDS

• Axial spondyloarthritis • Ankylosing spondylitis • Patient outcome assessment

KEY POINTS

- More than 20 separate studies in more than 12,000 patients have validated patient-reported outcome measures in axial spondyloarthritis over the past 30 years.
- Of the available patient-reported outcome measures available for axial spondyloarthritis, only 3 to 4 are currently used routinely.
- About half of North American rheumatologists with expertise in axial spondyloarthritis use formal patient-reported outcome measures in their practice.

Axial spondyloarthritis (axSpA) is a complex, debilitating inflammatory condition characterized by involvement of the joint of the spine and the sacroiliac joints. Ankylosing spondylitis (AS)—a severe and prototypic form of axial spondyloarthritis—includes fibrous or bony bridging of joints in the spine, frequently involving multiple intervertebral discs. Although the history of AS, as the most obvious presentation of axSpA, extends back several centuries, its cause and pathophysiology have yet to be fully defined. The delineation of patient-reported outcomes (PROs) in axSpA and AS has been a longstanding challenge, due to the lack of data from longitudinal epidemiologic studies and the nonspecific nature of inflammatory laboratory markers to monitor disease activity. At least since the execution of therapeutic trials in the 1960s,[1] PROs have been increasingly used to better define this disorder. PRO measures provide a quantifiable and reproducible method of capturing data in the context of medical practice, allowing for efficient measures of quality of life and disease activity. An overview of current patient-reported measures and their validation are provided herein.

Support: D.T. Nhan was supported by NIAMS T32 AR007534-28.
[a] Veterans Affairs Medical Center (VAMC), Denver, CO, USA; [b] University of Colorado School of Medicine, Aurora, CO, USA
* Corresponding author. University of Colorado School of Medicine, PO Box 6511, Mail Stop B115, Denver, CO 80045.
E-mail address: liron.caplan@ucdenver.edu

Rheum Dis Clin N Am 42 (2016) 285–299
http://dx.doi.org/10.1016/j.rdc.2016.01.011
0889-857X/16/$ – see front matter Published by Elsevier Inc.

HISTORY OF AXIAL SPONDYLOARTHRITIS AND ANKYLOSING SPONDYLITIS

The diagnosis of AS traces back to Galen's initial differentiation from rheumatoid arthritis in 200 AD, but it was not until 1559 that the first historical description of AS appeared in the literature. In that year, Realdo Colombo described 2 skeletons with AS-like characteristics in his book, *De Re Anatomica*. Other clinical descriptions have been scattered since then, and AS has historically been synonymous with terms such as Bechterew's disease and Marie-Strumpell disease.[2,3] As radiographic and clinical reports began to more precisely depict the features of AS, umbrella terms—"spondyloarthropathy" and "spondyloarthritis"—were then introduced in the 1970s, to distinguish this family of related disorders from rheumatoid arthritis.[4] This group of conditions included AS, psoriatic arthritis, reactive arthritis, inflammatory bowel disease–associated arthritis, and undifferentiated spondyloarthritis.

In his 1977 landmark paper, rheumatologist Andrei Calin and colleagues[5] described modern diagnostic criteria for inflammatory back pain (IBP), which was a hallmark of AS, and later, axSpA. Their criteria included: (a) age at onset less than 40 years; (b) back pain greater than 3 months; (c) insidious onset; (d) morning stiffness; and (e) improvement with exercise.[5] A few years later, a simplified version of the concept of IBP was codified in the modified New York criteria, which gained rapid acceptance.[6] Although adequate for identifying the well-established disease represented by AS, these criteria did not capture more subtle and earlier forms of axSpA. Thus, 2 additional classification criteria were constructed in the 1990s that identified a broader disease concept, including early-stage disease and peripheral spondyloarthritis without axial involvement.[7,8] Finally, in 2009, the Assessment of SpondyloArthritis international Society (ASAS) Criteria were developed using more rigorous methodology to allow for the identification of axSpA by integrating clinical, laboratory, and imaging data.[9]

DIFFERENT PATIENT-REPORTED OUTCOME MEASURES

The emergence of each of these classification criteria has often ushered in a complementary set of PRO measures. As a result, outcome measures for describing spondyloarthritides have exploded within the last 15 to 20 years, with significant progress in documentation of PROs, clinical and physical assessments, and characterization of disease stages for treatment protocols.[10] The characterization of disease activity in axSpA, on the other hand, has been somewhat delayed by comparison.

The following discusses the current uses, critiques, and evidence of validation for the currently published series of axSpA measures. Basic information regarding the content, format, method of calculation, and both respondent burden and time to score is provided in **Table 1**.

Quality of Life

The Ankylosing Spondylitis Quality of Life (ASQoL) questionnaire was originally developed using a needs-based model of health from 3 hospitals in northern England and 3 hospitals in southern Netherlands to monitor the impact of AS on a patient's ability to satisfy their needs of sleep, motivation, activities of daily living, relationships, and social life. The investigators established a goal of using the information to provide practitioners with a tool to guide clinical decision-making and improve patient outcomes. Since its publication, the ASQoL has been the most frequently used disease specific measure of health quality of life in AS studies, including the assessment of tumor necrosis factor inhibitor (TNFi) therapy among AS patients.[11]

The ASQoL questionnaire was originally derived from interview transcripts in the field and ultimately condensed to an 18-item measure that uses dichotomous format

Table 1
Characteristics of common patient-reported outcome measures in axial spondyloarthritis

PRO	General Description/ Components	No. of Items Comprising the PRO	Format	Common Method of Calculation	Respondent Burden (min)	Time to Score (min)	Languages
ASDAS	Back pain, duration of AM stiffness, peripheral joint pain/swelling, general well-being, CRP/ESR	5	Likert: 0–7	ASDAS calculator	<1 min	<1 min	US English, Spanish, French, multiple+
ASQoL	Impact of disease on sleep, mood, motivation, coping, ADL, relationships, social life	18	Likert: Y/N	Summation	2–16 min	<1 min	US English, Canadian French/ English, German, Spanish, Chinese, multiple+
BASDAI	Back pain, fatigue, peripheral joint pain/ swelling, tenderness, disease and severity of AM stiffness	6	Numeric: 0–10 (AM stiffness = 0–2+ h); VAS, 0–10 cm	Mean of Q1-4 + (Mean of Q5/Q6)	30 s–2 min	<1 min	English, French, Swedish, German, Arabic, Spanish, multiple+
BASFI	Functional anatomy and coping with daily life	6	Numeric: 0–10; VAS (0–10 cm)	Mean of 6 subscores	<3	<1 min	English, French, German, Spanish, Chinese, multiple+
BAS-G	Well-being, over last week and last 6 mo	2	Numeric: 0–10	N/A	<1 min	<1 min	Dutch and Norwegian, few others
BASMI	Cervical rotation, tragus to wall, lumbar flexion, lumbar side flexion, intermalleolar distance	5	Numeric: 0–10; ROM	Mean of 5 subscores	5–10 min	<1 min	English, German, Finnish, multiple+
DFI	ADLs	20	Likert: 0(n)–2 (y)	Summation	>BASFI	<1 min	English, German, Spanish, German, multiple+
HAQ-S	Dressing, eating, walking, chores, neck function, and posture	25	Likert: 0(n)–3 (y)	Mean of 10 subscores	N/A	<1 min	English, Dutch, Spanish, Turkish, multiple+

Abbreviations: ADL, activities of daily living; AM stiffness, morning stiffness; N/A, not applicable; Q, question/item number; ROM, range of motion; VAS, visual analog score.

(yes/no) choices.[11] On average, the measure takes a median of 4 minutes (2- to 16-minute range) to complete and less than 1 minute to score. The results are then converted to a score by summation. The ASQoL has received wide acclaim as a validated disease-specific health-related quality-of-life measure among AS patients.[11] Further research is necessary to clarify the cutoff marks for clinically significant quality-of-life change, but overall psychometric evaluations have supported this measure because of its ease of use in research with little administrative or respondent burden.

Functional Status and Disability

A measure of disability in AS patients, the Bath Ankylosing Spondylitis Functional Index (BASFI), was created by a similar group of rheumatologists and physiotherapists as the Bath Ankylosing Spondylitis Disease Activity Index (BASDAI) in 1994 (see later discussion). It has since been the standard functional index for quantifying the impact of AS and corresponds to the Health Assessment Questionnaire equivalent for monitoring functional index in rheumatoid arthritis. Like the BASDAI, the questionnaire uses a visual analog scale (ranging from 0 to 10 cm) anchored by the descriptors "easy" and "impossible" to assess self-reported functioning in 8 activities of everyday life and 2 items documenting the patients' ability to cope with everyday life. Scores are averaged, and an overall index score is calculated. The measure takes less than 3 minutes to complete, and scoring is rapid.[12]

The BASFI has been supported by the ASAS community as a measure to monitor functional status; however, it may be insensitive to patients with milder disease due to its floor effect.[13] Despite this concern, the BASFI has empiric evidence supporting its implementation in the clinic and research setting.[14,15] It has since been incorporated into the formal recommendations by the ASAS as the PRO for assessing functional index.[16]

The Dougados Functional Index (DFI) provides an assessment of the functional abilities in AS patients. Although similar in outcome to the BASFI, the DFI implements a 5-point Likert response scale and includes 20 items assessing daily living. It has been endorsed by the ASAS as an alternative to the BASFI for assessment of core physical functioning in AS. The DFI was originally created by 3 rheumatologists but did not involve initial trial testing with patients in the development phase.[17]

Given its focus on axial and large joint functionality, the DFI has been recommended for use in individuals with predominantly axial involvement, and less so for patients with extra-articular involvement. Of note, it demonstrates a significant flooring effect, and some have questioned the simplistic nature of the Likert scale to capture subtle changes in functioning.[13] Its use is appropriate for research but probably less favored in the clinic due to its larger respondent burden compared with the shorter, equally valid BASFI.

Disease Activity

Originally published in 1994, the BASDAI represents a measure of patient-reported disease activity in patients with AS.[18] The questionnaire assesses patient-reported severities of back pain, fatigue, peripheral joint pain, localized tenderness, and both the duration and the severity of morning stiffness using a visual analog scale from 0 to 10 cm anchored with descriptors of "none" and "very severe." As the ASQoL has been the most widely used measure for assessing quality of life, the BASDAI has been the gold standard for measuring disease activity in clinical trials and has been recommended for use in provider by ASAS.[19]

The BASDAI was initially created in Bath, England by a team of rheumatologists and physiotherapists. On average, the measure takes 67 seconds to complete (generally

30–120 seconds for most respondents) and the scoring takes less than a minute. The questionnaire consists of 6 questions and is scored as the mean of 5 domains, with 2 morning stiffness items averaged. Scores of 4 or more suggest suboptimal control of disease activity, whereas scores greater than 4 are typically good candidates for either a change in their therapy or enrollment in clinical trials for new drug therapies for AS. Given its ease in administration and interpretation, and quick turnaround in results, the BASDAI has been successfully used in clinical practice.[18] However, ASAS has described issues with the use of the traditional visual analog scale (used to rate 5 of the 6 components of the score) and instead now advocates for a switch to a numeric rating scale.[13]

Another simple measure, the Bath Ankylosing Spondylitis Global score (BAS-G), was created by Jones and colleagues[20] in 1996 and provides a global assessment of the AS patient's health using 2 visual analog scales over 2 time periods: within the last week and over the last 6 months. The questions simply ask respondents, "how have you been over the last week?" and "how have you been over the last 6 months?" Scales range between 0 and 10 cm with anchors of "none" to "very severe." The BAS-G is also endorsed by ASAS as an effective measure of globally assessing the patient and has been recommended as part of the core set of measures for monitoring AS.[13] Higher scores indicate a more significant impact on health quality.

As the shortest of all the measures, the BAS-G may provide a good marker of self-reported global well-being in an efficient manner. However, by reducing multiple domains drastically, the instrument may represent very different patient experiences similarly.[20]

One of the most recently developed measures, the Ankylosing Spondylitis Disease Activity Score (ASDAS), was created in 2008 by integrating objective aspects of disease activity with traditional patient-reported items represented in the BASDAI.[21,22] The ASDAS reports a composite score relating to back pain, duration of morning stiffness, peripheral joint pain, and either erythrocyte sedimentation rate (ESR) or C-reactive protein (CRP) levels. Selected cutoffs to distinguish between disease states include less than 1.3 for inactive disease, 1.3 to 2.1 for moderate disease, 2.1 to 3.5 for high disease, and greater than 3.5 for very high disease activity. In terms of changes in ASDAS scores for monitoring improvement, a change greater than or equal to 1.1 is clinical important improvement, whereas a change greater than 2.0 represents major improvement.[21–23] Four different versions of the ASDAS were initially developed, but the standard used in practice has been the ASDAS-CRP (and less so, the ASDAS-ESR). As such, these 2 are the versions treated in this review.

The instrument was created without using any patients directly in a 3-round Delphi process. The ASDAS score is ultimately calculated using a fairly complicated equation that weights each of the 5 criteria. The time for completion is short, requiring less than 1 minute. Provided the formula and a calculator are available, the scoring is also quick and facilitated by the presence of dedicated online calculators. Thus far, the ASDAS has been used for use in axSpA and psoriatic arthritis.[21,23]

VALIDATION (INCLUDES ROLE OF PATIENT-REPORTED OUTCOME MEASURES IN PREDICTING OUTCOME)

On diagnosis of axSpA, ASAS actively recommends using a highly reliable and validated outcome measures for management of patients in clinical research and daily practice. Specifically, they recommend BASFI for assessing function, BASMi for spinal mobility, and BASDAI or ASDAS for disease activity.[24] Although numerous instruments have been developed, poor standardization and assessment of their validity have made their selection in practice difficult. Consequently, it is imperative to assess the validity and reliability of these measures in the evaluation of axSpA patients and whether these remain quality measures for practice. Because each PRO has a designated purpose in clinical practice, comparisons of validation will be organized according to 3 domains: quality of life, functional status, and disease activity (**Table 2**).

Quality of Life

Although functional indices, discussed later, provide a practical assessment of activities impacted by axSpA, quality-of-life measures theoretically provide a more comprehensive method of depicting the consequences of the disease on daily functioning. The ASQoL was developed to serve this purpose and represents the current standard for understanding quality-of-life outcomes in AS, with the potential to extrapolate to axSpA. As such, it has been thoroughly validated in the literature across different AS patient populations and languages.[25]

The initial validation studies achieved Spearman's ρ of 0.91 and 0.92 for cohorts from the Netherlands and the United Kingdom, with internal consistencies of 0.89 to 0.90 and 0.91 to 0.92, respectively.[11] Test-retest probabilities ranged from 0.77 in the German and Spanish versions to 0.85 in the United States and 0.96 in the French versions of the questionnaire performed over a 2-week interval. Interobserver reliabilities are also consistently strong with ranges from 0.79 to 0.86 at baseline to 0.81 to 0.93 after 12 weeks in the same study.[25] In addition, Haywood and colleagues[26,27] have demonstrated the ASQoL's strong convergent validity with other established measures, including the BASDAI (Pearson's correlation coefficient of 0.79) and revised Leeds Disability Questionnaire (coefficient of 0.72).

Functional Index

The disease burden of axSpA is significant, and patients with spondyloarthritis frequently report as much or more pain and fatigue as individuals with rheumatoid arthritis.[28,29] Consequently, the ability to adequately capture functional outcome is imperative in assessing axSpA severity. Several functional indices have been developed over the past 20 years to characterize the impact of axSpA on functional anatomy and capacity. The most well-established measure has been the BASFI.[19] It has been validated more frequently than any of the other functional PROs, including the BAS-G, DFI, and the Health Assessment Questionnaire for the Spondyloarthropathies (HAQ-S).[30] Inclusion of the Bath Ankylosing Spondylitis Metrology Index (BASMI) among functional indices is somewhat debatable, because this only assesses spinal mobility rather than the more general notion of functional status.[31]

The BASFI's internal consistency resembles that of the BASDAI, with Cronbach's α reported as 0.94[32,33] and a ρ of 0.87 to 0.89.[34] In addition, the test-retest reliability was 0.89 after 24 hours[12] and as high as 0.92 to 0.94 within the week.[33,34] In addition, the BASFI demonstrates discriminability with a standardized mean difference (SMD) of 1.10 for distinguishing high (6/10) versus low (4/10) physician global assessments of disease and a 1.94 for distinguishing between patient's own assessment of high and low disease activity.[35,36] Effect sizes also range from 0.36 to 0.70, and standardized response mean (SRM) have been reported between 0.46 and 0.72 across 2 studies comparing the use of celecoxib and TNFi inhibitors as treatment.[17,37]

Another measure of functional index, the BAS-G, has been verified with test-retest probabilities of 0.84 within the week[38] and 0.93 within 6 months of assessment. One study has reported a Cronbach's α of 0.90,[33] which places it on par with the BASFI. An SRM of 1.54 has been identified between assessments 2 weeks apart.[20,38] Although promoted as a simpler alternative to the BASFI, the correlation between these instruments has been only modest (ρ = 0.30–0.69).[20,33,38] Its closer correlation

($\rho = 0.70–0.73$) with BASDAI[20,33,38] may justify its inclusion as a core PRO for AS. Validation work in the broader population of axSpA does not yet exist, to the authors' knowledge.

The DFI, another alternative to the BASFI, has undergone limited validation with regards to test-retest, interobserver reliability, and discriminability. For test-retest probability, correlations have been documented as $\rho = 0.96$ within the first 24 hours[12] and 0.99 within the first week. The interobserver reliability has been almost as impressive with a range of 0.85 to 0.91 across 3 studies.[12,39,40] The DFI has shown an effect size of 0.30 and SRM of 0.30[41] in identifying clinical improvement and an effect size of 0.47 and SRM of 0.59 for deterioration using a randomized responsiveness model. Aside from a study reporting a ρ of 0.64[42] for correlation with the HAQ-S, the literature is limited regarding the correlation of the DFI with the other major assessments of functional index.

Last, the HAQ-S provides another option for PRO measures of functionality in patients with spondyloarthritis. Similar to most of the functional indices, little information is available in the literature regarding its validation across multiple languages and in diverse patient populations. A study of the Turkish version of the HAQ-S and a few additional studies comparing the HAQ-S with the DFI have shown a test-retest probability of about 0.92 and a Cronbach α ranging from 0.94 to 0.98 for individual questions and 0.99 for the entire measure.[42,43] In terms of discriminability, its values are slightly lower than the DFI for assessing improvement and deterioration. A placebo-controlled randomized controlled trial of 39 patients calculated an effect size of 0.20 and SRM of 0.28 for improvement and an effect size of 0.29 and SRM of 0.72 for deterioration.[41] However, the HAQ-S does correlate more closely with the BASFI compared with the BASMI and BAS-G (data unavailable for the DFI).[33,43] The ρ of 0.88 implies it may be superior as a BASFI alternative compared with other PROs, while requiring less time for completion and scoring than the BASFI itself.[30,43,44]

Disease Activity

As the traditional gold standard to assess disease activity, the BASDAI has been well validated and has demonstrated good face validity and reliability across its different language versions and among different patient cohorts.[32,45,46] The BASDAI has demonstrated good internal consistency with Cronbach's α ranging from 0.78 to 0.87 across several studies.[26,47,48] Test-retest probabilities have also been good, with a range of 0.87 to 0.93[26,33,47] irrespective of whether the interval between test was 24 hours or 1 week. Interobserver reliabilities ranged from 0.78 to 0.87 when aggregating data from different language measures.[32,33,45–47,49] SMDs for the BASDAI have been reported as 2.38 for patient global scores and 1.01 for physician global scores.[35]

A more recent PRO for disease activity, the ASDAS, has repeated assessed for validity within the past 5 years. Several studies have validated the ASDAS' power to discriminate between high (greater than or equal to 6 on a 10-point scale) compared with low (less than or equal to 4/10) physician and patient global disease scores.[23,35] SMDs are comparable with the BASDAI with scores ranging from 1.33 to 2.18 for patient scores and 1.10 to 1.96 for physician assessments across 4 studies.[21,23,35,50] Although not surprising given the newness of the ASDAS, the literature is relatively sparse with regards to the ASDAS' test-retest probability and interobserver reliabilities. In addition, studies of the ASDAS' validity have been conducted principally in English-speaking populations.

Since the creation of the ASDAS in 2009, several studies have documented the correlations between BASDAI and ASDAS. Pearson's ρ's have ranged from 0.74 to 0.79

Table 2
Parameters of validity for patient-reported outcome measures in ankylosing spondylitis

PRO	Total of Patients Across Studies (N)	Reliability: Test-Retest Probability or Intraobserver Reliability (ρ vs ICC)	Reliability: Interobserver Reliability or Internal Consistency or Cronbach's α (Spearman's ρ)	Discriminability (SMD)[a]	Correlations with Other PROs: BASDAI (ρ)	Correlations with Other PROs: BASFI (ρ)	Correlations with Other PROs: BASMI (ρ)
ASDAS	1354	—	—	ES = 2.04 SRM = 1.45 PtGL after 6 mo = 1.65–2.35 PtGL at baseline = 1.33–1.55 PrGL = 1.10–1.48	0.74–0.80	0.57–0.66	0.48
ASQoL	1243	ρ = 0.73–0.96 ICC = 0.89	Interobserver reliability = 0.79–0.86 (baseline) Interobserver reliability = 0.81–0.93 (after 12 wk) Internal consistency = 0.89–0.92	SRM = −0.73–0.44 for improvement SRM = 0.48–0.68 for deterioration	0.521–0.79	0.57–0.75	0.37
BASDAI	5223	ρ = 0.93 ICC = 0.74–0.93	Interobserver reliability = 0.78–0.87	ES = 1.5–1.86 SRM = −1.02–1.36 for improvement SRM = 0.74 for deterioration PtGL = 2.38 PrGL = 1.01	0.62–0.83	0.60–0.75	—
BASFI	2725	ρ = 0.89 ICC = 0.92–0.94	Interobserver reliability = 0.87–0.94 Stability index = 0.98	PtGL = 1.94 PrGL = 1.10 Sensitivity for high vs low disease activity = 76–94% Specificity for high vs low disease activity = 66–87% ES = 0.36–0.70 SRM = 0.46–0.72	0.59–0.72	—	0.46–0.51

BAS-G	1168	$\rho = 0.84–0.93$ ICC = 0.94	Interobserver reliability = 0.9	SRM = 1.54	0.70–0.73	0.30–0.69	−0.16
BASMI	668	$\rho = 0.98–0.99$	Interobserver reliability = 0.94–0.99	ES = 0.95 (BASMI-10) ES = 1.04 (BASMI linear) SRM = 0.47	—	0.46	—
DFI	460	ICC = 0.86–0.99 $\rho = 0.96$	0.85–0.908	ES = 0.30; SRM = 0.33 for improvement ES = 0.47; SRM = 0.59 for deterioration	—	—	—
HAQ-S	271	$\rho = 0.92$	0.998 Cronbach $\alpha = 0.943–0.99$ in total	ES = 0.20; SRM = 0.28 for improvement ES = 0.28; SRM = 0.72 for deterioration	0.69	0.88	0.42

References for the above data available from the authors by request.

Abbreviations: ES, effect size; ICC, intraclass correlation coefficient; PrGL, provider global assessment of disease; PtGL, patient global assessment of disease.

[a] All results report SMD, unless otherwise indicated.

according to 2 studies, 1 with 676 patients from the Esperanza database and the other with 60 patients from a 1-year study of patients treated with TNFi.[35,50] The literature has suggested that the BASDAI correlates better with the BASFI compared with the ASDAS, although this is not surprising, given that both BASDAI and BASFI are purely patient-reported measures, whereas the ASDAS includes laboratory results.[50]

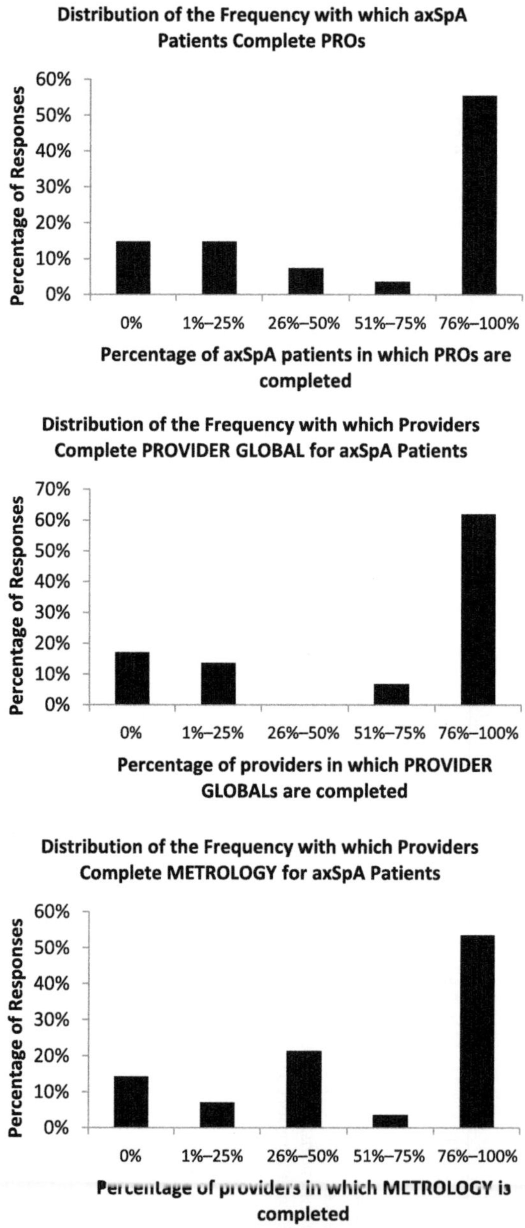

Fig. 1. Frequency with which PRO measures, provider global assessments, and metrology is completed in North American axSpA patients (N = 31 providers).

Others have verified its moderate correlation with the BASDAI (ρ = 0.52–0.79)[26,51–53] and relatively similar correlations with BASFI (ρ = 0.57–0.75).[11,25,51,52]

UTILIZATION OF PATIENT-REPORTED OUTCOMES IN CLINICAL PRACTICE

To provide the first indication of PRO use among North American rheumatologists interested in spondyloarthritis, surveys were conducted at the 2015 Annual Research and Education Meeting of SPARTAN (Spondyloarthritis Research and Treatment Network) in Denver, Colorado, July 25th and 26th. **Fig. 1** includes data from 31 private practitioners and investigators at academic centers across North America. Based on the results present in panel 1, slightly more than 50% of providers currently administer PROs to their patients at least 75% of the time. In turn, panels 2 and 3 illustrate that at least 60% of these providers completed a provider global questionnaire, and more than 50% completed a systematic metrology (validated physical examination measurements) at least 75% of the time as part of their clinical practice. These data suggest that PROs are common in patient care and a component in daily practice among those with special interest in spondyloarthritis, but that even in this highly selective group, approximately 40% of providers do not frequently use PROs in axSpA patients.

FUTURE DIRECTIONS

The ASQoL, BASDAI, and BASFI are now standardized measures that have been fairly thoroughly validated with sufficient reliability and face validity in AS patients.[13] Their performance in axSpA appears similar, although further investigation is necessary to more definitively address this question. The BASDAI has shown moderate correlation with biomarkers, such as the CRP and ESR, but more reliable biomarkers might facilitate the refinement of PROs in axSpA, including AS.[19] In addition, the BASDAI has been predictive of disease course, as demonstrated in the spondyloarthropathy methodology and research therapeutics cohort of 225 AS patients in the United Kingdom.[19] In this study, BASDAI scores remained greater than 4 on a 10-point scale or increased over a 5-year period, suggesting that AS may be progressive and that the field contains either inadequate therapies or nonoptimal use of existing therapies. The assessment of disease activity using the BASDAI has been well validated in several studies that have now been incorporated into current standard guidelines for AS treatment with TNFi.[54,55] The authors suggest that treatments should achieve at least a 50% improvement in the BASDAI score in order to be deemed successful. The ASDAS incorporates biomarkers and thus may help to move the field toward PROs that provide a more comprehensive and accurate reflection of the patient's status. It will be imperative to confirm the validity of using PROs in various axSpA subgroups and, in the coming years, to assess the validity of emerging PROs as they are developed.

REFERENCES

1. Simpson MR, Simpson NR, Scott BO, et al. A controlled study of flufenamic acid in ankylosing spondylitis. A preliminary report. Ann Phys Med 1966;Suppl: 126–8.
2. Ernst Adolph G.G. von Strümpell (1852-1925). Marie-Stmpell spondylitis. JAMA 1970;212(5):875–6.
3. Ebringer A. History of the origin of ankylosing spondylitis. Springer-Verlag (London): Ankylosing spondylitis and klebsiella. 2013. p. 7–13. Available at: http://www.springer.com/us/book/9781447142997.

4. Moll JM, Haslock I, Macrae IF, et al. Associations between ankylosing spondylitis, psoriatic arthritis, Reiter's disease, the intestinal arthropathies, and Behcet's syndrome. Medicine (Baltimore) 1974;53(5):343–64.
5. Calin A, Porta J, Fries JF, et al. Clinical history as a screening test for ankylosing spondylitis. JAMA 1977;237(24):2613–4.
6. van der Linden S, Valkenburg HA, Cats A. Evaluation of diagnostic criteria for ankylosing spondylitis. A proposal for modification of the New York criteria. Arthritis Rheum 1984;27(4):361–8.
7. Amor B, Dougados M, Mijiyawa M. Criteria of the classification of spondylarthropathies. Rev Rhum Mal Osteoartic 1990;57(2):85–9 [in French].
8. Dougados M, van der Linden S, Juhlin R, et al. The European Spondylarthropathy Study Group preliminary criteria for the classification of spondylarthropathy. Arthritis Rheum 1991;34(10):1218–27.
9. Rudwaleit M, van der Heijde D, Landewe R, et al. The development of Assessment of SpondyloArthritis International Society classification criteria for axial spondyloarthritis (part II): validation and final selection. Ann Rheum Dis 2009; 68(6):777–83.
10. Haywood KL, Garratt AM, Dawes PT. Patient-assessed health in ankylosing spondylitis: a structured review. Rheumatology (Oxford) 2005;44(5):577–86.
11. Doward LC, Spoorenberg A, Cook SA, et al. Development of the ASQoL: a quality of life instrument specific to ankylosing spondylitis. Ann Rheum Dis 2003;62(1):20–6.
12. Calin A, Garrett S, Whitelock H, et al. A new approach to defining functional ability in ankylosing spondylitis: the development of the bath ankylosing spondylitis functional index. J Rheumatol 1994;21(12):2281–5.
13. Zochling J. Measures of symptoms and disease status in ankylosing spondylitis: Ankylosing Spondylitis Disease Activity Score (ASDAS), Ankylosing Spondylitis Quality of Life scale (ASQoL), Bath Ankylosing Spondylitis Disease Activity Index (BASDAI), Bath Ankylosing Spondylitis Functional Index (BASFI), Bath Ankylosing Spondylitis Global score (BAS-G), Bath Ankylosing Spondylitis Metrology Index (BASMI), Dougados Functional Index (DFI), and Health Assessment Questionnaire for the Spondylarthropathies (HAQ-S). Arthritis Care Res (Hoboken) 2011;63(Suppl 11):S47–58.
14. Boonen A, de VH, van der Heijde D, et al. Work status and its determinants among patients with ankylosing spondylitis. A systematic literature review. J Rheumatol 2001;28(5):1056–62.
15. van Weely SF, van Denderen CJ, van der Horst-Bruinsma IE, et al. Reproducibility of performance measures of physical function based on the BASFI, in ankylosing spondylitis. Rheumatology (Oxford) 2009;48(10):1254–60.
16. Zochling J, van der Heijde D, Burgos-Vargas R, et al. ASAS/EULAR recommendations for the management of ankylosing spondylitis. Ann Rheum Dis 2006; 65(4):442–52.
17. Dougados M, Behier JM, Jolchine I, et al. Efficacy of celecoxib, a cyclooxygenase 2-specific inhibitor, in the treatment of ankylosing spondylitis: a six-week controlled study with comparison against placebo and against a conventional nonsteroidal antiinflammatory drug. Arthritis Rheum 2001;44(1):180–5.
18. Garrett S, Jenkinson T, Kennedy LG, et al. A new approach to defining disease status in ankylosing spondylitis: the bath ankylosing spondylitis disease activity index. J Rheumatol 1994;21(12):2286–91.
19. Sengupta R, Stone MA. The assessment of ankylosing spondylitis in clinical practice. Nat Clin Pract Rheumatol 2007;3(9):496–503.

20. Jones SD, Steiner A, Garrett SL, et al. The bath ankylosing spondylitis patient global score (BAS-G). Br J Rheumatol 1996;35(1):66–71.
21. Lukas C, Landewe R, Sieper J, et al. Development of an ASAS-endorsed disease activity score (ASDAS) in patients with ankylosing spondylitis. Ann Rheum Dis 2009;68(1):18–24.
22. Machado PM, Landewe RB, van der Heijde DM. Endorsement of definitions of disease activity states and improvement scores for the ankylosing spondylitis disease activity score: results from OMERACT 10. J Rheumatol 2011;38(7): 1502–6.
23. van der Heijde D, Lie E, Kvien TK, et al. ASDAS, a highly discriminatory ASAS-endorsed disease activity score in patients with ankylosing spondylitis. Ann Rheum Dis 2009;68(12):1811–8.
24. Sieper J, Rudwaleit M, Baraliakos X, et al. The Assessment of SpondyloArthritis International Society (ASAS) handbook: a guide to assess spondyloarthritis. Ann Rheum Dis 2009;68(Suppl 2):ii1–44.
25. Doward LC, McKenna SP, Meads DM, et al. Translation and validation of non-English versions of the ankylosing spondylitis quality of life (ASQOL) questionnaire. Health Qual Life Outcomes 2007;5:7.
26. Haywood KL, Garratt M, Jordan K, et al. Disease-specific, patient-assessed measures of health outcome in ankylosing spondylitis: reliability, validity and responsiveness. Rheumatology (Oxford) 2002;41(11):1295–302.
27. Haywood KL, Garratt AM, Jordan K, et al. Spinal mobility in ankylosing spondylitis: reliability, validity and responsiveness. Rheumatology (Oxford) 2004;43(6): 750–7.
28. Rupp I, Boshuizen HC, Jacobi CE, et al. Impact of fatigue on health-related quality of life in rheumatoid arthritis. Arthritis Rheum 2004;51(4):578–85.
29. Stebbings SM, Treharne GJ, Jenks K, et al. Fatigue in patients with spondyloarthritis associates with disease activity, quality of life and inflammatory bowel symptoms. Clin Rheumatol 2014;33(10):1467–74.
30. Daltroy LH, Larson MG, Roberts NW, et al. A modification of the health assessment questionnaire for the spondyloarthropathies. J Rheumatol 1990;17(7): 946–50.
31. Jenkinson TR, Mallorie PA, Whitelock HC, et al. Defining spinal mobility in ankylosing spondylitis (AS). The Bath AS Metrology Index. J Rheumatol 1994;21(9): 1694–8.
32. Biasi D, Carletto A, Caramaschi P, et al. An update on the Bath Ankylosing Spondylitis Disease Activity and Functional Indices (BASDAI, BASFI): excellent Cronbach's alpha scores. J Rheumatol 1996;23(2):407–8.
33. Wei JC, Wong RH, Huang JH, et al. Evaluation of internal consistency and re-test reliability of Bath Ankylosing Spondylitis Indices in a large cohort of adult and juvenile spondylitis patients in Taiwan. Clin Rheumatol 2007;26(10):1685–91.
34. Eyres S, Tennant A, Kay L, et al. Measuring disability in ankylosing spondylitis: comparison of Bath Ankylosing Spondylitis Functional Index with revised Leeds Disability Questionnaire. J Rheumatol 2002;29(5):979–86.
35. Fernandez-Espartero C, de ME, Loza E, et al. Validity of the Ankylosing Spondylitis Disease Activity Score (ASDAS) in patients with early spondyloarthritis from the Esperanza programme. Ann Rheum Dis 2014;73(7):1350–5.
36. Spoorenberg A, van der Heijde D, de KE, et al. A comparative study of the usefulness of the Bath Ankylosing Spondylitis Functional Index and the Dougados Functional Index in the assessment of ankylosing spondylitis. J Rheumatol 1999;26(4):961–5.

37. Gorman JD, Sack KE, Davis JC Jr. Treatment of ankylosing spondylitis by inhibition of tumor necrosis factor alpha. N Engl J Med 2002;346(18):1349–56.
38. Landewe R, Dougados M, Mielants H, et al. Physical function in ankylosing spondylitis is independently determined by both disease activity and radiographic damage of the spine. Ann Rheum Dis 2009;68(6):863–7.
39. Ruof J, Sangha O, Stucki G. Evaluation of a German version of the Bath Ankylosing Spondylitis Functional Index (BASFI) and Dougados Functional Index (D-FI). Z Rheumatol 1999;58(4):218–25.
40. Ozer HT, Sarpel T, Gulek B, et al. Evaluation of the Turkish version of the Dougados Functional Index in ankylosing spondylitis. Rheumatol Int 2005;25(5):368–72.
41. Ruof J, Sangha O, Stucki G. Comparative responsiveness of 3 functional indices in ankylosing spondylitis. J Rheumatol 1999;26(9):1959–63.
42. Ward MM, Kuzis S. Validity and sensitivity to change of spondylitis-specific measures of functional disability. J Rheumatol 1999;26(1):121–7.
43. Ozcan E, Yilmaz O, Tutoglu A, et al. Validity and reliability of the Turkish version of the health assessment questionnaire for the spondyloarthropathies. Rheumatol Int 2012;32(6):1563–8.
44. Jones SD, Porter J, Garrett SL, et al. A new scoring system for the Bath Ankylosing Spondylitis Metrology Index (BASMI). J Rheumatol 1995;22(8):1609.
45. Brandt J, Westhoff G, Rudwaleit M, et al. Adaption and validation of the Bath Ankylosing Spondylitis Disease Activity Index (BASDAI) for use in Germany. Z Rheumatol 2003;62(3):264–73 [in German].
46. Claudepierre P, Sibilia J, Goupille P, et al. Evaluation of a French version of the Bath Ankylosing Spondylitis Disease Activity Index in patients with spondyloarthropathy. J Rheumatol 1997;24(10):1954–8.
47. Calin A, Nakache JP, Gueguen A, et al. Defining disease activity in ankylosing spondylitis: is a combination of variables (Bath Ankylosing Spondylitis Disease Activity Index) an appropriate instrument? Rheumatology (Oxford) 1999;38(9):878–82.
48. Cardiel MH, Londono JD, Gutierrez E, et al. Translation, cross-cultural adaptation, and validation of the Bath Ankylosing Spondylitis Functional Index (BASFI), the Bath Ankylosing Spondylitis Disease Activity Index (BASDAI) and the Dougados Functional Index (DFI) in a Spanish speaking population with spondyloarthropathies. Clin Exp Rheumatol 2003;21(4):451–8.
49. Waldner A, Cronstedt H, Stenstrom CH. The Swedish version of the Bath Ankylosing Spondylitis Disease Activity Index. Reliability and validity. Scand J Rheumatol Suppl 1999;111:10–6.
50. Pedersen SJ, Sorensen IJ, Hermann KG, et al. Responsiveness of the Ankylosing Spondylitis Disease Activity Score (ASDAS) and clinical and MRI measures of disease activity in a 1-year follow-up study of patients with axial spondyloarthritis treated with tumour necrosis factor alpha inhibitors. Ann Rheum Dis 2010;69(6):1065–71.
51. Jenks K, Treharne GJ, Garcia J, et al. The ankylosing spondylitis quality of life questionnaire: validation in a New Zealand cohort. Int J Rheum Dis 2010;13(4):361–6.
52. Zhao LK, Liao ZT, Li CH, et al. Evaluation of quality of life using ASQoL questionnaire in patients with ankylosing spondylitis in a Chinese population. Rheumatol Int 2007;27(7):605–11.
53. Pham T, van der Heijde DM, Pouchot J, et al. Development and validation of the French ASQoL questionnaire. Clin Exp Rheumatol 2010;28(3):379–85.

54. Braun J, Pham T, Sieper J, et al. International ASAS consensus statement for the use of anti-tumour necrosis factor agents in patients with ankylosing spondylitis. Ann Rheum Dis 2003;62(9):817–24.
55. Keat A, Barkham N, Bhalla A, et al. BSR guidelines for prescribing TNF-alpha blockers in adults with ankylosing spondylitis. Report of a working party of the British Society for Rheumatology. Rheumatology (Oxford) 2005;44(7):939–47.

Patient-Reported Outcome Measures in Systemic Sclerosis (Scleroderma)

Russell E. Pellar, BESc[a], Theresa M. Tingey, B Arts Sc[a], Janet Elizabeth Pope, MD, MPH, FRCPC[b,c,*]

KEYWORDS

- Scleroderma • Systemic sclerosis • Patient-reported outcomes
- Health-related quality of life • Patient-reported outcome measures

KEY POINTS

- Systemic sclerosis (scleroderma) is a rare, chronic, connective tissue disease with fibrosis of the skin and many organs, vascular damage, and production of autoantibodies leading to many heterogeneous signs and symptoms.
- Systemic sclerosis is one of the most severe connective tissue diseases with disability; altered appearance; organ damage of skin, gastrointestinal tract, lungs, pulmonary arteries, kidneys, and other organs; digital ulcers; and amputation, with significant emotional and social impact.
- Patient-reported outcome measures provide a patient-centered method of assessing the impact of various problems in systemic sclerosis.
- Patient-reported outcome measures in systemic sclerosis can be general measures or tools that are unique to SSc.
- Commonly used patient-reported outcome measures include the Health Assessment Questionnaire Disability Index, Scleroderma Health Assessment Questionnaire, pain assessments, patient global assessments, Raynaud's Condition Score, and University of California, Los Angeles, Scleroderma Clinical Trials Consortium Gastrointestinal Scale 2.0.

Disclosure Statement: J.E. Pope consults and has performed research trials by Actelion, BMS, Celgene, Genentech, Pfizer, Roche. R.E. Pellar and T.M. Tingey have nothing to disclose.
[a] Faculty of Medicine, SJHC, Schulich School of Medicine and Dentistry, University of Western Ontario, c/o Rheumatology, 268 Grosvenor Street, London, Ontario N6A 4V2, Canada; [b] University of Western Ontario, London, Ontario, Canada; [c] Rheumatology, Department of Medicine, St. Joseph's Health Care, 268 Grosvenor Street, London, Ontario N6A 4V2, Canada
* Corresponding author. St. Joseph's Health Care, London, Ontario N6A 4V2, Canada.
E-mail address: janet.pope@sjhc.london.on.ca

Rheum Dis Clin N Am 42 (2016) 301–316
http://dx.doi.org/10.1016/j.rdc.2016.01.003 rheumatic.theclinics.com
0889-857X/16/$ – see front matter

INTRODUCTION

Systemic sclerosis (SSc), also known as scleroderma, is a chronic, rare autoimmune disease involving the connective tissues of several organs in a progressive manner.[1] SSc classically is associated with fibrosis of the skin and internal organs, the production of autoantibodies, and vascular disruption and damage. Depending on the severity of the disease and the organs affected, patients with SSc have different clinical features.[2] Scleroderma is considered one of the most severe of the connective tissue diseases with significant morbidity and mortality.[3–5]

SSc is classified according to the amount of skin involvement. In limited cutaneous SSc, the skin distal to the elbows and knees is involved, but the skin of the face and neck may also be fibrosed. In the more severe diffuse cutaneous SSc (dcSSc) subset, skin fibrosis occurs both proximally and distally. The diffuse form is more progressive and has earlier visceral organ involvement.[6–9]

SSc usually causes fibrosis of the tissues of the face and hands, leading to disability and disfigurement.[10–12] However, many other manifestations of SSc can affect a patient's quality of life (QoL) and prognosis.[4,13,14] For example, SSc patients often experience pain from many features of their disease, including Raynaud's phenomenon, digital ulcers, gastrointestinal tract involvement, and inflammatory arthritis.[15,16] Moreover, SSc patients may experience severe pruritus, which can interfere with function and sleep.[17,18] Pulmonary involvement can include pulmonary arterial hypertension (PAH) and interstitial lung disease (ILD), resulting in symptoms such as dyspnea, fatigue, cough, and chest pain.[15,19] Chest pain in SSc may also be related to cardiac involvement and pleural and pericardial effusions. Gastrointestinal tract fibrosis can lead to dysmotility, severe gastroesophageal reflux disorder (GERD), early satiety, cramps, bloating, diarrhea and incontinence.[15,19] Scleroderma may affect the kidneys, leading to scleroderma renal crisis, or the heart, leading to cardiomyopathy, arrhythmias, and constrictive pericarditis.[19]

One of the most common symptoms in SSc is fatigue, which occurs in 90% of patients.[19] Other symptoms, including depressive symptoms, sexual dysfunction, fear of disease progression and death, issues with body image, and work disability all affect the QoL of patients with SSc.[19–25] Approximately half become work disabled.[12,23] Altered facial appearance and abnormal hands disfigure SSc patients, affecting self-esteem. Moreover, SSc patients suffer psychologically because of the progressive nature of SSc and lack of a cure.[24,25] There may be reduced oral opening and dry mouth, and combined with reflux this can result in problems eating, halitosis, and poor oral hygiene.

Treatment of SSc is generally complicated, including a combination of symptomatic treatment and disease- or organ-specific treatment. There are scant guidelines for nonpharmacologic management of SSc. Patient-reported outcome (PRO) measurements (PROMs) give patients the opportunity to express the effects of their disease experience. PROMs are unique in that they do not measure the same thing as biologic parameters and physician-assessed outcomes, even though there can be correlations between various measurements.[26]

Although objective measurements of disease characteristics related to SSc exist, such as pulmonary function tests or digital ulcer counts, which may overlap with PROS, they do not fully quantify the patient's experience. Physicians may view major internal organ involvement as extremely important, whereas patients may be more concerned with symptoms that reduce their QoL, such as intense pain, pruritus, or fatigue.[27] PROs allow for the measurement of health outcomes according to the patient, which reflect the goal of improving their QoL and health care. Most trials in SSc include outcomes reflecting laboratory, physician, and patient measures.

KEY ELEMENTS OF PATIENT-REPORTED OUTCOME MEASUREMENTS IN SYSTEMIC SCLEROSIS

Performing a physical examination to assess skin disease or obtaining blood work to measure hemoglobin, renal function, and pulmonary function are well established and relatively easy ways to measure some aspects of SSc. However, it is not as simple to capture the patient experience. PROMs are tools that attempt to address this issue. The development and validation of these patient-centered instruments requires a rigorous process.

SSc is heterogeneous and can involve nearly every organ system. Accordingly, patients may be affected in every domain of their life, so a variety of tools are required to capture their experience. PROMs need to be reliable, valid, accurate, and ideally responsive to change. SSc has unique traits compared with other chronic illnesses, so some tools may be specific to SSc.

PROMs should be accessible, easy to use and score, relevant, and meaningful to the population in question. SSc affects individuals with varying levels of education, languages, and backgrounds, so PROMs should be straightforward and easily understood by patients. Many rheumatologists operate busy clinics, so for tools to gain widespread acceptance in practice, they should be easily integrated into daily routine. This fact is true for the Health Assessment Questionnaire (HAQ) and patient global assessments of overall disease, pain, and fatigue. On the other hand, some PROMs are solely used in clinical trials in which specific research is addressed (such as performing a Raynaud's Condition Score [RCS] daily during a Raynaud's phenomenon trial).[14]

The most commonly used PROs in SSc are the HAQ, the Scleroderma HAQ (SHAQ), pain assessments, patient global assessments, the RCS, and the University of California, Los Angeles, Scleroderma Clinical Trials Consortium Gastrointestinal Scale 2.0 (UCLA SCTC GIT 2.0). Tools that are newly being applied to SSc such as the Patient Reported Outcomes Measurement Information System (PROMIS) are also of interest. These instruments are the focus of this article, but there are numerous other PROMs that have been developed for or are used in SSc. **Fig. 1** illustrates the multitude of symptoms that frequently occur in SSc.

General Measures

Health Assessment Questionnaire

One of the earliest PROs used in rheumatic disease, the HAQ is a quick, easy, and inexpensive way to assess a patient's health status. Originally published in 1980, the HAQ focuses on 5 core domains: death, discomfort, disability, drug toxicity, and cost.[28] Items in the HAQ are scored from 0 to 3, with 3 indicating greater disability. An overall average score is then calculated using the totals for completed sections.[28] Although the HAQ was originally used in rheumatoid arthritis (RA), the disability section of the HAQ (HAQ-DI) is one of the most commonly used assessments of function in SSc. The HAQ-DI focuses on daily activities including eating, arising, hygiene, gripping, walking, and dressing.[26,28] The tool is reliable and responsive to change; has good predictive, concurrent, and construct validity; and predicts mortality in early dcSSc.[26,29–32] The HAQ-DI does, however, have limitations. For example, the HAQ-DI focuses mainly on musculoskeletal disability rather than other forms of disability that patients with SSc may encounter, such as dyspnea, fatigue, and gastrointestinal complaints. Moreover, it was suggested that including assistive devices in the scoring may overestimate the disability of the respondent.[33] Because the HAQ was published in 1980, there are also concerns that it may be outdated and may have certain items only applicable to some

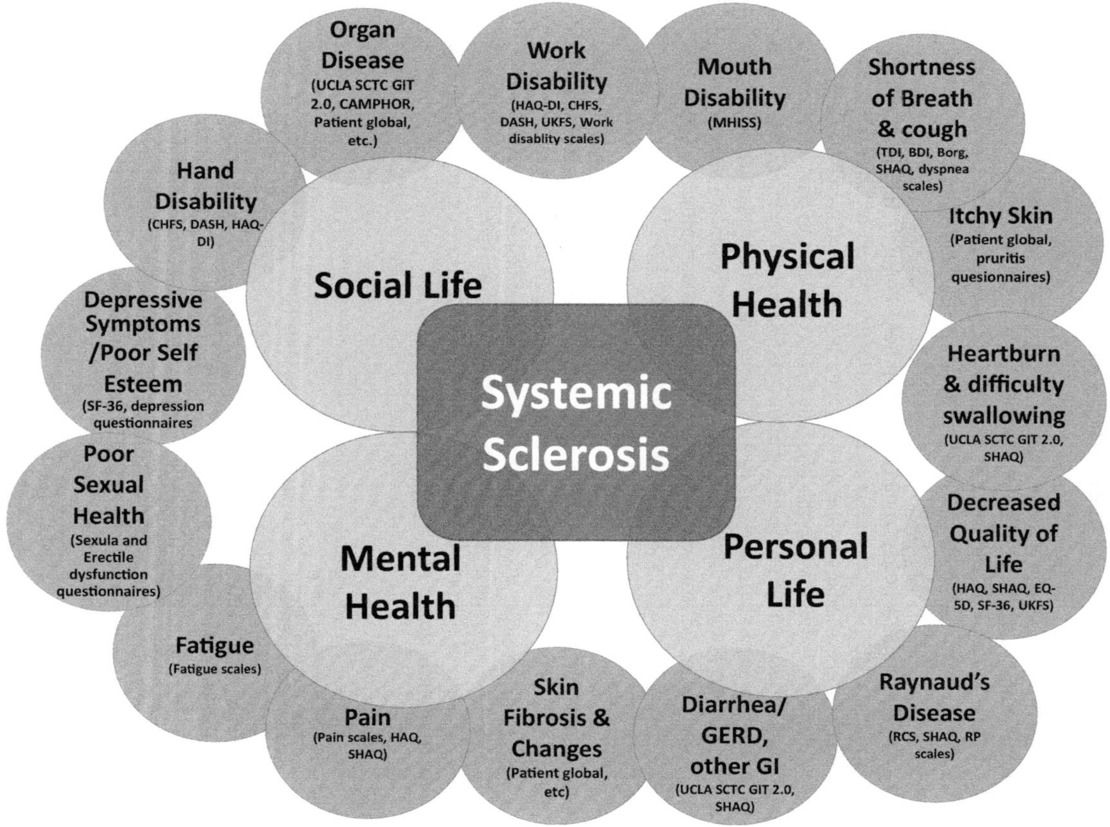

Fig. 1. Patient-related outcomes in systemic sclerosis. This figure represents the domains of health that SSc can affect and a variety of common symptoms that may occur. Examples of some applicable PROMs have been included to show the variety of tools that are used. Borg, Borg Dyspnea Index; CHFS, Cochin Hand Function Scale.

patients, such as opening a carton of milk.[26] It does not include current hand function such as keyboarding or using a cell phone.

Scleroderma Health Assessment Questionnaire

To make a more SSc-specific measurement than the generic HAQ, Steen and Medsger[32] published the SHAQ in 1997. The SHAQ is the HAQ-DI and also includes visual analog scales (VAS) for pain, digital ulcers, vascular problems, gastrointestinal symptoms, lung symptoms, and overall disease severity[32]; thus, it has features beyond function that commonly affect SSc patients. For each VAS symptom, a patient indicates on a 15-cm line how much the symptom interferes with their function. Each centimeter indicated is converted to 0.2 points, or the total distance in centimeters is measured and divided by 5 to give a score from 0 to 3. Each VAS score is displayed individually in addition to the HAQ-DI score.[32]

The SHAQ is also fast and easy to use with better face validity in SSc than the HAQ-DI.[29] Moreover, the SHAQ is responsive to change and is found to have reliability and convergent, predictive and concurrent validity.[11,26,30,32] The HAQ-DI is still more widely used than the SHAQ, and the SHAQ is sometimes improperly scored by those using it, as each VAS scale is to be scored separately.[26]

Global assessments

Global assessments are fast, easy-to-score tools that can be completed by a patient or others (eg, physicians or blinded assessor in trials). As with many other PRO measures, global assessments are useful because they allow patients to express their disease impact through one or more measures. Several different questions can be used in various global assessments. Global assessments may have one representative score or they may consist of a variety of subscales. Because physicians and patients rate disease differently, there are often differences in their individual global assessments. For example, patients often rate their disease severity higher than their physicians do.[34] Global assessments have been found to be valid and sensitive to change.[35–37] There is no standard question that is asked, and often scales are numerical or continuous. Global assessments may be for overall SSc disease activity, severity, and damage or be organ/symptom specific, such as for the impact of gastrointestinal problems, Raynaud's Phenomenon, pain, or fatigue. It is important to note that a single question may give enough information compared with a longer questionnaire, and it depends on what one wants to measure. A long questionnaire may be more comprehensive, but a visual analog scale may be just as sensitive to change when health status improves or worsens.

Other general measures

A variety of other PROs have been used as measures of health-related QoL (HRQoL) in SSc. The EuroQol-5D (EQ-5D) is one of the earliest of these PROs, developed in 1987.[38,39] The EQ-5D is found to correlate with the HAQ-DI, SHAQ, and the Short Form-6D (SF-6D) and is valid for patients with SSc.[40–43]

The Short-Form Health Survey (SF-36) is another PROM that has been applied to assess the HRQoL of patients with SSc.[44] The SF-36 strongly correlates to the HAQ-DI for SSc and has adequate validity, although reliability of this tool in SSc has yet to be determined.[37,45,46] The importance of general QoL measures is that they can potentially compare the impact of various diseases, but they may not be completely relevant or may not capture the totality of a specific disease.

General measures of well-being and HRQoL developed specifically for SSc include the Symptom Burden Index (SBI)[47] and the United Kingdom SSc Functional Score (UKFS).[48] Neither, however, is widely used in SSc studies. **Table 1** compares general and SSc-specific common PROMs.

Table 1
PROMs used in SSc

	Score	Features	Specific to SSc?
HRQoL and general measures	Health Assessment Questionnaire (HAQ)[28]	• Reliable, responsive to change, and has good concurrent, construct, and predictive validity[29,30] • Predictive of mortality in early diffuse SSc[31,32]	—
	SHAQ[32]	• Concurrent, convergent, and predictive validity, reliability, and responsiveness to change[11,30,32] • Incremental content and face validity over the HAQ-DI[29]	✓
	EQ-5D[38]	• Correlates well with the HAQ-DI, SHAQ, SF-6D, and other disease factors for SSc[40–43] • Valid for patients with SSc[40]	—
	SF-36[44]	• Valid in SSc, correlates well with the HAQ-DI[37,45,92] • Correlates with fatigue in SSc[96] • Reliability in SSc not fully determined[46]	—
	SBI[47]	• Good reliability between items, moderate to high interitem and item-total score correlations per domain, high internal consistency reliability estimates[47] • Correlates to the HAQ and SF-36[47] • Construct validity[47]	✓
	UKFS[48]	• Reliable, valid with acceptable test-retest reliability[11,48,93] • Correlates with the HAQ-DI and sensitive to change[11,94,95]	✓
Health status in chronic disease	FACIT[88]	• FACIT-dyspnea has been validated in SSc[90,91]	—
	PROMIS[86]	• PROMIS-29 static scale has been validated in SSc[90,91] • There is feasibility and construct validity of CAT-administered PROMIS[89]	—
Pulmonary involvement	Borg Dyspnea Index[83]	• Partially validated in ILD and PAH[83]	—
	Baseline Dyspnea Index and Transition Dyspnea Index[79]	• Reliability has not been fully tested in SSc • Construct and face validity have been partially shown in SSc[81,82]	—
	CAMPHOR[84]	• Not validated for SSc-associated PAH • Very good internal consistency, convergent and divergent validity, and good reproducibility for idiopathic PAH[47,84]	—

Hand involvement and disability	Cochin Hand Function Scale/Duruoz Hand Index[49]	• Content validity, construct validity, convergent validity, and test-retest reliability[50–54] • Ability to detect change not determined in SSc	—
	HAQ and HAQ-DI[28]	• Reliable, responsive to change, and has good concurrent, construct, and predictive validity[29,30] • Predictive of mortality in early diffuse SSc[31,32]	—
	DASH[58]	• Validated in Hungarian SSc patients[60] • Correlates to HAQ-DI and SF-36[60]	—
	ABILHAND[56]	• Reliable, valid, and reproducible in SSc[57]	—
	Michigan Hand Questionnaire[61]	—	—
Gastrointestinal involvement	SSc-GIT 1.0[67]	• Reliable and valid in SSc[67]	✓
	UCLA SCTC GIT 2.0[68]	• Acceptable reliability (test-retest and internal consistency) and validity[26,68,69] • Can describe disease burden[68] • Responsive to change[46,68,70]	✓
Mouth disability	MHISS[62]	• Excellent test-retest reliability, good construct validity and divergent validity[62]	✓
Raynaud's phenomenon	RCS[30]	• Reliable with construct, content, criterion, and discriminant validity[30,77] • Sensitive to change[30,76]	—

This is not an exhaustive list of PROMs used in SSc, but rather a list of commonly used tools.

Specific Organ Measures

Hand and upper limb

The hands and upper extremities are frequently involved in SSc because of fibrosis, musculoskeletal manifestations, flexion contractures, Raynaud's phenomenon, and digital ulcers, leading to functional disability among day-to-day tasks.

The Cochin Hand Function Scale (Duruoz Hand Index) is a simple questionnaire that determines functional ability of the hands; it has validity (content, construct, and convergent) and reliability (test-retest) and is responsive to change for osteoarthritis and RA.[49–54] However, it may need to be updated to assess more modern daily activities, such as using a cellular phone.[55]

The ABILHAND questionnaire is a valid and reliable instrument with reproducible scores that assesses a patient's ability to use their hands; it was developed for RA but adapted to SSc.[56,57]

The Disabilities of the Arm, Shoulder and Hand (DASH) and the shorter QuickDASH are validated PROMs that more broadly assess disability of the entire upper limbs.[58–60] The scores from both scales reflect SF-36 and HAQ-DI results, highlighting that considerable disability is owing to upper limb involvement.[60]

Other PROMs that can be used to investigate disability of the hand and upper limb include the Michigan Hand Questionnaire (MHQ),[61] UKFS,[48] HAQ-DI, and SHAQ, although the MHQ may not be useful in SSc, as it has not been extensively investigated for use in this condition.[26] One study examining the use of the MHQ for 94 SSc patients found that the MHQ does have reliability and validity.[62]

Mouth

SSc frequently involves the mouth, affecting eating, chewing, and swallowing and causing symptoms such as dryness and poor oral hygiene. Furthermore, SSc can affect the mouth, aesthetically resulting in thin lips, tight skin, and decreased mouth opening. The Mouth Handicap Scale in SSc (MHISS) created by Mouthon and colleagues[63] is the only SSc-specific patient-reported questionnaire regarding mouth-related concerns. The MHISS has acceptable validity (construct and divergent) and reliability (test-retest). The MHISS only moderately influences HAQ scores, suggesting that the measure of self-reported SSc-related mouth disease is likely important and not redundant to the HAQ.[63]

Gastrointestinal tract

Gastrointestinal organ disease occurs in approximately 90% of SSc patients and can be a source of great impact on the patient's HRQoL.[63–65] Many gastrointestinal conditions can arise, as SSc affects both the upper and lower gastrointestinal tract, leading to a potentially complicated clinical picture that is difficult to evaluate.[66,67] GERD is nearly universal and often more severe than in the general population who experience reflux.

Until 2007, there were no specific tools to assess HRQoL in SSc patients with regard to gastrointestinal disease. To properly assess gastrointestinal disease impact, Khanna and colleagues[68] created the SSc Gastrointestinal Tract 1.0 (SSc-GIT 1.0), which was an extensive, reliable, and valid 52-item questionnaire.

Despite the value of the SSc-GIT 1.0, it took too long to complete and, thus, was condensed and updated in 2009 to produce the University of California, Los Angeles, Scleroderma Clinical Trials Consortium Gastrointestinal Tract Scale 2.0 (UCLA SCTC GIT 2.0) instrument.[69] The UCLA SCTC GIT 2.0 contains 34 items organized into 7 multi-item scales assessing impact of GERD, diarrhea, distention/bloating, fecal soilage, constipation, emotional well-being, and social functioning. It is a feasible tool that is quick and easy to score. Most items are scored on a scale ranging from 0 to 3 (more severe). An aggregate score from 0 to 3 is calculated by taking the average of all scales except constipation.[26,46,69]

The UCLA SCTC GIT 2.0 is reliable (test-retest and internal consistency) and valid.[26,69,70] SSc patients who reported having mild gastrointestinal disease generated lower scores on all 7 scales. Furthermore, the total score can be used to ascertain global disease burden and improves ability to delineate between mild, intermediate, and severe gastrointestinal involvement.[69] The scale can differentiate gastrointestinal diagnoses, and the scores respond to change with respect to severity as indicated by the patient.[46,69,71] The UCLA SCTC GIT 2.0 is important because it is the only PROM specific to gastrointestinal tract disease in SSc. However, it likely has a ceiling effect, wherein a patient with considerable frequent daily diarrhea or GERD who then moderately improves may not see a change in their score.

As an alternative, the gastrointestinal tract visual analog scale from the SHAQ can be used but represents a less comprehensive measure of SSc-related gastrointestinal disease and has not been evaluated in comparison with the UCLA SCTC GIT 2.0 tool. The Gastrointestinal Quality of Life Index is a nonspecific measure that may be administered in SSc.[72]

Specific Symptom Measures

Pain

Pain occurs in more than 80% of SSc patients and can originate from many aspects of SSc. Many scales assess pain from specific disease features such as Raynaud's phenomenon or overall pain for any reason attributable to SSc (general pain measure).[26] Pain is incorporated into general tools in SSc, such as the SBI, the HAQ pain question and the SHAQ. The RCS also contains questions about pain related to Raynaud's phenomenon.

In general, scoring for pain is fast, as completion of most pain scales should be less than 1 minute.[26] Pain scales are valid within other PROM tools and when used alone.[16,30,32] Pain scales correlate well with disease manifestations, such as the modified Rodnan skin score[73] and alteration in body image.[74] There is face validity as pain is usually worse in dcSSc than limited cutaneous SSc, in which the latter is usually more mild.[16] Finally, pain scales can detect change with the use of some treatments[75] and have good test-retest reliability.[76] There are problems such as attribution when measuring pain.[14] This is true for other inflammatory rheumatic conditions. If a patient has concomitant fibromyalgia or sciatica, and the patient is asked about the severity of their pain from SSc, they may answer the question with respect to overall pain and not their disease that is being studied. There is also adaptation that occurs in which many patients with SSc have a pain level of 4 of 10 at any visit,[14] so pain may not reflect disease activity, but a change in pain can be important to a patient's QoL.

Raynaud's phenomenon and digital ulcers

Raynaud's phenomenon is associated with many rheumatic diseases but is most frequent and severe in SSc compared with other connective tissue diseases. A specific PROM developed to measure the frequency, severity, impact, and duration of Raynaud's phenomenon attacks is the RCS. The RCS uses a daily self-report on an 11-point scale averaged over a predetermined period.[30] The RCS has demonstrated validity (construct, criterion, content, and discriminant),[30,77] sensitivity to change, and reliability.[30,78] The RCS can also discriminate between those with and without digital ulcers (DUs), showing predictive validity.[30] Otherwise, outcomes of DUs have not been standardized in SSc, and no agreed-upon measurement of DUs is commonly used in research. Assessments of DUs may include PROMS such as within the SHAQ, patient and physician global assessments, DU pain scales, and other outcomes not assessed by the patient such as size, number, burden, and healing.[26,32,79]

Dyspnea

Many questionnaires for shortness of breath were developed in other diseases such as chronic obstructive lung disease but are used in other conditions such as pulmonary fibrosis. Dyspnea can be experienced by SSc patients suffering from ILD/pulmonary fibrosis and PAH, cardiac involvement, deconditioning, and myopathy of the diaphragm. Although there are no dyspnea scales specific to SSc, the Baseline Dyspnea Index and Transition Dyspnea Index have been partially validated in SSc.[80–83] The Modified Borg Dyspnea Scale, made from the Borg Dyspnea Index, can be used to measure the severity of dyspnea.[26,84]

Pulmonary arterial hypertension

The Cambridge Pulmonary Hypertension Outcome Review (CAMPHOR) can assess HRQoL for patients with PAH.[85] The CAMPHOR has not been validated specifically in SSc-associated PAH, although it has been for idiopathic PAH.[26,85] Usually in PAH, a dyspnea scale and functional class are used as PROMs, although the latter may be assigned by a clinician or a patient.

Other symptoms

SSc can result in a variety of conditions and symptoms, many of which do not have SSc-specific PROMs for them. Some common and problematic symptoms that negatively impact HRQoL for SSc patients include pruritus, fatigue, depressive symptoms, and sexual dysfunction.[19,20] Many of these symptoms are common in SSc.[14,86] Some aspects may be assessed through measures such as the HAQ, HAQ-DI, SHAQ, and global assessments but can also be measured using scales for depression, fatigue, sexual health, and erectile dysfunction.

Emerging Patient-reported Outcome Measures in Systemic Sclerosis

Patient Reported Outcomes Measurement Information System and systemic sclerosis

Health care providers are incorporating more advanced and modern methods of clinical and experimental assessment. The popularity is increasing for tools that use computer adaptive testing (CAT) to adapt and select questions specific to the patient, such as the PROMIS.[87] PROMIS is a unified system of dynamic item banks that addresses concerns common to many chronic conditions. Along with the flexible CAT-administered PROMIS, there are also static scales that can be used, such as the PROMIS-29. The PROMIS in SSc will be important for enabling interdisease and interstudy comparisons, which may be helpful to support underresearched aspects of SSc.[88]

Additionally, there is the Functional Assessment of Chronic Illness Therapy (FACIT) system, which is a collection of questionnaires regarding HRQoL that makes use of the CAT technology. It can be used along with PROMIS.[89]

PROMIS and FACIT have been studied in SSc patients. Khanna and colleagues[90] found feasibility and construct validity of CAT-administered PROMIS for 11 health domains in SSc. Patients took on average no more than 2 minutes to complete the assessment.[90] Hinchcliff and colleagues[91,92] further validated the static PROMIS-29 scale and FACIT-dyspnea measurement in SSc patients and suggested the use of these tools over other instruments owing to their simplicity and availability.

SUMMARY

SSc is a chronic, debilitating multifaceted disease. PROs in SSc are used in both clinical practice and research to measure the patient's experience. The HAQ-DI has the patient rate function and is validated in many rheumatic diseases. More specific measures of HRQoL in SSc include the SHAQ, SBI, and UKFS. These tools offer the patient the opportunity to express their experience with disease, beyond the objective measures that can be collected by a physician. There are also many symptom-specific PROs that further help characterize and quantify various symptoms in SSc. PROMs provide a holistic assessment of the patient and measure something different than physician measures and clinical tests. PROMs are especially helpful in research trials, because a treatment that improves an SSc symptom in a meaningful way to the patient is important to measure, and conversely a treatment that a patient considers not helpful or in fact worsens QoL is also noteworthy. Further research is indicated to refine SSc tools and investigate validity of measures in SSc. Moreover, with the use of new technologies, PROMs have the potential to have streamlined measures that are patient specific.

REFERENCES

1. Schnitzer M, Hudson M, Baron M, et al, Canadian Scleroderma Research Group. Disability in systemic sclerosis - a longitudinal observational study. J Rheumatol 2011;38(4):685–92.
2. Pattanaik D, Brown M, Postlethwaite BC, et al. Pathogenesis of systemic sclerosis. Front Immunol 2015;6:272.
3. Allanore Y, Avouac J, Kahan A. Systemic sclerosis: an update in 2008. Joint Bone Spine 2008;75(6):650–5.
4. Johnson SR, Glaman DD, Schentag CT, et al. Quality of life and functional status in systemic sclerosis compared to other rheumatic diseases. J Rheumatol 2006;33(6):1117–22.
5. Mayes MD, Lacey JV Jr, Beebe-Dimmer J, et al. Prevalence, incidence, survival, and disease characteristics of systemic sclerosis in a large US population. Arthritis Rheum 2003;48:2246–55.
6. Leroy EC, Black C, Fleischmajer R, et al. Scleroderma (systemic sclerosis): classification, subsets and pathogenesis. J Rheumatol 1988;15:202–5.
7. Seibold J. Connective tissue diseases characterized by fibrosis. In: Ruddy S, Harris ED Jr, Sledge CB, editors. Textbook of rheumatology. Philadelphia: WB Saunders Co; 2001. p. 1133–59.
8. Wigley F, Systemic Sclerosis B. Clinical features. In: Klippel JH, editor. Primer on the rheumatic diseases. Atlanta (GA): The Arthritis Foundation; 2001. p. 357–64.
9. Medsger TA Jr. Natural history of systemic sclerosis and the assessment of disease activity, severity, functional status, and psychologic well-being. Rheum Dis Clin North Am 2003;29:255–73.
10. Paquette DL, Falanga V. Cutaneous concerns of scleroderma patients. J Dermatol 2003;30:438–43.
11. Smyth AE, MacGregor AJ, Mukerjee D, et al. A cross-sectional comparison of three self-reported functional indices in scleroderma. Rheumatology (Oxford) 2003;42(6):732–8.
12. Ouimet JM, Pope JE, Gutmanis I, et al. Work disability in scleroderma is greater than in rheumatoid arthritis and is predicted by high HAQ scores. Open Rheumatol J 2008;2:44–52.

13. Hudson M, Thombs BD, Steele R, et al, Canadian Scleroderma Research Group. Quality of life in patients with systemic sclerosis compared to the general population and patients with other chronic conditions. J Rheumatol 2009;36:768–72.
14. Sekhon S, Pope J, Canadian Scleroderma Research Group (CSRG), et al. The minimally important difference (MID) for patient centered outcomes including Health Assessment Questionnaire (HAQ), Fatigue, Pain, Sleep, Global VAS and SF-36 in Scleroderma (SSc). J Rheumatol 2010;37(3):591–8.
15. Varga J, Denton CP, Wigley FM, editors. Scleroderma: from pathogenesis to comprehensive management. New York: Springer Science Business Media, LLC; 2012. http://dx.doi.org/10.1007/978-1-4419-5774-0_7.
16. Schieir O, Thombs BD, Hudson M, et al. Prevalence, severity, and clinical correlates of pain in patients with systemic sclerosis. Arthritis Care Res (Hoboken) 2010;62(3):409–17.
17. El-Baalbaki G, Razykov I, Hudson M, et al. Association of pruritus with quality of life and disability in systemic sclerosis. Arthritis Care Res (Hoboken) 2010;62(10): 1489–95.
18. Zucker I, Yosipovitch G, David M, et al. Prevalence and characterization of uremic pruritus in patients undergoing hemodialysis: uremic pruritus is still a major problem for patients with end-stage renal disease. J Am Acad Dermatol 2003;49: 842–6.
19. Bassel M, Hudson M, Taillefer SS, et al. Frequency and impact of symptoms experienced by patients with systemic sclerosis: results from a Canadian National Survey. Rheumatology (Oxford) 2010;50:762–7.
20. Thombs BD, Hudson M, Taillefer SS, et al, Canadian Scleroderma Research Group. Prevalence and clinical correlates of symptoms of depression in patients with systemic sclerosis. Arthritis Rheum 2008;59(4):504–9.
21. Jewett LR, Hudson M, Malcarne VL, et al, Canadian Scleroderma Research Group. Sociodemographic and disease correlates of body image distress among patients with systemic sclerosis. PLoS One 2012;7(3):e33281.
22. Knafo R, Thombs BD, Jewett L, et al. (Not) talking about sex: a systematic comparison of sexual impairment in women with systemic sclerosis and other chronic disease samples. Rheumatology (Oxford) 2009;48(10):1300–3.
23. Hudson M, Steele R, Lu Y, et al, Canadian Scleroderma Research Group. Work disability in systemic sclerosis. J Rheumatol 2009;36(11):2481–6.
24. Malcarne VL, Fox RS, Mills SD, et al. Psychosocial aspects of systemic sclerosis. Curr Opin Rheumatol 2013;25:707–13.
25. Thombs BD, van Lankveld W, Bassel M, et al. Psychological health and well-being in systemic sclerosis: State of the science and consensus research agenda. Arthritis Care Res (Hoboken) 2010;62:1181–9.
26. Pope J. Measures of systemic sclerosis (Scleroderma). Arthritis Care Res 2011; 63(S11):S98–111.
27. Suarez-Almazor ME, Kallen MA, Roundtree AK, et al. Disease and symptom burden in systemic sclerosis: a patient perspective. J Rheumatol 2007;34:171826.
28. Fries JF, Spitz P, Kraines RG, et al. Measurement of patient outcome in arthritis. Arthritis Rheum 1980;23:137–45.
29. Johnson SR, Hawker GA, Davis AM. The health assessment questionnaire disability index and scleroderma health assessment questionnaire in scleroderma trials: an evaluation of their measurement properties. Arthritis Rheum 2005;53: 256–62.

30. Merkel PA, Herlyn K, Martin RW, et al. Measuring disease activity and functional status in patients with scleroderma and Raynaud's phenomenon. Arthritis Rheum 2002;46:2410–20.
31. Clements PJ, Wong WK, Hurwitz EL, et al. The disability index of the health assessment questionnaire is a predictor and correlate of outcome in the high-dose versus low-dose penicillamine in systemic sclerosis trial. Arthritis Rheum 2001;44(3):653–61.
32. Steen VD, Medsger TA Jr. The value of the Health Assessment Questionnaire and special patient-generated scales to demonstrate change in systemic sclerosis patients over time. Arthritis Rheum 1997;40(11):1984–91.
33. Khanna D, Clements PJ, Postlethwaite AE, et al. Does incorporation of aids and devices make a difference in the score of the health assessment questionnaire-disability index? Analysis from a scleroderma clinical trial. J Rheumatol 2008; 35:466–8.
34. Hudson M, Impens A, Baron M, et al. Discordance between patient and physician assessments of disease severity in systemic sclerosis. J Rheumatol 2010;37: 2307–12.
35. Clements PJ, Hurwitz EL, Wong WK, et al. Skin thickness score as a predictor and correlate of outcome in systemic sclerosis: high-dose versus low-dose penicillamine trial. Arthritis Rheum 2000;43:2445–54.
36. Sultan N, Pope JE, Clements PJ, Scleroderma Trials Study Group. The Health Assessment Questionnaire (HAQ) is strongly predictive of good outcome in early diffuse scleroderma: results from an analysis of two randomized controlled trials in early diffuse scleroderma. Rheumatology (Oxford) 2004;43:472–8.
37. Khanna D, Furst DE, Clements PJ, et al. Responsiveness of the SF-36 and the Health Assessment Questionnaire disability index in a systemic sclerosis clinical trial. J Rheumatol 2005;32:832–40.
38. The EuroQol Group. EuroQol-a new facility for the measurement of health-related quality of life. Health Policy 1990;16:199–208.
39. Rabin R, de Charro F. EQ-5D: a measure of health status from the EuroQol Group. Ann Med 2001;33:337–43.
40. Gualtierotti R, Scalone L, Ingegnoli F, et al. Health related quality of life assessment in patients with systemic sclerosis. Reumatismo 2010;62(3):210–4.
41. Muller H, Rehberger P, Gunther C, et al. Determinants of disability, quality of life and depression in dermatological patients with systemic scleroderma. Br J Dermatol 2011;166(2):343–53.
42. Strickland G, Pauling J, Cavill C, et al. Predictors of health-related quality of life and fatigue in systemic sclerosis: evaluation of the EuroQol-5D and FACIT-F assessment tools. Clin Rheumatol 2012;31:1215–22.
43. Kwakkenbos L, Fransen J, Vonk MC, et al. A comparison of the measurement properties and estimation of minimal important differences of the EQ-5D and SF-6D utility measures in patients with systemic sclerosis. Clin Exp Rheumatol 2013;31(2 Suppl 76):50–6.
44. Ware JE Jr, Sherbourne CD. The MOS 36-item short health survey (SF-36) I. Conceptual framework and item selection. Med Care 1992;30:473–83.
45. McHorney CA, Ware JE, Raczek AE. The MOS 36-Item Short-Form Health Survey (SF-36): II. Psychometric and clinical validity in measuring physical and mental health constructs. Med Care 1993;31(3):247–63.
46. Khanna D. Measuring disease activity and outcomes in clinical trials. In: Varga J, Denton CP, Wigley FM, editors. Scleroderma: from pathogenesis to comprehensive management. New York: Springer Science Business Media; 2012. p. 661–72.

47. Kallen MA, Mayes MD, Kriseman YL, et al. The symptom burden index: development and initial findings from use with patients with systemic sclerosis. J Rheumatol 2010; 37:1692–8.
48. Silman A, Akesson A, Newman J, et al. Assessment of functional ability in patients with scleroderma: a proposed disability assessment instrument. J Rheumatol 1998;25(1):79–83.
49. Duruoz MT, Poiraudeau S, Fermanian J, et al. Development and validation of a rheumatoid hand functional disability scale that assesses functional handicap. J Rheumatol 1996;23:1167–72.
50. Brower LM, Poole JL. Reliability and validity of the Duruoz Hand Index in persons with systemic sclerosis (scleroderma). Arthritis Rheum 2004;51:805–9.
51. Rannou F, Poiraudeau S, Berezne A, et al. Assessing disability and quality of life in systemic sclerosis: construct validities of the Cochin Hand Function Scale, Health Assessment Questionnaire (HAQ), Systemic Sclerosis HAQ, and Medical Outcomes Study 36-Item Short Form Health Survey. Arthritis Rheum 2007;57: 94–102.
52. Poiraudeau S, Chevalier X, Conrozier T, et al. Reliability, validity, and sensitivity to change of the Cochin Hand Functional Disability Scale in hand osteoarthritis. Osteoarthritis Cartilage 2001;9:570–7.
53. Lefevre-Colau MM, Poiraudeau S, Fermanian J, et al. Responsiveness of the Cochin rheumatoid disability scale after surgery. Rheumatology (Oxford) 2001; 40:843–50.
54. Poiraudeau S, Lefevre-Colau MM, Fermanian J, et al. The ability of the Cochin Rheumatoid Arthritis Hand Functional Scale to detect change during the course of disease. Arthritis Care Res 2000;13:296–303.
55. Poole JL. Measures of hand function. Arthritis Care Res (Hoboken) 2011;63: S189–99.
56. Penta M, Thonnard JL, Tesio L. ABILHAND: a Rasch-built measure of manual ability. Arch Phys Med Rehabil 1998;79:1038–42.
57. Vanthuyne M, Smith V, Arat S, et al. Validation of a manual ability questionnaire in patients with systemic sclerosis. Arthritis Rheum 2009;61(5):695–703.
58. Hudak PL, Amadio PC, Bombardier C. Development of an upper extremity outcome measure: the DASH (Disabilities of the Arm, Shoulder and Hand). Am J Ind Med 1996;29:602–8.
59. Gabel CP, Yelland M, Melloh M, et al. A modified QuickDASH-9 provides a valid outcome instrument for upper limb function. BMC Musculoskelet Disord 2009;10: 161.
60. Varju C, Balint Z, Solyom AI, et al. Cross-cultural adaptation of the disabilities of the arm, shoulder, and hand (DASH) questionnaire into Hungarian and investigation of its validity in patients with systemic sclerosis. Clin Exp Rheumatol 2008; 26(5):776–83.
61. Chung KC, Pillsbury MS, Walters MR, et al. Reliability and validity testing of the Michigan hand outcomes questionnaire. J Hand Surg Am 1998;23:575–87.
62. Impens AJ, Chung KC, Buch MH, et al. Validation of the Michigan Hand Outcomes Questionnaire (MHQ) in Systemic Sclerosis (SSc). Poster. Ann Arbor (MI): University of Michigan; 2004. Available at: http://www.med.umich.edu/scleroderma/images/MHQValidationAbstract.pdf.
63. Mouthon L, Rannou F, Berezne A, et al. Development and validation of a scale for mouth handicap in systemic sclerosis: the Mouth Handicap in Systemic Sclerosis scale. Ann Rheum Dis 2007;66:1651–5.

64. Sjogren RW. Gastrointestinal motility disorders in scleroderma [review]. Arthritis Rheum 1994;37:1265–82.
65. Lock G, Holstege A, Lang B, et al. Gastrointestinal manifestations of progressive systemic sclerosis. Am J Gastroenterol 1997;92:763–71.
66. Nietert PJ, Mitchell HC, Bolster MB, et al. Correlates of depression, including overall and gastrointestinal functional status, among patients with systemic sclerosis. J Rheumatol 2005;32:51–7.
67. Gliddon AE, Dore CJ, Maddison PJ, the QUINS Trial Study Group. Influence of clinical features on the health status of patients with limited cutaneous systemic sclerosis. Arthritis Rheum 2006;55:473–9.
68. Khanna D, Hays RD, Park GS, et al. Development of a preliminary scleroderma gastrointestinal tract 1.0 quality of life instrument. Arthritis Rheum 2007;57:1280–6.
69. Khanna D, Hays RD, Maranian P, et al. Reliability and validity of the University of California, Los Angeles Scleroderma clinical trial consortium gastrointestinal tract instrument. Arthritis Rheum 2009;61:1257–63.
70. Baron M, Hudson M, Steele R, et al, Canadian Scleroderma Research Group. Validation of the UCLA Scleroderma Clinical Trial Gastrointestinal Tract Instrument version 2.0 for systemic sclerosis. J Rheumatol 2011;38(9):1925–30.
71. Frech TM, Khanna D, Maranian P, et al. Probiotics for the treatment of systemic sclerosis-associated gastrointestinal bloating/distention. Clin Exp Rheumatol 2011;29(2 Suppl 65):S22–5.
72. Eypasch E, Williams JI, Wood-Dauphinee S, et al. Gastrointestinal Quality of Life Index: development, validation and application of a new instrument. Br J Surg 1995;82:216–22.
73. Malcarne VL, Hansdottir I, McKinney A, et al. Medical signs and symptoms associated with disability, pain, and psychosocial adjustment in systemic sclerosis. J Rheumatol 2007;34:359–67.
74. Benrud-Larson LM, Heinberg LJ, Boling C, et al. Body image dissatisfaction among women with scleroderma: extent and relationship to psychosocial function. Health Psychol 2003;22:130–9.
75. Thompson AE, Shea B, Welch V, et al. Calcium channel blockers for Raynaud's phenomenon in progressive systemic sclerosis. Arthritis Rheum 2001;44:1841–7.
76. Stevens A, Pope JE. Retest reliabilities and variability among scleroderma patients for 4 tests of disability: support for a better measure. Presented at the Canadian Rheumatology Association Meeting, 1995. J Rheumatol 1995;22:1603.
77. Khanna PP, Maranian P, Gregory J, et al. The minimally important difference and patient acceptable symptom state for the Raynaud's condition score in patients with Raynaud's phenomenon in a large randomised controlled clinical trial. Ann Rheum Dis 2010;69:588–91.
78. Shenoy PD, Kumar S, Jha LK, et al. Efficacy of tadalafil in secondary Raynaud's phenomenon resistant to vasodilator therapy: a double-blind randomized crossover trial. Rheumatology (Oxford) 2010;49:2420–8.
79. Matucci-Cerinic M, Seibold JR. Digital ulcers and outcomes assessment in scleroderma [review]. Rheumatology (Oxford) 2008;47(Suppl 5):v46–7.
80. Mahler DA, Weinberg DH, Wells CK, et al. The measurement of dyspnea: contents, interobserver agreement and physiologic correlates of two new clinical indexes. Chest 1984;85:751–8.
81. Tashkin DP, Elashoff R, Clements PJ, et al. Cyclophosphamide versus placebo in scleroderma lung disease. N Engl J Med 2006;354:2655–66.

82. Khanna D, Clements PJ, Furst DE, et al. Correlation of the degree of dyspnea with health-related quality of life, functional abilities, and diffusing capacity for carbon monoxide in patients with systemic sclerosis and active alveolitis: results from the Scleroderma Lung Study. Arthritis Rheum 2005;52:592–600.
83. Khanna D, Yan X, Tashkin DP, et al. Impact of oral cyclophosphamide on health-related quality of life in patients with active scleroderma lung disease: results from the scleroderma lung study. Arthritis Rheum 2007;56:1676–84.
84. Borg G. Psychophysical basis of perceived exertion. Med Sci Sports Exerc 1982; 14:377–81.
85. McKenna SP, Doughty N, Meads DM, et al. The Cambridge Pulmonary Hypertension Outcome Review (CAMPHOR): a measure of health-related quality of life and quality of life for patients with pulmonary hypertension. Qual Life Res 2006;15: 103–15.
86. Hong P, Pope JE, Ouimet JM, et al. Erectile dysfunction associated with scleroderma: a case-control study of men with scleroderma and rheumatoid arthritis. J Rheumatol 2004;31(3):508–13.
87. Cella D, Yount S, Rothrock N, et al. The patient-reported outcomes measurement information system (PROMIS): progress of an NIH roadmap cooperative group during its first two years. Med Care 2007;45(5):S3–11.
88. Hinchcliff M, Cella D. Patient-reported outcomes. In: Varga J, Denton CP, Wigley FM, editors. Scleroderma: from pathogenesis to comprehensive management. New York: Springer Science Business Media; 2012. p. 673–8.
89. Webster K, Cella D, Yost K. The Functional Assessment of Chronic Illness Therapy (FACIT) measurement system: properties, applications, and interpretation. Health Qual Life Outcomes 2003;1:79.
90. Khanna D, Maranian P, Rothrock N, et al. Feasibility and Construct Validity of PROMIS and "Legacy" Instruments in an Academic Scleroderma Clinic. Value Health 2012;15:128–34.
91. Hinchcliff M, Beaumont JL, Thavarajah K, et al. Validity of two new patient-reported outcome measures in systemic sclerosis: Patient-Reported Outcomes Measurement Information System 29-item Health Profile and Functional Assessment of Chronic Illness Therapy-Dyspnea short form. Arthritis Care Res (Hoboken) 2011;63(11):1620–8.
92. Hinchcliff M, Beaumont JL, Carns MA, et al. Longitudinal evaluation of PROMIS-29 and FACIT-dyspnea short forms in systemic sclerosis. J Rheumatol 2015; 42(1):64–72.
93. Cosutta R, Zeni S, Soldi A, et al. Evaluation of quality of life in patients with systemic sclerosis by the SR-36 questionnaire. Rheumatismo 2002;54:122–7 [In Italian].
94. Poole JL, Brower L. Validity of the scleroderma functional assessment questionnaire. J Rheumatol 2004;31:402–3.
95. Serednicka K, Smyth AE, Black CM, et al. Using a self-reported functional score to assess disease progression in systemic sclerosis. Rheumatology (Oxford) 2007;46(7):1107–10.
96. Harel D, Thombs BD, Hudson M, et al, on behalf of the Canadian Scleroderma Research Group. Measuring fatigue in SSc: a comparison of the Short Form-36 Vitality subscale and Functional Assessment of Chronic Illness Therapy – Fatigue Scale. Rheumatology (Oxford) 2012;51(12):2177–85.

Patient-Reported Outcomes and Fibromyalgia

David A. Williams, PhD[a,b,c,d,*], Anna L. Kratz, PhD[e]

KEYWORDS

• Fibromyalgia • Diagnosis • Phenotyping • Multimodal assessment • Self-report • Pain

KEY POINTS

- Physicians and/or patient-reported outcomes (PROs) remain the most sensitive and specific means of diagnosing fibromyalgia (FM) in clinical or research settings.
- The primary uses of PROs for FM include diagnostics, disease monitoring, phenotyping/characterization, and as outcomes for clinical trials.
- FM is a multifaceted condition requiring a multifaceted assessment if the complexity of the condition is to be represented in a reliable and valid manner.

INTRODUCTION

Fibromyalgia (FM) is considered to be a chronic pain condition characterized by chronic widespread pain along with accompanying symptoms of fatigue, sleep difficulties, diminished physical functioning, mood disturbances, and cognitive

Funding Sources: Dr D.A. Williams, NIDDK/NIH U01DK82345; U01 DK82345, Multidisciplinary Approach to the Study of Chronic Pelvic Pain (MAPP) Research Network. National Institutes of Diabetes and Digestive and Kidney Disease (NIDDK/NIH). A. Kratz was supported during article preparation by a grant from the National Institute of Arthritis and Musculoskeletal and Skin Diseases (1K01AR064275).
Conflict of Interest: Dr D.A. Williams serves as a consultant to Community Health Focus Inc and to Pfizer Inc He is also on the Board of Directors and President-elect of the American Pain Society. There is no conflict associated with the content or preparation of this article.
[a] Department of Anesthesiology, University of Michigan Health System, University of Michigan, 24 Frank Lloyd Wright Drive, PO Box 385, Lobby M, Ann Arbor, MI 48106, USA; [b] Department of Internal Medicine, University of Michigan, 3110 Taubman Center, SPC 5368, 1500 East Medical Center Drive, Ann Arbor, MI 48109, USA; [c] Department of Psychiatry, University of Michigan, F6327 UH South, SPC 5295, 1500 East Medical Center Drive, Ann Arbor, MI 48109, USA; [d] Department of Psychology, University of Michigan, F6327 UH South, SPC 5295, 1500 East Medical Center Drive, Ann Arbor, MI 48109, USA; [e] Department of Physical Medicine and Rehabilitation, University of Michigan, North Campus Research Complex, 2800 Plymouth Road, Building NCRC B14, Room G218, Ann Arbor, MI 48109-2800, USA
* Corresponding author. Department of Anesthesiology, University of Michigan Health System, University of Michigan, 24 Frank Lloyd Wright Drive, PO Box 385, Lobby M, Ann Arbor, MI 48106.
E-mail address: daveawms@umich.edu

Rheum Dis Clin N Am 42 (2016) 317–332
http://dx.doi.org/10.1016/j.rdc.2016.01.009 rheumatic.theclinics.com
0889-857X/16/$ – see front matter

dysfunction that can include problems with memory, concentration, and mental clarity.[1,2] Globally, the mean prevalence of FM is 2.7% with females having a global mean prevalence of 4.2% and males having a mean prevalence of 1.4% (female to male ratio of 3:1).[3] Individuals with FM often report diminished quality of life,[4] diminished functional status,[5] and greater than expected health care use.[6]

FM is currently considered to be a central pain state suggesting that, although peripheral input may be playing a role, central factors (eg, central sensitization) likely account for much of the symptomatology.[7] In FM, aberrant activity in both central afferent[8] as well as descending modulatory mechanisms[9] contribute to symptoms and can be targeted therapeutically with some success.[10–12]

Currently, self-report measures, increasingly referred to as patient-reported outcomes (PROs), remain the best method for characterizing the multiple facets of FM. Although numerous attempts to identify biomarkers have produced mixed results (eg, genetics, autoantibodies, cytokines, hematologic findings, oxidative stress, neuroimaging, neuropathology),[13] pathophysiologic indices with sufficient sensitivity and specificity to serve as an FM biomarker remain elusive.[14] The use of PROs in the context of FM can take several forms, depending on the purpose of assessment: (a) diagnostics, (b) symptom monitoring, (c) phenotyping/characterization, and (d) as outcomes for clinical trials. The remainder of this paper focuses on these 4 uses of PROs for FM and describes instruments that can be used to support each use.

DIAGNOSTICS

In 1990, the American College of Rheumatology developed research classification criteria so that standardized selection of individuals likely to have FM could be identified in support of conducting research on the condition. These criteria required the presence of tender points and widespread pain over a prolonged period of time.[15] Although the American College of Rheumatology 1990 criteria were useful in promoting research, the tender point concept was flawed as a means of identifying FM.[16] Women generally report more musculoskeletal tenderness compared with men and thus defining FM by tenderness lead to the erroneous conclusion that FM was predominantly a "female" condition. When tenderness was replaced with widespread pain, the distribution still favored females but not nearly as much.[17]

In 2010, the American College of Rheumatology released for the first time their Clinical Diagnostic Criteria for FM. These new criteria retained the need to have widespread pain, but eliminated the tender point concept for the reasons discussed. The new diagnostic criteria included other symptoms in addition to pain that are commonly experienced by people with FM, such as cognitive dysfunction, fatigue, and sleep problems. These new criteria also require a physician to rule out a number of other diagnoses that could account for the symptoms.[18]

Again, in the interest of conducting research on FM with the new clinical criteria, a PRO survey containing most of the diagnostic criteria was published in 2011.[19] There are a number of practical differences between the actual diagnostic criteria and the survey criteria in that the survey can be mailed to people, completed online via an Internet-based platform, and/or completed in a research setting without a physician present. The survey criteria also permit the calculation of a continuously scaled Fibromyalgia Score (0–31) allowing an individual to have a lot or a little of FM, consistent with the experience reported by individuals with FM that FM tends to be variable over time and with the observation that some individuals have greater disease (symptom) burden compared with others. Scores on this continuous measure can provide an indication of "fibromyalgianess," or degree of augmented sensory (most prominently pain sensation) processing.[20,21]

DISEASE MONITORING

Until the mid-1990s, there was little uniformity in the assessment of pain in clinical settings. In his presidential address to the American Pain Society, Jim Campbell observed that, "if pain were assessed with the same zeal as other vital signs are, it would have a much better chance of being treated properly." After this address, the American Pain Society advanced the concept of pain being the fifth vital sign. In subsequent years, both the Veteran's Administration and the Joint Commission (formerly the Joint Commission on Accreditation of Healthcare Organizations) adopted the concept of pain being the fifth vital sign. In clinical settings, this is often operationalized by having patients rate their pain on a 0 to 10 numeric rating scale (NRS), which then gets transferred to the electronic medical record. Typically, pain greater than 4 on a scale of 10 triggers more comprehensive pain assessment and management.

Given that pain is only 1 aspect of FM, use of the NRS as a means of monitoring the condition is likely to be insufficient.[22] One instrument that has been used to monitor diverse FM symptomatology and impact overtime has been the Fibromyalgia Impact Questionnaire-Revised.[23] The Fibromyalgia Impact Questionnaire-Revised, one of the few PROs developed specifically for FM, covers 3 domains relevant to FM: function, overall impact, and multidimensional symptomatology. Containing 21 items, this questionnaire can be given weekly (ie, recall period is defined as 1 week), and only takes 3 to 5 minutes to administer. Its development was rigorous and numerous studies support its validation (for review see Ref.[24]). Whether used to monitor disease or as an outcome in clinical trials, a 14% change in the Fibromyalgia Impact Questionnaire-Revised total score, which is the sum of the 3 domain scores, seems to represent a clinically meaningful change in FM.[25] Although more recently developed, the survey criteria for FM described for epidemiologic purposes[19] can also be used to monitor disease variability when the continuous FM scale (as described) is used.

PHENOTYPING AND FIBROMYALGIA CHARACTERIZATION

Despite pain being the cardinal symptom of FM, to be "well" with FM requires far more than pain improvement. When characterizing FM it is helpful to think in terms of 6 assessment domains: (1) pain, (2) comorbidities, (3) affective vulnerability, (4) beliefs and attitudes, (5) behavior, and (6) environmental/social. Next we provide a nonexhaustive listing of standardized PRO instruments that can be used to assess these domains in the context of FM.

Pain

Historically only pain intensity was assessed routinely for FM using visual analogue scales, NRS, or a "faces" approach.[26] There are, however, other aspects of pain that can hold relevance to FM. These include the quality of pain, its location (eg, how widespread it is), and its temporality (eg, constant vs intermittent; **Table 1**). One of the first measures of pain quality was the McGill Pain Questionnaire (MPQ).[27] This questionnaire provided 78 pain descriptors grouped into 20 categories indicative of various types of pain (eg, "stinging," "aching," "pounding") that could be scored along 3 dimensions of painful experiences: sensation, affect, and evaluative components of pain. The MPQ also offers a body map to assess pain location and captures an NRS for present pain. The Brief Pain Inventory (BPI)[28] is another commonly used pain question that captures both pain intensity and pain interference

Table 1
Assessment of the pain domain

Domain	Instrument		Items	Score Range
Pain				
Intensity	VAS and NRS[26]		1	0–10
Quality, intensity, and distribution	McGill Pain Questionnaire (MPQ)[27]		78	0–78
Intensity, distribution, and interference	Brief Pain Inventory (BPI)[28]		16	—
	Subscales	Pain intensity	4	0–10
		Pain interference	7	0–10
Quality, intensity, distribution, and temporality	painDETECT[30]		9	−1–38

Abbreviations: NRS, numerical rating scales; VAS, visual analog scale.

(ie, elements of functional status). Like the MPQ, it uses a body map to assess location and queries about the effectiveness of treatment. Body maps are becoming increasingly important in the identification of single versus multiple comorbid pain conditions and are helping to identify individuals with just a primary condition versus multiple overlapping pain conditions. For example,[29] a newer questionnaire, the painDETECT,[30] combines many of the important elements of pain assessment by offering an index of pain intensity assessment similar to the BPI, an abbreviated assessment of pain quality similar to the MPQ, a body map like both the MPQ and the BPI, as well as assessment of pain temporality. The painDETECT can also be scored to help differentiate the presence of musculoskeletal versus neuropathic pain, which in FM can present in the same individual to differing degrees.

Comorbidities

Comorbidities refer to both diagnosable conditions as well as to coaggregated symptoms that tend to accompany chronic pain[31] (**Table 2**). The concept of coexisting chronic pain conditions was mentioned in the 2011 Institute of Medicine report on *Relieving Pain in America*[32] and is now recognized by both the National Institutes of Health and the US Congress as a set of coaggregating disorders that share symptomatology and putatively common mechanisms despite residing in anatomically distinct regions of the body. Currently labeled as chronic overlapping pain conditions (COPCs), this collective of pain conditions includes but is not limited to FM, temporomandibular disorders, irritable bowel syndrome, chronic tension type headache, migraine, chronic low back pain, myalgic encephalomyelitis/chronic fatigue syndrome, interstitial cystitis/painful bladder syndrome, endometriosis, and vulvodynia.[33] Currently, one of the best means of assessing for the presence of 1 or more COPCs in a given individual is through the use of the Complex Multi-Symptom Inventory (CMSI).[34] The CMSI contains 2 parts,[1] a 41-item symptom screener and[2] the published diagnostic criteria for 6 of the 10 COPCs listed. Rather than administering all diagnostic criteria to all patients, patients first complete the screener, which contains specific items that trigger the administration of the full diagnostic criteria for COPCs that are relevant for that individual, effectively limiting response burden by only administering relevant questions. An updated version of the CMSI is in development that includes all 10 COPCs. The CMSI symptom screener can also be used as a tally of functional somatic burden much like a similar measure, the Pennebaker Inventory of Limbic Languidness[35] or the FM survey criteria described.[19] Such coaggregated symptom tallies have demonstrated usefulness in predicting both the onset and chronification of COPCs.[36]

Table 2
Assessment of the comorbidities domain

Domain	Instrument		Items	Score Range
Comorbidities				
Symptom burden, chronic overlapping pain conditions (COPC) diagnostics	Complex Medical Symptom Inventory (CMSI)[34] (screener and measure of symptom burden) Includes diagnostic criteria for COPCs		41	0–41
Symptom burden	Pennebaker Inventory of Limbic Languidness (PILL)[35]		54	0–54
Fibromyalgia diagnostics	Fibromyalgia survey criteria[19]		7	—
Fibromyalgia-ness	"Fibromyalgianess" as a continuous construct		—	0–31
Waking	PROMIS Sleep-Related Impairment Short Form 8[37]		8	8–40
Sleep	PROMIS Sleep Disturbance Short Form 8a[37]		8	8–40
	Medical Outcome Study (MOS) sleep scale[38]		12	—
	Subscales	Sleep disturbance	4	1–6
		Snoring	1	1–6
		Shortness of breath	1	1–6
		Sleep adequacy	2	1–6
		Somnolence	3	1–6
		Sleep quantity (h)	1	—
	Pittsburgh Sleep Quality Index (PSQI)[39]		19	—
	Subscales	Sleep quality	1	0–3
		Sleep latency	2	0–3
		Sleep duration	1	0–3
		Sleep efficiency	2	0–3
		Sleep disturbances	9	0–3
		Use of sleep medication	1	0–3
		Daytime dysfunction	2	0–3
		Global score	18	0–21
Fatigue	PROMIS Fatigue Short Form 8a[37]		8	8–40
	Multidimensional fatigue Inventory (MFI)[40]		20	—
	Subscales	General fatigue	4	4–20
		Physical fatigue	4	4–20
		Mental fatigue	4	4–20
		Reduced motivation	4	4–20
		Reduced activity	4	4–20
Dyscognition	Multiple Ability Self-Report Questionnaire (MASQ)[41]		38	38–190
	Subscales	Language	8	8–40
		Visual–perceptual ability	6	6–30
		Verbal memory	8	8–40
		Visual–spatial memory	8	8–40
		Attention/concentration	8	8–40
	Multidimensional Inventory of Subjective Cognitive Impairment (MISCI)[43]		10	10–50

Despite pain being the cardinal symptom of FM, an Internet-based survey of 2596 individuals with FM revealed that the intensity of fatigue, sleep problems, and difficulties with memory, concentration, and mental clarity (ie, dyscognition) are often more severe and problematic than pain.[1] Brief instruments for assessing both sleep quality and sleep-related impairment can be obtained through the Patient Reported Outcomes Measurement Information System (PROMIS) administration and information website, AssessmentCenter.[37] Other measures of sleep disturbances that have been more commonly used with FM populations include the Medical Outcomes Study sleep scale[38] or the Pittsburg Sleep Quality Index.[39] Fatigue can also be assessed via PROMIS measures that provide a single fatigue score reflecting a combination of fatigue intensity and fatigue interference/impact,[37] or with the Multidimensional Fatigue Inventory.[40] The Multidimensional Fatigue Inventory allows for the assessment of general fatigue, physical fatigue, mental fatigue, reduced motivation, and reduced activity. To assess perceived cognitive difficulties across several dimensions, the Multiple Ability Self-Report Questionnaire[41] has been used with FM samples.[42] This questionnaire assesses perceived cognitive difficulties across several dimensions: language ability, visual–perceptual ability, verbal memory, visual memory, and attention/concentration. One drawback of this questionnaire, however, is its length. At 38 items, it can represent considerable response burden to patients. Recently, a new measure of perceived dyscognition, based on the PROMIS item banks, was developed via classical and item response theory methods specifically for FM and widespread pain conditions. Entitled the Multidimensional Inventory of Subjective Cognitive Impairment,[43] this 10-item inventory provides indices for cognitive concerns in the areas of mental clarity, memory, attention/concentration, executive functioning, and language, and is highly correlated ($r = 0.82$) with the lengthier Multiple Ability Self-Report Questionnaire.

Affective Vulnerability

Pain is defined as both a sensory and an affective experience.[44] Thus, emotion is not a confounder or downstream byproduct of pain, but is central to the very experience. Historically, the phenotype of FM included the high prevalence of comorbid affective disorders in individuals with FM.[45,46] As such, it became common to identify the presence of negative affective symptoms using such measures as the Beck Depression Inventory-II,[47,48] the Center for Epidemiologic Studies Depression Scale,[49,50] or the PHQ-9[51] for depression and the State-Trait Anxiety Inventory[52] or General Anxiety Disorder-7[53] for anxious affect. Some measures such as the Hospital Anxiety and Depression Scale[54] assess both constructs. Each of these measures can be scored to reveal either a probable diagnosis of an effective disorder or a continuous measure of negative affect. One need not be psychiatrically ill, however, to have FM, which is why the continuous measurement of emotion is preferable when assessing the role of affect in a pain condition. Other measures of negative affect (ie, not diagnostic of disorders) include the PROMIS negative emotions scales (eg, depressed affect, anxious affect, and anger).[37] and the Positive and Negative Affect Scale.[55] In addition to characterizing pain by negative affect, the Positive and Negative Affect Scale introduces the ability to assess positive emotion, which is thought to represent an element of resilience that can serve to buffer or even diminish the perception of pain[56]; deficits in the balance between positive and negative affect in FM have been discovered and highlight the importance of a comprehensive assessment of affect in this condition.[57,58] The Positive and Negative Affect Scale can be scored to derive an index of affect balance, a ratio between positive and negative emotion that is associated with well-being in FM.[59]

Constructs related to affective vulnerability also include stress/trauma and personality. Stress is a statelike phenomena with influences on pain perception that can be assessed with measures such as the Perceived Stress Scale.[60] Longer and more stable affective influences on pain can emerge from trauma (eg, assessed with measures such as the Childhood and Recent Traumatic Events Scales[61] or personality characteristics. The latter, personality characteristics, often use measures that assess the big 5 personality domains: neuroticism, extroversion, openness, conscientiousness, and agreeableness (eg, NEO Personality Inventory, NEO Personality Inventory[62,63]), the International Personality Item Pool,[64–66] or the Ten-Item Personality Inventory[67] (**Table 3** reviews Affective scales).

Beliefs/Attitudes

Beliefs and attitudes about pain can directly influence a patient's affect and functional status.[68] Further, a single detrimental belief such as "catastrophizing" has

Table 3
Assessment of the affective vulnerability domain

Domain	Instrument		Items	Score Range
Affective Vulnerability				
Depression	Beck Depression Inventory-II (BDI-II)[47,48]		21	0–63
	Center for Epidemiologic Studies of Depression Scale Revised (CED-R)[49]		20	0–60
	Patient Health Questionnaire – 9 (PHQ-9)[51]		9	0–27
	PROMIS Depression Short Form 8a[37]		8	8–40
Anxiety	State-Trait Anxiety Inventory (STAI)[52]		40	—
	Subscales	State anxiety scale	20	20–80
		Trait anxiety scale	20	20–80
	Generalized Anxiety Disorder -7 (GAD-7)[53]		7	0–21
	PROMIS Anxiety Short Form 8a[37]		8	0–32
Anxiety and depression	Hospital Anxiety Depression Scale (HADS)[54]		14	0–42
	Subscales	Anxiety	7	0–21
		Depression	7	0–21
Stress	Perceived Stress Scale (PSS)[60]		10	0–40
Trauma	Childhood Traumatic Events Scale (CTES)/Recent Traumatic Events Scale (RTES)[61] (single items are scored separately)		13	—
Personality	NEO Personality Inventory–Revised (NEO-PI-R)[62,63]; Full scale has 243 items including 3 validity items		240	—
	Subscales	Extraversion	48	0–192
		Agreeableness	48	0–192
		Conscientiousness	48	0–192
		Neuroticism	48	0–192
		Openness to experience	48	0–192
	International Personality Item Pool (IPIP)[64–66]		120	—
	Subscales	Extraversion	—	—
		Agreeableness	—	—
		Conscientiousness	—	—
		Neuroticism	—	—
		Openness to experience	—	—
	TIPI (67)		10	—
	Subscales	Extraversion	2	1–7
		Agreeableness	2	1–7
		Conscientiousness	2	1–7
		Neuroticism	2	1–7
		Openness to experience	2	1–7
Positive and negative affect	Positive and Negative Affect Schedule (PANAS)[55]		20	—
	Subscales	Positive Affect	10	10–50
		Negative Affect	10	10–50

been shown to account for up to 47% of the variance in chronification in low back pain[69] and is a common cognitive style for individuals with FM.[70] Several measures are used to assess catastrophizing; the Pain Catastrophizing Scale[71] and the Catastrophizing subscale of the Coping Strategies Questionnaire.[72] Other beliefs and attitudes associated with pain and subsequent outcomes in FM include locus of control (ie, assessed by the Beliefs in Pain Control Questionnaire),[73] self-efficacy to control pain (ie, assessed by the Perceived Self-Efficacy Scale),[74] coping resources (eg, the full version of the above mentioned Coping Strategies Questionnaire[72]), and multidimensional measures of pain beliefs (eg, the Survey of Pain Attitudes[75] or the Pain Belief and Perceptions Inventory[76]; **Table 4** lists belief/attitudes scales).

Table 4
Assessment of the beliefs/attitudes domain

Domain	Instrument		Items	Score Range
Beliefs/Attitudes				
Catastrophizing	Pain Catastrophizing Scale (PCS)[71]		13	0–52
	Subscales	Rumination	4	0–16
		Magnification	3	0–12
		Helplessness	6	0–24
Locus of control	Beliefs About Pain Control Questionnaire (BPCQ)[73]		13	—
	Subscales	Internal control	5	5–30
		Powerful others	4	4–24
		Chance	4	4–24
Self-efficacy	Arthritis Self Efficacy Scales (ASE)[74]		20	—
	Subscales	Self-efficacy pain	5	1–10
		Self-efficacy function	9	1–10
		Self-efficacy other symptoms	6	1–10
Coping strategies	Coping Strategies Questionnaire (CSQ)[72]		50	—
	Subscales	Diverting attention	6	0–36
		Reinterpreting pain sensations	6	0–36
		Coping self-statements	6	0–36
		Ignoring pain sensations	6	0–36
		Praying/hoping	6	0–36
		Catastrophizing	6	0–36
		Increasing behavioral activity	6	0–36
		Ability to control pain	1	0–6
		Ability to decrease pain	1	0–6
Pain beliefs	Survey of Pain Attitudes (SOPA)[75]		57	—
	Subscales	Control	10	0–40
		Emotion	8	0–32
		Disability	10	0–40
		Harm	8	0–32
		Medication	6	0–24
		Solicitude	6	0–24
		Medical cure	9	0–36
	Pain Beliefs and Perceptions Inventory (PBPI)[76]		16	—
	Subscales	Mystery	4	−2 – +2
		Constant	4	−2 – +2
		Permanent	4	−2 – +2
		Self-blame	4	−2 – +2

Behavior

There are a number of behavioral domains that can hold relevance for individuals with FM, but perhaps the most common is physical functioning (**Table 5**). In many studies, the Short Form-36[77] (or one of the shorter versions of this instrument) has been used for assessment.[78] Other measures of physical functioning with relevance for FM include the PROMIS physical functioning scales,[37] the Pain Disability Index,[79] and, as mentioned previously, the pain interference scale from the BPI.[28] Underscoring the importance of assessing behavioral responses to pain, outcomes such as health care use have shown stronger relationships with demand for services and disability than with indices more specifically tied to symptomatology, such as illness severity, prognosis, or treatment status.[80]

Environmental/Social

For rheumatologic forms of pain, both the quality and quantity of social support at the initial diagnosis of a condition can be predictive of pain and functional status 3 to 5 years later.[81] For this reason, social factors are often considered in the phenotypic assessment of FM. Measures of family functioning (eg, the Dyadic Adjustment Scale[82]), work place activities (eg, Workplace Productivity and Activity Impairment[83]), and measures of social engagement with friends and others (eg, Participation Enfranchisement[84]) capture 3 highly relevant components of individuals' social world. A more general multidimensional measure, the West Haven-Yale Multidimensional Pain Inventory[85] also provides multidimensional indices of constructs relevant to the social/environmental influences on pain: interference, support, pain severity, life-control, affective distress, negative responses, solicitous responses, distracting responses, household chores, outdoor work, activities away from home, social activities, and general activities (**Table 6**).

Table 5
Assessment of the behavior domain

Domain	Instrument		Items	Score Range
Behavior				
Physical and mental function	Medical Outcomes Study Short Form Health Survey-36 (SF-36)[77]		36	—
	Subscales	Physical functioning	10	0–100
		Role physical	4	0–100
		Bodily pain	2	0–100
		General health	5	0–100
		Vitality	4	0–100
		Social functioning	2	0–100
		Role emotional	3	0–100
		Mental health	5	0–100
Physical function	PROMIS Physical Function Short Form 10a[37]		10	10–50
Disability	Pain Disability Index (PDI)[79]		7	0–70
Pain interference	Brief Pain Inventory – Interference subscale (BPI)[28]		7	0–10
Physical function and multimodal fibromyalgia	Fibromyalgia Impact Questionnaire–Revised (FIQR)[23]		21	0–100
	Subscales	Function	9	0–30
		Symptoms	10	0–50
		Overall impact	2	0–20

Table 6
Assessment of the social/environmental domain

Domain	Instrument		Items	Score Range
Social/environmental				
Home	Dyadic Adjustment Scale (DAS)[82]		32	0–151
	Subscales	Dyadic consensus	13	0–65
		Dyadic satisfaction	10	0–50
		Dyadic cohesion	5	0–12
		Affectional expression	4	0–24
Work	Work Productivity and Activity Impairment (WPAI)[83]		6	—
	Subscales	Percent work missed owing to health	—	0–100
		Percent impairment while working owing to health	—	0–100
		Percent overall work impairment owing to health	—	0–100
		Percent activity impairment owing to health	—	0–100
Friends	Participation Enfranchisement (PE)[84]		19	—
Multimodal	West Haven-Yale Multidimensional Pain Inventory (WHYMPI)[85]		54	—
	Subscales	Pain interference	9	0–6
		Support	3	0–6
		Pain severity	3	0–6
		Life control	2	0–6
		Affective distress	3	0–6
		Negative responses	4	0–6
		Solicitous responses	6	0–6
		Distracting responses	4	0–6
		Household chores	5	0–6
		Outdoor work	5	0–6
		Activities away from home	4	0–6
		Social activities	4	0–6
		General activity	18	0–6

CLINICAL TRIALS

The Outcome Measures in Rheumatology Clinical Trials (OMERACT) is an organization that seeks to refine outcomes measurement issues in part by identifying core sets of variables that should be collected and reported in any clinical trial involving rheumatologic conditions.[86] Dating back to 2004, a task force within OMERACT focused on FM, conducted 2 Delphi studies so as to establish consensus regarding the most relevant domains of assessment for clinical trials involving FM. One of these studies involved individuals with FM[87] and the second involved clinicians treating FM.[88] Despite some differences in the ordering of symptom priority between patients and clinicians (eg, patients seemed more concerned with dyscognition than were clinicians), there was considerable consensus about the domains of relevance for clinical trials.[2] These OMERACT domains included pain, fatigue, functional status, sleep, mood, tenderness, stiffness, and dyscognition (eg, memory and concentration).

The Initiative on Methods, Measurement, and Pain Assessment in Clinical Trials (IMMPACT) has similarly identified the domains of relevance for any clinical trial of a painful condition. IMMPACT recommends that 4 core areas be assessed: (1) pain intensity, (2) physical functioning, (3) emotional functioning, and (4) overall improvement/well-being.[89–91] Despite OMERACT and IMMPACT being 2 independent organizations, there was substantial agreement between organizations as to what domains to assess. It should be noted that, although each organization identified relevant domains, neither organization dictated the specific instruments that needed to be used in the assessment of each domain, leaving that up to individual investigators.

To date, clinical trials in FM have used many different questionnaires to assess the relevant domains.[24,78] Although this may seem problematic, at least 1 published study that combined datasets from across large clinical trials, assessment approaches, and differing pharmacologic agents, empirically identified the phenotype of an "FM treatment responder." This study suggested that regardless of the assessment instrument used, an FM treatment responder would demonstrate (1) a 30% improvement in pain, (2) a 10% improvement in physical functioning, and (3) a 30% improvement in at least 2 of the following domains: fatigue, sleep, depression, anxiety, or dyscognition.[78]

SUMMARY

PROs remain the best approach for assessing the multiple facets of FM for the purposes of diagnosis, disease monitoring, phenotyping, and clinical trials. Through the use of PROs, it is possible to classify individuals as having FM for both clinical and research purposes. Given that FM is a highly variable condition with a variety of symptomatic manifestations, PROS that capture the waxing and waning of FM's multifaceted symptomatology are necessary for monitoring the condition. To better understand the mechanisms underlying FM, it is necessary to characterize individuals with FM comprehensively. Depending on the research question, this can require extensive exploration of putative mechanisms interacting across multiple domains of assessment. Assessments can be briefer in the context of clinical trials given that the "discovery" is related to the intervention rather than to the underlying mechanisms of FM. Still, a multifaceted assessment is needed to adequately identify the potential of the intervention to impact multiple domains of relevance to FM. Although researchers continue to explore biomarkers for FM, it is likely that PROs will continue to be informative to this field for years to come.

REFERENCES

1. Bennett RM, Jones J, Turk DC, et al. An internet survey of 2,596 people with fibromyalgia. BMC Musculoskelet Disord 2007;8:27.
2. Mease PJ, Arnold LM, Crofford LJ, et al. Identifying the clinical domains of fibromyalgia: contributions from clinician and patient Delphi exercises. Arthritis Rheum 2008;59(7):952–60.
3. Queiroz LP. Worldwide epidemiology of fibromyalgia. Curr Pain Headache Rep 2013;17(8):356.
4. Forseth KK, Gran JT. Management of fibromyalgia: what are the best treatment choices? Drugs 2002;62(4):577–92.
5. Hoffman DL, Dukes EM. The health status burden of people with fibromyalgia: a review of studies that assessed health status with the SF-36 or the SF-12. Int J Clin Pract 2008;62(1):115–26.
6. Berger A, Dukes E, Martin S, et al. Characteristics and healthcare costs of patients with fibromyalgia syndrome. Int J Clin Pract 2007;61(9):1498–508.
7. Clauw DJ. Fibromyalgia: a clinical review. JAMA 2014;311(15):1547–55.
8. Harris RE, Napadow V, Huggins JP, et al. Pregabalin rectifies aberrant brain chemistry, connectivity, and functional response in chronic pain patients. Anesthesiology 2013;119(6):1453–64.

9. Hauser W, Wolfe F, Tolle T, et al. The role of antidepressants in the management of fibromyalgia syndrome: a systematic review and meta-analysis. CNS Drugs 2012; 26(4):297–307.
10. Tzellos TG, Toulis KA, Goulis DG, et al. Gabapentin and pregabalin in the treatment of fibromyalgia: a systematic review and a meta-analysis. J Clin Pharm Ther 2010;35(6):639–56.
11. Arnold LM, Clauw DJ, Wohlreich MM, et al. Efficacy of duloxetine in patients with fibromyalgia: pooled analysis of 4 placebo-controlled clinical trials. Prim Care Companion J Clin Psychiatry 2009;11(5):237–44.
12. Geisser ME, Palmer RH, Gendreau RM, et al. A pooled analysis of two randomized, double-blind, placebo-controlled trials of milnacipran monotherapy in the treatment of fibromyalgia. Pain Pract 2011;11(2):120–31.
13. Ablin JN, Buskila D, Clauw DJ. Biomarkers in fibromyalgia. Curr Pain Headache Rep 2009;13(5):343–9.
14. Giacomelli C, Sernissi F, Rossi A, et al. Biomarkers in fibromyalgia: a review. Current Biomarker Findings 2014;4:35–41.
15. Wolfe F, Smythe HA, Yunus MB, et al. The American College of Rheumatology 1990 criteria for the classification of fibromyalgia. Report of the Multicenter Criteria Committee. Arthritis Rheum 1990;33(2):160–72.
16. Petzke F, Gracely RH, Park KM, et al. What do tender points measure? Influence of distress on 4 measures of tenderness. J Rheumatol 2003;30(3):567–74.
17. Macfarlane GJ, Croft PR, Schollum J, et al. Widespread pain: is an improved classification possible? J Rheumatol 1996;23(9):1628–32.
18. Wolfe F, Clauw DJ, Fitzcharles MA, et al. The American College of Rheumatology preliminary diagnostic criteria for fibromyalgia and measurement of symptom severity. Arthritis Care Res (Hoboken) 2010;62(5):600–10.
19. Wolfe F, Clauw DJ, Fitzcharles MA, et al. Fibromyalgia criteria and severity scales for clinical and epidemiological studies: a modification of the ACR preliminary diagnostic criteria for fibromyalgia. J Rheumatol 2011;38(6):1113–22.
20. Smith HS, Harris R, Clauw D. Fibromyalgia: an afferent processing disorder leading to a complex pain generalized syndrome. Pain Physician 2011;14(2): E217–45.
21. Phillips K, Clauw DJ. Central pain mechanisms in chronic pain states–maybe it is all in their head. Best Pract Res Clin Rheumatol 2011;25(2):141–54.
22. Alves AM, Natour J, Assis MR, et al. Assessment of different instruments used as outcome measures in patients with fibromyalgia. Rev Bras Reumatol 2012;52(4): 501–6.
23. Bennett RM, Friend R, Jones KD, et al. The Revised Fibromyalgia Impact Questionnaire (FIQR): validation and psychometric properties. Arthritis Res Ther 2009; 11(4):R120.
24. Williams DA, Arnold LM. Measures of fibromyalgia: Fibromyalgia Impact Questionnaire (FIQ), Brief Pain Inventory (BPI), Multidimensional Fatigue Inventory (MFI-20), Medical Outcomes Study (MOS) Sleep Scale, and Multiple Ability Self-Report Questionnaire (MASQ). Arthritis Care Res 2011;63(Suppl 11):S86–97.
25. Bennett RM, Bushmakin AG, Cappelleri JC, et al. Minimal clinically important difference in the fibromyalgia impact questionnaire. J Rheumatol 2009;36(6): 1304–11.
26. Jensen MP, Karoly P. Self-report scales and procedures for assessing pain in adults. In: Turk DC, Melzack R, editors. Handbook of pain assessment. New York: Guilford Press; 2011. p. 19–44.

27. Melzack R. The McGill Pain Questionnaire: major properties and scoring methods. Pain 1975;1(3):277–99.
28. Cleeland C. The brief pain inventory: user guide. Houston (TX): MD Anderson Cancer Center; 2009.
29. Nickel JC, Tripp DA. International Interstitial Cystitis Study Group. Clinical and psychological parameters associated with pain pattern phenotypes in women with interstitial cystitis/bladder pain syndrome. J Urol 2015;193(1):138–44.
30. Freynhagen R, Baron R, Gockel U, et al. painDETECT: a new screening questionnaire to identify neuropathic components in patients with back pain. Curr Med Res Opin 2006;22(10):1911–20.
31. Aaron LA, Buchwald D. A review of the evidence for overlap among unexplained clinical conditions. Ann Intern Med 2001;134:868–81.
32. IOM. Relieving pain in America: a blueprint for transforming prevention, care education, and research. Washington, DC: The National Academies Press; 2011.
33. Veasley C, Clare D, Clauw DJ, et al. Impact of chronic overlapping pain conditions on public health and the urgent need for safe and effective treatment: 2015 analysis and policy recommendations. The Chronic Pain Research Alliance 2015.
34. Williams DA, Schilling S. Advances in the assessment of fibromyalgia. Rheum Dis Clin North Am 2009;35(2):339–57.
35. Pennebaker JW. The psychology of physical symptoms. New York: Springer-Verlag; 1982.
36. Fillingim RB, Ohrbach R, Greenspan JD, et al. Psychological factors associated with development of TMD: the OPPERA prospective cohort study. J Pain 2013; 14(Suppl 12):T75–90.
37. Cella D, Riley W, Stone A, et al. The Patient-Reported Outcomes Measurement Information System (PROMIS) developed and tested its first wave of adult self-reported health outcome item banks: 2005-2008. J Clin Epidemiol 2010;63(11): 1179–94.
38. Allen RP, Kosinski M, Hill-Zabala CE, et al. Psychometric evaluation and tests of validity of the medical outcomes study 12-item sleep scale (MOS sleep). Sleep Med 2009;10(5):531–9.
39. Buysse DJ, Reynolds CF III, Monk TH, et al. The Pittsburgh sleep quality index: a new instrument for psychiatric practice and research. Psychiatry Res 1989;28(2): 193–213.
40. Smets EM, Garssen B, Bonke B, et al. The Multidimensional Fatigue Inventory (MFI) psychometric qualities of an instrument to assess fatigue. J Psychosom Res 1995;39(3):315–25.
41. Seidenberg M, Haltiner A, Taylor MA, et al. Development and validation of a multiple ability self-report questionnaire. J Clin Exp Neuropsychol 1994;16(1): 93–104.
42. Williams DA, Clauw DJ, Glass JM. Perceived cognitive dysfunction in fibromyalgia syndrome. J Musculoskelet Pain 2011;19(2):66–75.
43. Kratz AL, Schilling SG, Goesling J, et al. Development and initial validation of a brief self-report measure of cognitive dysfunction in fibromyalgia. J Pain 2015; 16(6):527–36.
44. International Association for the Study of Pain (IASP). IASP taxonomy 2015. Available at: www.IASP-Pain.org/taxonomy. Accessed January 9, 2015.
45. Goldenberg DL. Psychological symptoms and psychiatric diagnosis in patients with fibromyalgia. J Rheumatol Suppl 1989;19:127–30.

46. Alfisi S, Sigal M, Landau M. Primary fibromyalgia syndrome - a variant of depressive disorder? Psychother Psychosom 1989;51(3):156–61.
47. Beck AT, Steer RA, Garbin MG. Psychometric properties of the beck depression inventory: twenty-five years of evaluation. Clin Psychol Rev 1988;8:77–100.
48. Beck AT, Steer RA, Ball R, et al. Comparison of beck depression inventories-IA and -II in psychiatric outpatients. J Pers Assess 1996;67(3):588–97.
49. Radloff LS. The CES-D scale: a self-report depression scale for research in the general population. Applied Psychological Measurement 1977;1(3):385–401.
50. Eaton WW, Muntaner C, Smith C, et al. Center for Epidemiologic Studies Depression Scale: Review and revision (CESD and CESD-R). In: Maruish ME, editor. The use of psychological testing for treatment planning and outcomes assessment. 3rd edition. Mahwah (NJ): Lawrence Erlbaum; 2004. p. 363–77.
51. Kroenke K, Spitzer RL, Williams JB. The PHQ-9: validity of a brief depression severity measure. J Gen Intern Med 2001;16(9):606–13.
52. Spielberger CD, Gorsuch RC, Lushene RE, et al. Manual for the state-trait anxiety inventory (Form Y): ("Self-evaluation questionnaire"). Palo Alto (CA): Consulting Psychologists; 1983. p. 36.
53. Spitzer RL, Kroenke K, Williams JB, et al. A brief measure for assessing generalized anxiety disorder: the GAD-7. Arch Intern Med 2006;166(10):1092–7.
54. Snaith RP. The hospital anxiety and depression scale. Health Qual Life Outcomes 2003;1:29.
55. Watson D, Clark LA, Tellegen A. Development and validation of brief measures of positive and negative affect: the PANAS scales. J Pers Soc Psychol 1988;54(6): 1063–70.
56. Zautra AJ, Johnson LM, Davis MC. Positive affect as a source of resilience for women in chronic pain. J Consult Clin Psychol 2005;73(2):212–20.
57. Zautra AJ, Fasman R, Reich JW, et al. Fibromyalgia: evidence for deficits in positive affect regulation. Psychosom Med 2005;67(1):147–55.
58. Finan PH, Zautra AJ, Davis MC. Daily affect relations in fibromyalgia patients reveal positive affective disturbance. Psychosom Med 2009;71(4):474–82.
59. Hassett AL, Simonelli LE, Radvanski DC, et al. The relationship between affect balance style and clinical outcomes in fibromyalgia. Arthritis Rheum 2008; 59(6):833–40.
60. Cohen S, Kamarck T, Mermelstein R. A global measure of perceived stress. J Health Soc Behav 1983;24(4):385–96.
61. Pennebaker JW, Susman JR. Disclosure of traumas and psychosomatic processes. Soc Sci Med 1988;26(3):327–32.
62. Costa PT Jr, McCrae RR. Revised NEO Personality Inventory (NEO PI-R) and NEO Five-Factor Inventory (NEO-FFI) professional manual. Odessa (FL): Psychological Assessment Resources; 1992.
63. Costa PT, Mcrea RR. NEO PI-R professional manual. Odessa (FL): Psychological Assessment Resources, Inc.; 1992.
64. Goldberg LR, Johnson JA, Eber HW, et al. The International Personality Item Pool and the future of public-domain personality measures. J Res Pers 2006;40:84–96.
65. Maples JL, Guan L, Carter NT, et al. A test of the international personality item pool representation of the revised NEO personality inventory and development of a 120-item IPIP-based Measure of the five-factor model. Psychol Assess 2014;26(4):1070–84.
66. Johnson JA. Development of a short form of the IPIP-NEO personality inventory. Association for Research in Personality. Riverside, CA, June 17, 2011.

67. Gosling SD, Rentfrow PJ, Swann WB Jr. A very brief measure of the Big-Five personality domains. J Res Pers 2003;37:504–28.
68. Turner JA, Jensen MP, Romano JM. Do beliefs, coping, and catastrophizing independently predict functioning in patients with chronic pain? Pain 2000;85(1–2): 115–25.
69. Burton AK, Tillotson KM, Main CJ, et al. Psychosocial predictors of outcome in acute and subchronic low back trouble. Spine (Phila Pa 1976) 1995;20(6):722–8.
70. Edwards RR, Bingham CO 3rd, Bathon J, et al. Catastrophizing and pain in arthritis, fibromyalgia, and other rheumatic diseases. Arthritis Rheum 2006; 55(2):325–32.
71. Sullivan MJ, Bishop S, Pivik J. The pain catastrophizing scale: development and validation. Psychol Assess 1995;7:524–32.
72. Rosenstiel AK, Keefe FJ. The use of coping strategies in chronic low back pain patients: relationship to patient characteristics and current adjustment. Pain 1983;17(1):33–44.
73. Skevington SM. A standardized scale to measure beliefs about controlling pain (BPCQ): a preliminary study. Psychol Health 1990;4:221–32.
74. Lorig K, Chastain RL, Ung E, et al. Development and evaluation of a scale to measure perceived self-efficacy in people with arthritis. Arthritis Rheum 1989;32(1): 37–44.
75. Jensen MP, Turner JA, Romano JM. Pain beliefs assessment: a comparison of the short and long versions of the survey of pain attitudes. J Pain 2000;1:138–50.
76. Williams DA, Robinson ME, Geisser ME. Pain beliefs: assessment and utility. Pain 1994;59(1):71–8.
77. Ware JE, Kosinski M, Dewey J. How to score version two of the SF-36 health survey. Lincoln (RI): QualityMetric, Inc.; 2000.
78. Arnold LM, Williams DA, Hudson JI, et al. Development of responder definitions for fibromyalgia clinical trials. Arthritis Rheum 2012;64(3):885–94.
79. Tait RC, Chibnall JT, Krause S. The pain disability index: psychometric properties. Pain 1990;40(2):171–82.
80. Browne GB, Arpin K, Corey P, et al. Individual correlates of health service utilization and the cost of poor adjustment to chronic illness. Med Care 1990;28(1): 43–58.
81. Evers AW, Kraaimaat FW, Geenen R, et al. Pain coping and social support as predictors of long-term functional disability and pain in early rheumatoid arthritis. Behav Res Ther 2003;41(11):1295–310.
82. Spanier GB. The measurement of marital quality. J Sex Marital Ther 1979;5(3): 288–300.
83. Reilly MC, Zbrozek AS, Dukes EM. The validity and reproducibility of a work productivity and activity impairment instrument. Pharmacoeconomics 1993;4(5): 353–65.
84. Heinemann AW, Lai JS, Magasi S, et al. Measuring participation enfranchisement. Arch Phys Med Rehabil 2011;92(4):564–71.
85. Kerns RD, Turk DC, Rudy TE. The West Haven-Yale Multidimensional Pain Inventory (WHYMPI). Pain 1985;23(4):345–56.
86. Tugwell P, Boers M, Brooks P, et al. OMERACT: an international initiative to improve outcome measurement in rheumatology. Trial 2007;8:38.
87. Arnold LM, Crofford LJ, Mease PJ, et al. Patient perspectives on the impact of fibromyalgia. Patient Educ Couns 2008;73(1):114–20.
88. Mease PJ, Clauw DJ, Arnold LM, et al. Fibromyalgia syndrome. J Rheumatol 2005;32(11):2270–7.

89. Dworkin RH, Turk DC, Wyrwich KW, et al. Interpreting the clinical importance of treatment outcomes in chronic pain clinical trials: IMMPACT recommendations. J Pain 2008;9(2):105–21.
90. Turk DC, Dworkin RH, Allen RR, et al. Core outcome domains for chronic pain clinical trials: IMMPACT recommendations. Pain 2003;106(3):337–45.
91. Turk DC, Dworkin RH, Revicki D, et al. Identifying important outcome domains for chronic pain clinical trials: an IMMPACT survey of people with pain. Pain 2008;137(2):276–85.

Using Patient-Reported Outcome Measures to Capture the Patient's Voice in Research and Care of Juvenile Idiopathic Arthritis

Aimee O. Hersh, MD[a,*], Parissa K. Salimian, BA[b],
Elissa R. Weitzman, ScD, MSc[c,d,e]

KEYWORDS

- Juvenile arthritis • Health outcomes • Patient-centered care • Self-report
- Quality of life • Pediatric rheumatology • Chronic disease
- Comparative effectiveness research

KEY POINTS

- Incorporating patient-reported outcome (PRO) measures into routine clinical care of patients with juvenile idiopathic arthritis can help facilitate movement from physician-centered to patient-centered care.
- PRO measures relevant to juvenile idiopathic arthritis provide information germane to evaluating treatment outcomes and comparative effectiveness of therapies.
- Valid and reliable PRO measures are available that capture the experience of juvenile idiopathic arthritis from the perspective of patients and parents.
- Length, age, potential discordance between parent and child responses, and clinical validity are among the issues that need to be considered when selecting PRO measures.

Research reported in this publication was supported by the National Library of Medicine and by the National Institute of Arthritis and Musculoskeletal and Skin Diseases of the National Institutes of Health under award numbers R01LM011185 and U19AR069522, respectively, to Dr E.R. Weitzman and the National Institute of Arthritis and Musculoskeletal and Skin Diseases of the National Institutes of Health under award number K23AR066064 to Dr A. Hersh. The content is solely the responsibility of the authors and does not necessarily represent the official views of the National Institutes of Health.

[a] Pediatric Rheumatology, University of Utah, 81 Mario Capecchi Way, 4th Floor, Salt Lake City, UT 84113, USA; [b] Division of Developmental Medicine, Boston Children's Hospital, 300 Longwood Avenue BCH3185, Boston, MA 02115, USA; [c] Division of Adolescent/Young Adult Medicine, Boston Children's Hospital, 300 Longwood Avenue BCH3187, Boston, MA 02115, USA; [d] Department of Pediatrics, Harvard Medical School, 300 Longwood Avenue BCH3187, Boston, MA 02115, USA; [e] Computational Health Informatics Program, Boston Children's Hospital, 300 Longwood Avenue BCH3187, Boston, MA 02115, USA
* Corresponding author.
E-mail address: aimee.hersh@hsc.utah.edu

Rheum Dis Clin N Am 42 (2016) 333–346
http://dx.doi.org/10.1016/j.rdc.2016.01.004 rheumatic.theclinics.com

INTRODUCTION

Juvenile idiopathic arthritis (JIA) is the most common cause of acquired disability in the United States and the fifth most common chronic childhood disease.[1] Children with JIA experience an unpredictable disease course, with periods of improved disease control intermixed with episodes of flare.[2–4] Over the past decade, assessing patient-reported outcomes (PROs) has become increasingly important in the context of clinical care and research centered on JIA.[5–7]

Several factors are driving the evolution of PRO measures and their adoption within pediatric health care and research efforts. Studies in the general population indicate that PROs are predictive of future health care utilization for adults and children.[8–10] Measures of health behaviors and mental health status—domains suitable to PRO assessment—can predict future disease activity, as may levels of stress, adequacy of sleep, and availability of coping supports.[11] These issues are often reported by patients; however, they are not captured by routine clinical measures. At a system level, capturing a broad range of information about symptoms, side effects, and treatment outcomes is thought to contribute to more patient-centered care, improved patient experience, and potentially better treatments, particularly when this information is used to assess comparative effectiveness. Recognizing this, infrastructure has been developed to support patient-centered outcomes research. In addition, the development and validation of PROs has been prioritized through federal initiatives and investment.[12,13] Capturing the knowledge and voice of patients through high-quality, standardized, and validated measures may provide information to guide interventions and improve disease trajectories.

In this review, the authors provide an overview of the major domains of PRO assessment in JIA (pain, health-related quality of life, physical functioning and medication side effects, and commonly used measures in these domains) and the rationale for incorporating PROs into JIA clinical care and research.

JUVENILE IDIOPATHIC ARTHRITIS

Currently there are 7 categories of JIA as defined by the International League of Associations for Rheumatology's classification criteria.[14] The JIA subtypes vary with regard to associated clinical features, laboratory studies, and severity of disease; however, the common clinical feature across the categories of JIA is arthritis in one or more joints presenting before 16 years of age. Like adult patients with arthritis, pediatric patients with arthritis experience inflammation of their joints leading to pain, swelling, stiffness, and loss of range of motion. Unique to pediatrics is the impact these symptoms can have on physical development (eg, learning to walk) and social development (eg, attending school, playing sports). Appropriate assessment of pediatric patients' experience with arthritis is crucial to understanding the impact of the disease on patients, their families, disease course, and outcomes.

DOMAINS OF PATIENT-REPORTED OUTCOME MEASURES

Examples of generic and JIA-specific PROs by measurement domain are provided in **Table 1**. When selecting a particular PRO measure for clinical or research use, in addition to considering whether a given domain is represented by a generic or disease-specific measure, factors such as length, target age for administration, response format, and recall period may be relevant.

Pain

Assessment of pain has been identified by patients and their parents as one of the most important outcome measures in JIA.[15] For youth with JIA, most patients experience near-daily pain and reports of severe pain are found in one in 4 patients.[16] Daily pain is significantly associated with increased functional disability and anxiety and other daily symptoms,[16] so understanding factors that contribute to pain and addressing pain may have high clinical benefits. Several psychological factors seem to influence the report of pain among patients with JIA with high pain but low disease activity, such as cognitive health beliefs regarding disability and physical harm.[17] Variability in pain among youth with JIA is highly associated with the ability to effectively cope with stress; however, it is only minimally related to changes in disease activity.[18,19] Pain in youth with JIA is a primary determinant of the extent of difficulties these children have with vital socio-emotional functioning, including in areas related to physical ability, social life, and academic performance.[18,19]

Because of the complexity of measuring pain, its assessment often includes evaluation of pain intensity and the extent to which the experience of pain interferes with life activities (pain interference). Common pain measures are shown in **Table 1**. Measures of pain intensity include the Wong-Baker FACES Pain Rating Scale, which can be used to assess pain in patients 3 years of age and older. Also frequently used is a numerical rating scale or a visual analog scale response to a simple question such as: How much pain has your child had because of his or her rheumatic condition in the past week? Respondents are asked to provide an ordinal numerical rating on a scale of 0 to 10 where 0 is *no pain* and 10 is *very severe pain*. The Pediatric Quality of Life Inventory, a quality-of-life measure, includes a Pediatric Pain Questionnaire.[20–22]

The results of pain assessment in JIA should be interpreted with some caution. Several studies have demonstrated that patients with JIA have a lower pain tolerance or threshold than healthy children or their peers.[23] It is not uncommon for patients whose arthritis is in remission on medications to continue to report pain.[24] Because of the challenge posed by subjectivity for evaluating pain, a trend has developed toward evaluating pain interference with measures such as the Child Activity Limitations Interview-21.[25] Another is the National Institutes of Health Patient Reported Outcomes Measurement Information System (NIH PROMIS) pain interference measure. This measure ascertains the extent to which the experience of pain interfered with daily activities and tasks in the past week.[26] Providing this type of context around the experience of pain is thought to help clinicians and researchers interpret reports about pain as these measures are grounded in the functional role and impact on activity.

Functional Status

The assessment of functional ability and mobility is important for a condition like JIA, which can directly impact activities of daily living. The most widely used measure for assessing functional status in JIA is the Childhood Health Assessment Questionnaire (C-HAQ), which assesses functional health status for pediatric patients 1 to 19 years of age with a chronic rheumatic disease.[27] This measure was originally validated for patients with JIA in 1994.[27] The C-HAQ assesses disability in 8 domains, including dressing and grooming, arising, eating, walking, hygiene, reach, grip, and activities with respondents selecting the amount of difficulty the child may have with a particular task, with 0 being *without any difficulty* and 3 being *unable to do*. Although the C-HAQ is still commonly used in clinical studies and trials for assessing functional impairment in JIA, its utility has been questioned because of its significant ceiling

Table 1
Pediatric PRO measures for JIA

Domain	Measure	Number of Items	Ages of Administration: Self-Report	Ages of Administration: Parent-Proxy Report	Time Frame
Pain interference	Child Activity Limitations Interview-21[25]	21	8–18 y	8–18 y	Past month
	PROMIS Short Form v1.0 – Pain Interference 8a[26,46]	8	8–17 y	5–17 y	Past week
Pain intensity	Faces scales (eg, Faces Pain Scale-Revised[57])[58]	1	≥5 y	not applicable	Current
	Numeral rating scales[59]	1	≥8 y	Any	Varies
	PedsQL Pediatric Pain Questionnaire[20–22]	3	8–18 y	5–18 y	Past week, current
	VAS[60]	1	>7 y	Any	Varies
Quality of life	Child Health Questionnaire[61,62]	87 (self-report version), 28 or 50 (parent versions)	10–18 y	5–18 y	Varies by question
	Children's Assessment of Participation and Enjoyment[31,63]	55	6–21 y	not applicable	Past 4 mo
	Juvenile Arthritis Quality of Life Questionnaire[64]	74	>9 y	2–18 y	Past 2 wk
	PedsQL 4.0 Generic Core Scales[65–67]	21–23, depending on age	5–18 y	2–18 y	Past month
	PedsQL 3.0 Rheumatology Module[66]	14–22, depending on age	5–18 y	2–18 y	Past month (standard version), past week (acute version)
	Pediatric Rheumatology Quality of Life Scale[68,69]	10	7–18 y	2–18 y	Past month

Physical function or activity	Activities Scale for Kids[70]	30	5–15 y	not applicable	Past week
	C-HAQ[27,71,72]	30 (simplified version assessing disability without aids/devices and help items[73]) 2 (VAS of pain and overall well-being)	9–19 y	1–8 y	Past week
	Juvenile Arthritis Functional Assessment Report[72,74]	23	7–18 y	7–18 y	Past week
	Juvenile Arthritis Self-Report Index[72,75,76]	100	8–18 y	not applicable	Current
	Physical Activity Questionnaire[77,78]	9–10, depending on age	Grades 4–12 (approx 8–20 y)	not applicable	Past week
	Pediatric Outcomes Data Collection Instrument[79,80]	83–86, depending on age	11–18 y	2–18 y	Varies by question
	PROMIS Short Form v1.0 Physical Function (Upper Extremity and Mobility instruments)[26]	8	8–17 y	5–17 y	Current
Medication side effects	Gastrointestinal Symptom Scale for Kids[41]	9 (GI symptoms) 1 (VAS of symptom severity)	8–18 y	2–18 y	Past week
	Methotrexate Intolerance Severity Score questionnaire[42,81]	12 (modified version)	12–18 y	1–18 y	Past month

Abbreviations: approx, approximately; C-HAQ, Childhood Health Assessment Questionnaire; PedsQL, Pediatric Quality of Life; PROMIS, Patient Reported Outcomes Measurement Information System; VAS, visual analog scale.

effect, particularly for patients with well-controlled JIA. Revised versions of the C-HAQ have been developed with only modest improvement in the discriminative validity between patients with JIA with minimal disease activity and healthy controls.[28,29]

Other measures of functional ability used in JIA include the Juvenile Arthritis Functional Assessment Report (JAFAR), Juvenile Arthritis Self-Report Index, Physical Activity Questionnaire, NIH PROMIS Physical Function Instruments, Pediatric Outcomes Data Collection Instrument, and Activities Scale for Kids (see **Table 1**).[30] The Children's Assessment of Participation and Enjoyment has been used to assess participation in leisure activities among patients with JIA.[31]

Quality of Life

Health-related quality of life (HRQoL) is a multidimensional concept that generally includes the self-assessment of a person's physical and mental health. Children with JIA report poorer HRQoL than their healthy peers, with decreased HRQoL, even in the setting of low disease activity and treatment with biological agents.[32–34] The impact of JIA is not confined to childhood as longitudinal, observational cohorts have reported nearly one-half of children with JIA have recurrent or ongoing disease activity on entry into adulthood, with active arthritis, progressive joint destruction, and decreased quality of life.[33,35–38] Early intervention to improve HRQoL may lessen morbidity and during childhood, possibly increasing the odds of successful participation in age-appropriate activities (eg, school, independence from parents, employment) with compounding benefit over the life course.[39] Both JIA-specific and non–disease-specific measures have been used to assess quality of life among patients with JIA (see **Table 1**).

Medication Side Effects

Many patients with JIA require treatment with systemic medications, including nonsteroidal antiinflammatories, disease-modifying antirheumatic drugs, such as methotrexate, and biological therapies. Depending on the severity of the illness, the medication burden can be high, which can impact adherence to the treatment regimen, HRQoL, and disease outcomes.[40] The patients' and families' experience with medication administration and potential side effects may impact adherence. This point is particularly important to understand as it relates to comparative effectiveness studies when it needs to be determined if a group of patients are not responding optimally to a medication because of inadequate response versus intolerance. Using the self-administered Gastrointestinal Symptom Scale for Kids tool, Brunner and colleagues found that more than half of patients with JIA on second-line medications have gastrointestinal (GI) symptoms. When compared to clinically similar patients without GI symptoms, patients with GI symptoms had a lower HRQoL.[41] Methotrexate intolerance also occurs frequently among patients with JIA.[42] A validated questionnaire called the Methotrexate Intolerance Severity Score has been developed to assess this common clinical issue (see **Table 1**).[42]

Composite Patient-Reported Outcome Measures Specific to Juvenile Idiopathic Arthritis

Most PROs previously discussed are disease generic and have been used to measure outcomes across rheumatic diseases. In contrast, the Juvenile Arthritis Multidimensional Assessment Report (JAMAR) relies solely on parent or patient reports to assess PROs in JIA. The JAMAR includes 15 parent- or patient-reported measures/items that assess functional status (using the JAFAR); pain; HRQoL (using the Pediatric Rheumatology Quality of Life scale); well-being; joint symptoms, including stiffness, pain, and swelling; assessment of extra-articular symptoms (fever and rash); level of disease activity; rating of disease status (remission, continued activity, relapse); rating of disease course as compared with the prior visit; listing of medications; description of medication side effects; difficulties with medication administration; school problems related to JIA; and satisfaction with the illness outcome.[43] The JAMAR can be completed by parent-proxy report or by patient report for patients 7 to 18 years of age. In a study of 940 patients with JIA, the JAMAR was found to be feasible and to have face and content validity. Parent and patient reports were concordant, and the measure performed well across age group and JIA categories. Although the investigators could not identify any studies describing the use of the JAMAR in routine clinical settings, it is being studied in a novel multinational collaborative effort to study JIA outcomes.[44]

Use of the Patient Reported Outcomes Measurement Information System Pediatric Measures in Juvenile Idiopathic Arthritis

The recently developed NIH PROMIS pediatric measures include several psychosocial and behavioral domains with relevance across a range of chronic diseases and conditions.[45] Pediatric measures with item banks and scoring algorithms are available in formats suitable for paper or computer-assisted administration so that patients can enter PROs electronically. Importantly, the PROMIS measures capture a range of domains relevant to JIA, including measures that assess physical, mental, and social health.[46] Not all PROMIS measures have been validated for JIA; but the system is growing, and considerable attention continues to be paid to validation of new measures against clinical anchors (to establish responsiveness) and other similar measures (to establish convergent validity). Investment in standardization and validation of PRO measures and integration of high-quality item banks for clinical epidemiology and postmarketing surveillance enables both scientific rigor and patient voice/annotation.[5,6] The available PROMIS measures can be obtained at http://www.nihpromis.org/measures/availableinstruments.

Potential Challenges with Pediatric Patient-Reported Outcomes for Juvenile Idiopathic Arthritis

There are several potential challenges to using PROs for JIA. One of the challenges is that patients with JIA can be affected across a wide age range. For example, oligoarticular JIA, which is the most common subtype of JIA, has a peak age of onset in the toddler and preschool years. In contrast, rheumatoid factor positive polyarticular JIA has its peak incidence in adolescence. The use of various PRO measures in JIA may vary depending on patient age and development and the appropriateness of patient versus parent/proxy report measures.

Rheumatology providers also need to be aware that the explanatory power and levels of PROs vary across the categories of JIA. A recent study by Taxter and colleagues[47] demonstrated that patients with enthesitis-related arthritis (ERA) and undifferentiated JIA reported higher pain and poorer quality of life than patients with other types of JIA, including polyarticular rheumatoid factor positive JIA, which is similar to adult rheumatoid arthritis. Poorer physical function was reported among patients with polyarticular JIA, ERA, and undifferentiated JIA. The variability of PROs based on JIA categories suggests that even within JIA, no one size fits all.

Another potential issue is that patients' experience of their disease state and HRQoL may be quite different from the perceptions of external observers.[48] Hence, care is needed when collecting and interpreting PROs. Some measures, including select PROs developed under the NIH PROMIS, provide versions that are calibrated and validated for patient versus parent-proxy report. Although dyadic reports may track each other, they may differ with regard to intensity, severity, or clinical implications of a problem.[49] Pediatric patients may provide a more favorable evaluation of their well-being than their parents because of the inherent resilience and optimism represented in a child's point of view.[50] Conversely, parents' worry, anxiety, and burden of health care decision making may lead them to describe their child's well-being, including disease state, symptoms, and experience of medications, in worse terms than their child reports. For treating clinicians, this can be a confusing picture. Similarly, investigators undertaking longitudinal cohort research may need to consider the potential for subtle reporting bias due to a change in the respondent, as when a child starts self-reporting on a measure that heretofore had been completed by a parent. A related issue is that patients/families may attend to and prioritize aspects of their illness and treatment experiences differently than their clinicians. Discordance between parent/patient- and physician-reported ratings of functional ability, pain, and assessment of inactive disease in JIA have been well described, with the physician tending to have a more optimistic view of these measures than the patients or families.[51–53] At this point it is not clear how to address these potential issues of discordance.

PATIENT-REPORTED OUTCOMES FOR THE MANAGEMENT AND STUDY OF JUVENILE IDIOPATHIC ARTHRITIS

Clinicians who want to integrate PROs into practice, and researchers aiming to include PROs in cohort studies and clinical trials, may need to consider nuanced issues related to measurement focus, burden (length), periodicity, point of view (parent and/or child report), developmental relevance, and clinical validity. Although the field is still evolving, an emerging body of literature offers insight into these issues.

Use of Patient-Reported Outcomes in Clinical Care

As work to clinically validate PRO measures matures, opportunities are increasing to use PROs as part of the routine clinical care of patients with JIA. Clinical validity has not been established for all PROs, however. The development of more robust electronic health records (EHRs) should allow for increased utilization of PROs in the clinical setting and for making real-time decisions regarding patient response to treatments and interventions. Similarly, opportunities are growing to add the voice of the patients to clinically reported measures through mHealth (mobile health) tools and Web-enabled information technologies that may interoperate with EHRs or complement them.[54] Interestingly, Dijkstra and colleagues[55] recently described the use of patient-reported joint counts in JIA; there was only moderate correlation between patient- and physician-reported joint counts as patients with JIA tended to overestimate the number of active joints. The investigators suggest that based on these results, self-reported joint counts should not be used in lieu of clinical assessment.

Use of Patient-Reported Outcomes in Various Research Settings

In pediatric rheumatology, clinical treatment trials and comparative effectiveness research using observational cohorts are frequently used to study medication efficacy and safety. Because the voices of patients are largely missing in these data sources, key efficacy end points, including aspects of HRQoL, may not factor into clinical decision making and policy recommendations regarding treatments. For JIA, psychosocial stress, functional status, and even experience of problems/side effects from medications and adverse events, including those that decrease below the threshold for a typical health care encounter, may influence adherence and treatment outcomes. Hence, measuring these factors may greatly enhance the knowledge of treatment efficacy, safety, and disease progression.

PROs are also important in clinical research, particularly for assessing long-term outcomes when a patient may not be able to be seen in a clinical setting and the assessment relies on a patient report. An example is a study by Swarup and colleagues,[56] which examined implant survival and patient-reported outcomes after total hip arthroplasty (THA) in patients with JIA. The patients were assessed a mean of 12 years after hip replacement using a survey that included a patient-reported hip disability and osteoarthritis outcomes score (HOOS). In multivariate analysis, the HOOS scores were associated with important patient characteristics (such as implant type and history of a THA revision) and outcomes.

Although inclusion of patients' perspective regarding response to therapy and symptoms through measuring PROs has gained increasing recognition by clinicians and researchers who strive to understand treatment outcomes and the comparative effectiveness of therapies, researchers still need to choose among the broad range of available PROs to measure these factors. Choice will be governed by the treatment model being explored, time available to collect data from patients (which may require parsimony), and the reporting period for various measures. For example, intervening to address depression, anxiety, and coping skills that contribute to the experience of pain may require a somewhat long-term time horizon for assessing outcomes because changes in these factors may take time to manifest. In contrast, detection of change in pain interference or inflammation may take a relatively short time to investigate with regard to effects of medications.

SUMMARY

Significant momentum exists for adopting PRO measures within JIA clinical care and research. Use of these measures may help advance patients' experiences by ensuring that the voice and knowledge of the patient and parent proxy are incorporated into problem and progress appraisal and health care decision making. Including PROs in studies of comparative effectiveness can capture the acceptability and impacts of therapies from the patients' point of view and, thus, lead to more meaningful patient outcomes. Although progress has been made, much remains to be learned about PRO usage, particularly in the areas of interpretation and clinical response in JIA. Not all PROs have been clinically validated, and responsiveness of a given measure to treatment changes and shifts in disease course may not be established. The choice of measures can be confusing where multiple measures for assessing pain, quality of life, and other domains exist. Nuance, sensitivity, and consideration of the developmental status of patients are needed when choosing between patient and parent-proxy report and when mounting longitudinal studies in which a shift from parent proxy to patient report over the course of a study can confound observations and introduce reporting bias. Although the use of PROs is a relatively new phenomenon, considerable investment in high-quality validation work, including testing against known clinical anchors and in relation to gold standard measures, offers the potential for greatly advancing meaningful integration of patients' voices and experience within health care and research settings. This idea may be particularly on point for a chronic disease like JIA, whereby lifelong patient engagement, adherence, and shared decision making are prerequisites for favorable outcomes.

REFERENCES

1. Sacks JJ, Helmick CG, Luo YH, et al. Prevalence of and annual ambulatory health care visits for pediatric arthritis and other rheumatologic conditions in the United States in 2001-2004. Arthritis Rheum 2007;57(8):1439–45.
2. Wallace CA, Huang B, Bandeira M, et al. Patterns of clinical remission in select categories of juvenile idiopathic arthritis. Arthritis Rheum 2005;52(11):3554–62.
3. Ringold S, Seidel KD, Koepsell TD, et al. Inactive disease in polyarticular juvenile idiopathic arthritis: current patterns and associations. Rheumatology (Oxford) 2009;48(8):972–7.
4. Magni-Manzoni S, Pistorio A, Labò E, et al. A longitudinal analysis of physical functional disability over the course of juvenile idiopathic arthritis. Ann Rheum Dis 2008;67(8):1159–64.
5. Khanna D, Krishnan E, Dewitt EM, et al. The future of measuring patient-reported outcomes in rheumatology: patient-reported outcomes measurement information system (PROMIS). Arthritis Care Res (Hoboken) 2011;63(Suppl 11):S486–90.
6. DeWitt EM. Outcomes research in childhood autoimmune diseases. Rheum Dis Clin North Am 2013;39(4):921–33.
7. Luca NJ, Feldman BM. Health outcomes of pediatric rheumatic diseases. Best Pract Res Clin Rheumatol 2014;28(2):331–50.
8. Parkerson GR Jr, Harrell FE Jr, Hammond WE, et al. Characteristics of adult primary care patients as predictors of future health services charges. Med Care 2001;39(11):1170–81.
9. Seid M, Varni JW, Segall D, et al. Health-related quality of life as a predictor of pediatric healthcare costs: a two-year prospective cohort analysis. Health Qual Life Outcomes 2004;2:48.
10. Riley AW, Forrest CB, Rebok GW, et al. The child report form of the CHIP-child edition: reliability and validity. Med Care 2004;42(3):221–31.
11. Ananthakrishnan AN, Long MD, Martin CF, et al. Sleep disturbance and risk of active disease in patients with Crohn's disease and ulcerative colitis. Clin Gastroenterol Hepatol 2013;11(8):965–71.
12. Selby JV. The patient-centered outcomes research institute: a 2013 agenda for "research done differently". Popul Health Manag 2013;16(2):69–70.
13. Bevans KB, Riley AW, Moon J, et al. Conceptual and methodological advances in child-reported outcomes measurement. Expert Rev Pharmacoecon Outcomes Res 2010;10(4):385–96.
14. Petty RE, Southwood TR, Manners P, et al. International League of Associations for Rheumatology classification of juvenile idiopathic arthritis: second revision, Edmonton, 2001. J Rheumatol 2004;31(2):390–2.
15. Guzman J, Gómez-Ramírez O, Jurencak R, et al. What matters most for patients, parents, and clinicians in the course of juvenile idiopathic arthritis? A qualitative study. J Rheumatol 2014;41(11):2260–9.
16. Schanberg LE, Anthony KK, Gil KM, et al. Daily pain and symptoms in children with polyarticular arthritis. Arthritis Rheum 2003;48(5):1390–7.
17. Thastum M, Herlin T, Zachariae R. Relationship of pain-coping strategies and pain-specific beliefs to pain experience in children with juvenile idiopathic arthritis. Arthritis Rheum 2005;53(2):178–84.
18. Schanberg LE, Sandstrom MJ, Starr K, et al. The relationship of daily mood and stressful events to symptoms in juvenile rheumatic disease. Arthritis Care Res 2000;13(1):33–41.

19. Schanberg LE, Gil KM, Anthony KK, et al. Pain, stiffness, and fatigue in juvenile polyarticular arthritis: contemporaneous stressful events and mood as predictors. Arthritis Rheum 2005;52(4):1196–204.
20. Gragg RA, Rapoff MA, Danovsky MB, et al. Assessing chronic musculoskeletal pain associated with rheumatic disease: further validation of the pediatric pain questionnaire. J Pediatr Psychol 1996;21(2):237–50.
21. Thompson KL, Varni JW, Hanson V. Comprehensive assessment of pain in juvenile rheumatoid arthritis: an empirical model. J Pediatr Psychol 1987;12(2):241–55.
22. Varni JW, Thompson KL, Hanson V. The Varni/Thompson pediatric pain questionnaire. I. Chronic musculoskeletal pain in juvenile rheumatoid arthritis. Pain 1987; 28(1):27–38.
23. Thastum M, Zachariae R, Herlin T. Pain experience and pain coping strategies in children with juvenile idiopathic arthritis. J Rheumatol 2001;28(5):1091–8.
24. Lomholt JJ, Thastum M, Herlin T. Pain experience in children with juvenile idiopathic arthritis treated with anti-TNF agents compared to non-biologic standard treatment. Pediatr Rheumatol Online J 2013;11(1):21.
25. Palermo TM, Lewandowski AS, Long AC, et al. Validation of a self-report questionnaire version of the child activity limitations interview (CALI): the CALI-21. Pain 2008;139(3):644–52.
26. Kashikar-Zuck S, Carle A, Barnett K, et al. Longitudinal evaluation of patient-reported outcomes measurement information systems (PROMIS) measures in pediatric chronic pain. Pain 2016;157:339–47.
27. Singh G, Athreya BH, Fries JF, et al. Measurement of health status in children with juvenile rheumatoid arthritis. Arthritis Rheum 1994;37(12):1761–9.
28. Groen W, Ünal E, Nørgaard M, et al. Comparing different revisions of the childhood health assessment questionnaire to reduce the ceiling effect and improve score distribution: data from a multi-center European cohort study of children with JIA. Pediatr Rheumatol Online J 2010;8:16.
29. Nørgaard M, Thastum M, Herlin T. The relevance of using the Childhood Health Assessment Questionnaire (CHAQ) in revised versions for the assessment of juvenile idiopathic arthritis. Scand J Rheumatol 2013;42(6):457–64.
30. Klepper SE. Measures of pediatric function: Child Health Assessment Questionnaire (C-HAQ), Juvenile Arthritis Functional Assessment Scale (JAFAS), Pediatric Outcomes Data Collection Instrument (PODCI), and Activities Scale for Kids (ASK). Arthritis Care Res (Hoboken) 2011;63(Suppl 11):S371–82.
31. Cavallo S, Majnemer A, Duffy CM, et al. Participation in leisure activities by children and adolescents with juvenile idiopathic arthritis. J Rheumatol 2015; 42(9):1708–15.
32. Gutierrez-Suarez R, Pistorio A, Cespedes Cruz A, et al. Health-related quality of life of patients with juvenile idiopathic arthritis coming from 3 different geographic areas. The PRINTO multinational quality of life cohort study. Rheumatology (Oxford) 2007;46(2):314–20.
33. Seid M, Opipari L, Huang B, et al. Disease control and health-related quality of life in juvenile idiopathic arthritis. Arthritis Rheum 2009;61(3):393–9.
34. Haverman L, Grootenhuis MA, van den Berg JM, et al. Predictors of health-related quality of life in children and adolescents with juvenile idiopathic arthritis: results from a web-based survey. Arthritis Care Res (Hoboken) 2012;64(5): 694–703.
35. Minden K, Niewerth M, Listing J, et al. Long-term outcome in patients with juvenile idiopathic arthritis. Arthritis Rheum 2002;46(9):2392–401.

36. Oen K, Malleson PN, Cabral DA, et al. Disease course and outcome of juvenile rheumatoid arthritis in a multicenter cohort. J Rheumatol 2002;29(9):1989–99.
37. Packham JC, Hall MA, Pimm TJ. Long-term follow-up of 246 adults with juvenile idiopathic arthritis: predictive factors for mood and pain. Rheumatology (Oxford) 2002;41(12):1444–9.
38. Zak M, Pedersen FK. Juvenile chronic arthritis into adulthood: a long-term follow-up study. Rheumatology (Oxford) 2000;39(2):198–204.
39. Fuchs CE, Van Geelen SM, Hermans HJ, et al. Psychological intervention for adolescents with juvenile idiopathic arthritis: for whom and when? J Rheumatol 2013;40(4):528–34.
40. Bugni VM, Ozaki LS, Okamoto KY, et al. Factors associated with adherence to treatment in children and adolescents with chronic rheumatic diseases. J Pediatr (Rio J) 2012;88(6):483–8.
41. Brunner HI, Johnson AL, Barron AC, et al. Gastrointestinal symptoms and their association with health-related quality of life of children with juvenile rheumatoid arthritis: validation of a gastrointestinal symptom questionnaire. J Clin Rheumatol 2005;11(4):194–204.
42. Bulatovic M, Heijstek MW, Verkaaik M, et al. High prevalence of methotrexate intolerance in juvenile idiopathic arthritis: development and validation of a methotrexate intolerance severity score. Arthritis Rheum 2011;63(7):2007–13.
43. Filocamo G, Consolaro A, Schiappapietra B, et al. A new approach to clinical care of juvenile idiopathic arthritis: the juvenile arthritis multidimensional assessment report. J Rheumatol 2011;38(5):938–53.
44. Consolaro A, Ruperto N, Filocamo G, et al. Seeking insights into the epidemiology, treatment and outcome of childhood arthritis through a multinational collaborative effort: introduction of the EPOCA study. Pediatr Rheumatol Online J 2012;10(1):39.
45. DeWalt DA, Gross HE, Gipson DS, et al. PROMIS((R)) pediatric self-report scales distinguish subgroups of children within and across six common pediatric chronic health conditions. Qual Life Res 2015;24(9):2195–208.
46. Jacobson CJ, Farrell JE, Kashikar-Zuck S, et al. Disclosure and self-report of emotional, social, and physical health in children and adolescents with chronic pain–a qualitative study of PROMIS pediatric measures. J Pediatr Psychol 2013;38(1):82–93.
47. Taxter AJ, Wileyto EP, Behrens EM, et al. Patient-reported outcomes across categories of juvenile idiopathic arthritis. J Rheumatol 2015;42(10):1914–21.
48. Eiser C, Morse R. A review of measures of quality of life for children with chronic illness. Arch Dis Child 2001;84(3):205–11.
49. Vetter TR, Bridgewater CL, McGwin G Jr. An observational study of patient versus parental perceptions of health-related quality of life in children and adolescents with a chronic pain condition: who should the clinician believe? Health Qual Life Outcomes 2012;10:85.
50. Ravelli A, Viola S, Migliavacca D, et al. Discordance between proxy-reported and observed assessment of functional ability of children with juvenile idiopathic arthritis. Rheumatology (Oxford) 2001;40(8):914–9.
51. Consolaro A, Vitale R, Pistorio A, et al. Physicians' and parents' ratings of inactive disease are frequently discordant in juvenile idiopathic arthritis. J Rheumatol 2007;34(8):1773–6.
52. Garcia-Munitis P, Bandeira M, Pistorio A, et al. Level of agreement between children, parents, and physicians in rating pain intensity in juvenile idiopathic arthritis. Arthritis Rheum 2006;55(2):177–83.

53. Palmisani E, Solari N, Pistorio A, et al. Agreement between physicians and parents in rating functional ability of children with juvenile idiopathic arthritis. Pediatr Rheumatol Online J 2007;5:23.
54. Padrez KA, Ungar L, Schwartz HA, et al. Linking social media and medical record data: a study of adults presenting to an academic, urban emergency department. BMJ Qual Saf 2015. [Epub ahead of print].
55. Dijkstra ME, Anink J, van Pelt PA, et al. Patient-reported joint count in juvenile idiopathic arthritis: the reliability of a manikin format. J Rheumatol 2015;42(3):527–33.
56. Swarup I, Lee YY, Christoph EI, et al. Implant survival and patient-reported outcomes after total hip arthroplasty in young patients with juvenile idiopathic arthritis. J Arthroplasty 2015;30(3):398–402.
57. Hicks CL, von Baeyer CL, Spafford PA, et al. The faces pain scale-revised: toward a common metric in pediatric pain measurement. Pain 2001;93(2): 173–83.
58. Tomlinson D, von Baeyer CL, Stinson JN, et al. A systematic review of faces scales for the self-report of pain intensity in children. Pediatrics 2010;126(5): e1168–98.
59. Ruskin D, Lalloo C, Amaria K, et al. Assessing pain intensity in children with chronic pain: convergent and discriminant validity of the 0 to 10 numerical rating scale in clinical practice. Pain Res Manag 2014;19(3):141–8.
60. Shields BJ, Cohen DM, Harbeck-Weber C, et al. Pediatric pain measurement using a visual analogue scale: a comparison of two teaching methods. Clin Pediatr (Phila) 2003;42(3):227–34.
61. Selvaag AM, Flatø B, Lien G, et al. Measuring health status in early juvenile idiopathic arthritis: determinants and responsiveness of the child health questionnaire. J Rheumatol 2003;30(7):1602–10.
62. Oliveira S, Ravelli A, Pistorio A, et al. Proxy-reported health-related quality of life of patients with juvenile idiopathic arthritis: the pediatric rheumatology international trials organization multinational quality of life cohort study. Arthritis Rheum 2007;57(1):35–43.
63. King GA, Law M, King S, et al. Measuring children's participation in recreation and leisure activities: construct validation of the CAPE and PAC. Child Care Health Dev 2007;33(1):28–39.
64. Duffy CM, Arsenault L, Duffy KN, et al. The juvenile arthritis quality of life questionnaire–development of a new responsive index for juvenile rheumatoid arthritis and juvenile spondyloarthritides. J Rheumatol 1997;24(4):738–46.
65. Varni JW, Seid M, Kurtin PS. PedsQL 4.0: reliability and validity of the pediatric quality of life inventory version 4.0 generic core scales in healthy and patient populations. Med Care 2001;39(8):800–12.
66. Varni JW, Seid M, Smith Knight T, et al. The PedsQL in pediatric rheumatology: reliability, validity, and responsiveness of the pediatric quality of life inventory generic core scales and rheumatology module. Arthritis Rheum 2002;46(3): 714–25.
67. Varni JW, Burwinkle TM, Seid M, et al. The PedsQL 4.0 as a pediatric population health measure: feasibility, reliability, and validity. Ambul Pediatr 2003;3(6): 329–41.
68. Weiss PF, Klink AJ, Faerber J, et al. The pediatric rheumatology quality of life scale: validation of the English version in a US cohort of juvenile idiopathic arthritis. Pediatr Rheumatol Online J 2013;11(1):43.

69. Filocamo G, Schiappapietra B, Bertamino M, et al. A new short and simple health-related quality of life measurement for paediatric rheumatic diseases: initial validation in juvenile idiopathic arthritis. Rheumatology (Oxford) 2010;49(7):1272–80.
70. Young NL, Williams JI, Yoshida KK, et al. Measurement properties of the activities scale for kids. J Clin Epidemiol 2000;53(2):125–37.
71. Pouchot J, Ecosse E, Coste J, et al. Validity of the childhood health assessment questionnaire is independent of age in juvenile idiopathic arthritis. Arthritis Rheum 2004;51(4):519–26.
72. Brown GT, Wright FV, Lang BA, et al. Clinical responsiveness of self-report functional assessment measures for children with juvenile idiopathic arthritis undergoing intraarticular corticosteroid injections. Arthritis Rheum 2005;53(6):897–904.
73. Saad-Magalhães C, Pistorio A, Ravelli A, et al. Does removal of aids/devices and help make a difference in the childhood health assessment questionnaire disability index? Ann Rheum Dis 2010;69(1):82–7.
74. Howe S, Levinson J, Shear E, et al. Development of a disability measurement tool for juvenile rheumatoid arthritis. The Juvenile Arthritis Functional Assessment Report for Children and Their Parents. Arthritis Rheum 1991;34(7):873–80.
75. Wright FV, Kimber JL, Law M, et al. The Juvenile Arthritis Functional Status Index (JASI): a validation study. J Rheumatol 1996;23(6):1066–79.
76. Wright FV, Law M, Crombie V, et al. Development of a self-report functional status index for juvenile rheumatoid arthritis. J Rheumatol 1994;21(3):536–44.
77. Biddle S, Gorely T, Pearson N, et al. An assessment of self-reported physical activity instruments in young people for population surveillance: project ALPHA. Int J Behav Nutr Phys Act 2011;8(1):1.
78. Crocker PR, Bailey DA, Faulkner RA, et al. Measuring general levels of physical activity: preliminary evidence for the physical activity questionnaire for older children. Med Sci Sports Exerc 1997;29(10):1344–9.
79. Misterska E, Adamczak K, Kaminiarczyk-Pyzałka D, et al. The Pediatric Outcomes Data Collection instrument for Polish sample with juvenile idiopathic arthritis: psychometric properties of proxy version. Int J Rheum Dis 2015. [Epub ahead of print].
80. Daltroy LH, Liang MH, Fossel AH, et al. The POSNA pediatric musculoskeletal functional health questionnaire: report on reliability, validity, and sensitivity to change. Pediatric Outcomes Instrument Development Group. Pediatric Orthopaedic Society of North America. J Pediatr Orthop 1998;18(5):561–71.
81. van Dijkhuizen EH, Bulatović Ćalasan M, Pluijm SM, et al. Prediction of methotrexate intolerance in juvenile idiopathic arthritis: a prospective, observational cohort study. Pediatr Rheumatol Online J 2015;13:5.

The Challenge and Opportunity of Capturing Patient Reported Measures of Rheumatoid Arthritis Disease Activity in Vulnerable Populations with Limited Health Literacy and Limited English Proficiency

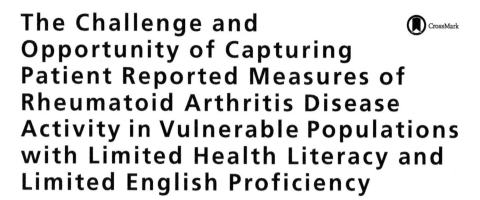

Joel M. Hirsh, MD

KEYWORDS

- Patient-reported outcome measures
- RA patient global assessment of disease activity • Rheumatoid arthritis
- Health outcomes • Limited health literacy • Limited English proficiency

KEY POINTS

- Limited health literacy (LHL) and limited English proficiency (LEP) are widely prevalent and contribute to rheumatoid arthritis (RA) health care disparities.
- The RA Patient Global Assessment of Disease Activity often introduces complexity to the health care encounters of patients and research subjects with LHL and LEP.
- Important work is being done to ensure that patient-reported outcome measures (PROM) are validated and appropriate for diverse and vulnerable populations.

INTRODUCTION

Earlier, more aggressive, and more effective treatments of rheumatoid arthritis (RA) have made remission a realistic target and have greatly improved outcomes compared with past decades.[1,2] Unfortunately, the therapeutic benefits of the biologic era have not been experienced equally by all patients. There is abundant evidence of ongoing racial and ethnic disparities in RA outcomes in both the United States and abroad (**Box 1**).[3]

Disclosures: None.

Division of Rheumatology, Department of Medicine, Denver Health, University of Colorado Denver School of Medicine, 777 Bannock Street, Mail Code 4000, Denver, CO 80204, USA
E-mail address: joel.hirshMD@dhha.org

Rheum Dis Clin N Am 42 (2016) 347–362
http://dx.doi.org/10.1016/j.rdc.2016.01.006 **rheumatic.theclinics.com**
0889-857X/16/$ – see front matter

Box 1
Care disparities in rheumatoid arthritis

- United States
  - More disability and worse global health among non-whites compared with whites[11]
  - Higher disease activity and worse functional status in non-whites, non-anglophones, and foreign born[12]
  - Men, non-whites, and persons of lower socioeconomic status are less likely to receive a disease modifying anti-rheumatic drug (DMARD)[13]
  - DMARD therapy is often delayed in ethnic minorities[14]
  - Income and ethnicity impact use of biologic therapies[15]
- Europe
  - Higher hospitalization rates for RA patients with lower socioeconomic status and manual labor employment[16]
  - Worse functional status in patients from deprived socioeconomic areas[17]
  - Negative association between disease activity and gross domestic product per capita[18]
  - Women are less likely to achieve remission[19]
- Latin America
  - Low socioeconomic status is related to high disease activity in early RA[20]

The widely accepted "treat-to-target" paradigm of RA management guided to remission or low disease activity mandates low scores along a visual analog scale (VAS) on one patient-reported outcome (PRO), the Patient Global Assessment of Disease Activity (PtGA-VAS).[4,5] PtGA-VAS scores are often discrepant with evaluator assessments of disease activity and may alone prevent patients from being classified in remission.[6–10] Vulnerable RA patients (defined as elderly, members of racial/ethnic minorities, those with limited health literacy, or non-English speakers) often have difficulty completing the PtGA-VAS. These same RA patients are at the complex intersection of being at risk for health care disparities and having their providers follow guidelines to treat them to a target of low disease activity or remission.

Limited health literacy (LHL) and limited English proficiency (LEP) are variables that may, in part, explain disparities in RA care. This article introduces the reader to these concepts and then reviews the research, which links LEP and LHL to outcomes in RA. The proposed causal pathways responsible for these associations will then be covered, followed by a discussion of the challenges vulnerable populations face completing PROs using the PtGA-VAS as an example. The article concludes with strategies to improve the PtGA-VAS and reduce complexity in the health care system for all patients.

LIMITED ENGLISH PROFICIENCY

Rheumatologists often encounter RA patients with LEP because more than 60 million US residents speak a language other English at home.[21] LEP is defined based on responses to the US Census and American Community Survey question, "How well do you speak English?" (**Box 2**). Persons that report "very well" are considered English proficient. Persons that report "well," "not well," or "not at all" are considered to have LEP.[21,22] Twenty-five million Americans were self-classified as LEP in the 2011 American Community Survey.[21]

Some of the challenges caring for patients with LEP may be avoidable through the use of professional interpreters as recommended by the Institute of Medicine as a quality and patient safety imperative.[23] Unfortunately, providers often eschew using professional interpreters and opt to "get by" rather than "get help" when caring for

Box 2
Questions on language from the 2011 American Community Survey

a. Does this person speak a language other than English at home?

b. What is that language?

____

c. How well does this person speak English?
- Very well
- Well
- Not well
- Not well at all

From Ryan C. Language use in the United States: 2011 American community survey reports. United States Cesus Bureau and Department of Commerce; 2013. Ref Type: Pamphlet.

patients with LEP.[24] A recent retrospective review in a well-resourced academic hospital showed that 66% of LEP patients never had documentation of interpreter use during their hospital stay.[25]

LEP has been shown to be a risk factor for suboptimal care in a myriad of nonrheumatologic diseases by disrupting the entire continuum of care. Accessing care is the first hurdle facing LEP patients. Insured patients with LEP make less use of preventive services and experiences suboptimal primary care access compared with patients without language barriers.[26,27] LEP patients are less likely to understand the diagnosis and treatment of their medical condition.[28] LEP patients are also less adherent to medications and less satisfied with the medical care they receive.[29,30] The impact of LEP has not been widely studied in RA, but there is emerging evidence to support plausible pathways by which it may promote deleterious RA outcomes (**Box 3**).

Box 3
Studies regarding associations of limited English proficiency in rheumatoid arthritis patients

- Suboptimal shared decision-making[31]
- Poor knowledge about Methotrexate[32]

LIMITED HEALTH LITERACY

Health literacy (HL) has been defined as "the degree to which individuals can obtain, process, and understand the basic health information and services they need to make appropriate health decisions."[33] A more nuanced conceptualization of HL not only focuses on the patient's skills but also takes into account the demand side of the equation and the complexity of the health care system.[34] Much like LEP, LHL is widely prevalent. Nearly one-half of the adults in the United States have limited HL, and low HL is more prevalent among the elderly and ethnic minorities.[35]

HL status is assessed in research studies using performance-based and self-reported measures (**Box 4**).[36] The Short Test of Functional Health in Adults (s-TOFHLA) is a 7-minute, 14-point-font cloze procedure, whereby words are deleted from 2 passages about medical subjects and respondents attempt to select the correct missing word.[37] Performance-based testing of patients in the clinical setting is not recommended because of the possibility of shaming or embarrassing patients with LHL.[38] There are several versions of Single-Item Literacy Screening (SILS) questions, which ask patients to self-rate their HL. Responses of sometimes, often, or always to

Box 4
Sample questions from Health Literacy Assessment Instruments

- Short Test of Functional Health in Adults (S-TOFHLA)

The x-ray will ____________ from 1-3 ___________ to do.

a. take	a. beds
b. view	b. brains
c. talk	c. hours
d. look	d. diets

- Single-Item Literacy Screening (SILS) questions

How often do you need to have someone help you when you read instructions, pamphlets, or other written material from your doctor or pharmacy?[40]
- ○ Never
- ○ Rarely
- ○ Sometimes
- ○ Often
- ○ Always

How confident are you filling out medical forms by yourself?
- ○ Not at all
- ○ A little bit
- ○ Somewhat
- ○ Quite a bit
- ○ Extremely

Adapted from Nurss JR, Parker R, Williams M, et al. TOFHLA: Test of functional health literacy in adults. Snow Camp, NC: Peppercorn Books, 2001; with permission; and Morris NS, MacLean CD, Chew LD, et al. The single item literacy screener: evaluation of a brief instrument to identify limited reading ability. BMC Fam Pract 2006;7:21.

the first SILS question in **Box 4** are classified as LHL. Responses of not at all, a little bit, or somewhat to the second SILS question in **Box 4** are classified as LHL. Most assessments of HL are limited to functional literacy and numeracy, but do not assess more complex aspects of HL, such as cognition, social skills, verbal fluency, proactive oral communication, and aural literacy.[39]

The emerging field of HL-related rheumatology research has clarified the HL skills of patients, the high literacy burden of written patient educational material, and the negative outcomes associated with LHL.[41] LHL has been associated with poor health outcomes in several RA studies (**Box 5**). Of note, research at Denver Health and with the National Data Bank for Rheumatic Diseases has shown a strong relationship between LHL as assessed by the SILS and RA functional status measured by the Multidimensional Health Assessment questionnaire and Health Assessment Questionnaire, respectively.[42,43] The latter study included more than 6,000 RA subjects and demonstrated that LHL was more strongly associated with poor functional status than

Box 5
Outcomes and associations of limited health literacy in rheumatoid arthritis patients

- Worse functional status[42]
- Increased pain and physical limitations[44]

prednisone use, smoking history, and biologic agent use. This relationship persisted even after modeling educational attainment.[41]

CAUSAL PATHWAYS LINKING LIMITED ENGLISH PROFICIENCY AND LIMITED HEALTH LITERACY WITH OUTCOMES

There are several causal pathways by which LHL might influence patient outcomes: access and utilization of health care, patient-provider interaction, and self-care (**Fig. 1**).[45] The importance of accessing care quickly and adroitly navigating the health care system is of great importance in RA given the wealth of data regarding the importance of timely diagnosis and early aggressive treatment of RA.[46] Patients with LHL have been shown to delay seeking care and have difficulty with access in nonarthritic diseases.[47] Delays in obtaining RA care may explain the research findings, showing preserved disease activity scores, but worse functional status presumably stemming from disease damage accumulated early in the disease course. The RA research linking LHL with the causal pathways of adverse health outcomes is illustrated in **Box 6**.

System factors include the complexity of the process of receiving care and how this can influence the access and utilization of health care. Patients with LHL have difficulty completing forms and paperwork. The challenges that PROs present will be covered in great detail in the next section. At one US urban rheumatology clinic, it has been shown that nearly 1 in 3 patients responded to one of the SILS questions, indicating that they do not feel confident filling out medical forms without help.[43,48]

Poor communication between providers and patients is another mechanism by which LHL likely impacts RA outcomes. Patients with LHL and RA may be less

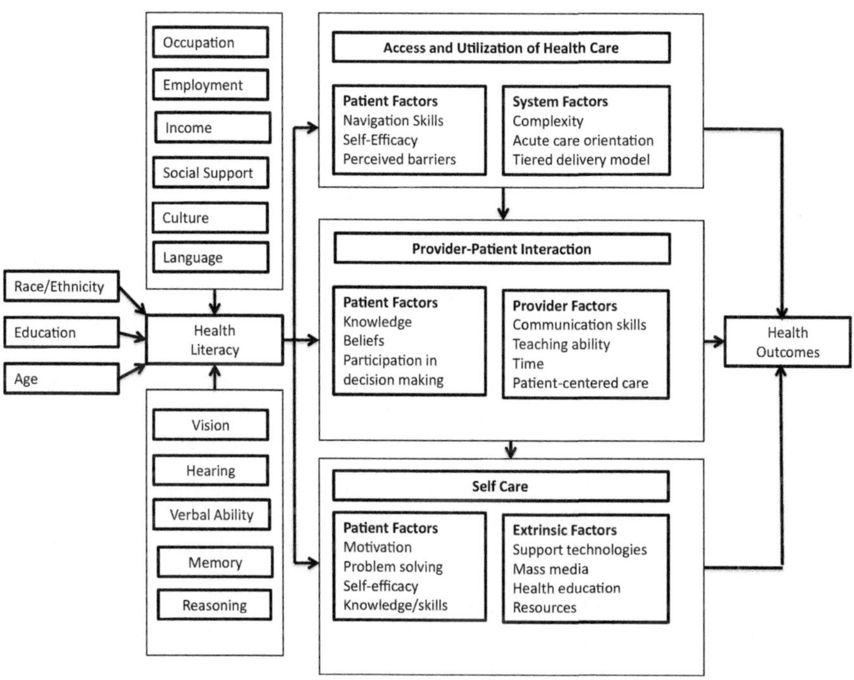

Fig. 1. Causal pathways linking LEP and limited HL with outcomes. (*From* Paasche-Orlow MK, Wolf MS. The causal pathways linking health literacy to health outcomes. Am J Health Behav 2007;31(Suppl 1):S21; with permission.)

Box 6
Support of limited health literacy's causal pathways in rheumatoid arthritis

- Suboptimal shared decision-making[31]
- Poor understanding of written prescribing instructions regarding rheumatology medication use[55]
- Less likely to access their electronic medical records via a Web portal[49]
- Less knowledge about rheumatology medications[56]
- Lower medication adherence[42]
- Higher risk perception and less willingness to take a DMARD[54]
- Discrepancy between patient and provider global assessments of RA activity[7]
- Increased anxiety[53]
- Self-reported difficulty completing forms[43]
- Self-reported difficulty understanding written instructions from doctors and pharmacists[42]

prepared for visits than patients with adequate HL, given research documenting that LHL RA patients are less likely to log-on and view the electronic medical records via a Web portal.[49] Limited verbal fluency and proactive oral communication have been demonstrated in other chronic diseases.[47,50–52] LHL RA patients' increased anxiety[53] and lower knowledge about RA and its treatment also interfered with optimal patient-provider interaction. In addition, patients with LHL and RA have higher risk perception and less willingness to take a disease-modifying antirheumatic drug (DMARD) than patients with adequate HL.[54] LHL is strongly associated with suboptimal shared decision-making in patients with RA.[31] The author's research at Denver Health has demonstrated that LHL is associated with the discrepancy between patient and provider global assessments of RA activity.[7]

Self-care is another causal pathway by which LHL can influence adverse health outcomes. Self-management requires both knowledge and the capacity to carry out the plan decided on with the provider. RA patients with LHL have poor understanding of written prescribing instructions regarding rheumatology medication use.[55] LHL as measured by one of the SILS questions has also been associated with lower medication adherence in RA.[42] Little is known in RA regarding the role of problem-solving skills and self-efficacy in mediating poor outcomes in RA patients.

THE CHALLENGES OF OBTAINING PATIENT-REPORTED OUTCOMES IN PATIENTS WITH LIMITED ENGLISH PROFICIENCY AND LIMITED HEALTH LITERACY—THE PATIENT GLOBAL ASSESSMENT OF DISEASE ACTIVITY–VISUAL ANALOGUE SCALE

The RA PtGA-VAS is a salient example of the great challenge PROs can pose to patients with LHL.[57] The PtGA has a complicated history that is necessary to review before a discussion of the complexity it introduces to the health care encounters for patients with LHL and LEP. The PtGA-VAS plays a major role in RA clinical practice and research trials.[8] Current disease management recommendations from the American College of Rheumatology (ACR) and European League Against Rheumatism (EULAR) recommend either low disease activity or remission as acceptable management goals—both mandate a low PtGA-VAS score (**Box 7**). The target of remission by the stricter ACR/EULAR or Simplified Disease Activity Index (SDAI) criteria has become preferred as data showing that radiographic progression can continue unabated in patients in remission by the less strict Disease Activity score in 28 joints (DAS28) remission criteria.[58]

Booleen-based Definition

In order to fulfill the Booleen-based definition, a patient must satisfy all of the following: tender joint count (TJC) $\leq$1, swollen joint count (SJC) $\leq$1, C-reactive protein (CRP) $\leq$1 mg/dL, and PtGA-VAS $\leq$1 (on a 1–10 scale).

Index-based Definition

In order to fulfill the index-based definition, a patient must satisfy all of the following: SDAI score of $\leq$3.3 (SDAI = TJC [0–28] + SJC [0–28] + PtGA-VAS [0–10] + physician global assessment [0–10] + CRP in mg/dL).

This present prominent position of the PtGA-VAS is surprising given its somewhat obscure and opaque origins.[59] Original publications regarding composite RA disease activity indices did not solicit patient input, or specify the question's wording, time-frame queried, or the content of the double anchors bracketing the VAS line.[60] Although no guidance was offered regarding standardized language for explaining to patients what exact domains the PtGA is intended to capture, the authors of the ACR/EULAR remission criteria did attempt to alleviate some of this confusion by defining standard language and format for the question:

> *Format: a horizontal 10-cm visual analog or Likert scale with the best anchor and lowest score on the left side and the worst anchor and highest score on the right side. Wording of the question and anchors: For patient global assessment, 'considering all the ways your arthritis has affected you, how do you feel your arthritis is today?' (anchors: very well-very poor)*[5]

The PtGA-VAS is highly complex and confusing to patients with LHL. Research at Denver Health has demonstrated that nearly 1 in 4 subjects had missing or noninterpretable PtGA-VAS responses.[57] This finding mirrors other studies that have shown missing VAS data in RA patients with LEP.[61] Writing along the VAS line or circling an anchor were examples of responses that could not be scored. In multivariate regression that included education, LHL as defined by the S-TOFHLA was independently associated with missing and noninterpretable PtGA-VAS responses.[57] There are many aspects of the PtGA-VAS that may engender confusion: its high literacy burden and wording, the scope of the question, high numeracy burdens, and anchors.

The various versions of the PtGA-VAS demand a high level of literacy for comprehension. The Gunning Fog Index of the reading grade level required for comprehension of 2 versions of the PtGA-VAS were 11.47 and 14.06.[7] This is consistent with research showing that high literacy levels are required to complete many other frequently used rheumatology PROs.[62] In addition to the information discussed regarding the high prevalence of LHL, it is worth noting that 15 of the 337 subjects that were screened for a recent RA HL study at Denver Health were excluded because of complete functional illiteracy.[57]

The wording of the various PtGA-VAS versions may also be a source of confusion. The "Disease activity" version of the PtGA-VAS asks patients, "How active has your disease been this week?"[60] RA patients likely understand better than their providers the conceptualization of RA as an entity that has different levels of severity that wax and wane. The term "activity" is problematic, however, because the patient may confuse the query and its anchors, "not active at all" and "extremely active" to be assessing the level of physical activity that their RA allows. The Arthritis Impact

Measurement Scales version of the PtGA-VAS recommended by the ACR asks the patient to consider all of the ways that arthritis has affected them in the past, but then makes the surprising and perhaps confusing request for the patient to be the mouthpiece of their adversary and respond regarding how the *arthritis* is today. It is also interesting that the patient is asked to report her disease activity in the context of past experience. For example, a patient with a history of very severe disease that was under poor control might say that having 6 rather than 20 swollen joints is close to the anchor of very well if interpreting the question in a strictly literal fashion.

Patients are also unsure which dimensions of RA the PtGA-VAS is intended to capture.[63] This uncertainty is reflected by the fact that the PtGA-VAS is highly influenced by factors other than inflammatory pain and as such is often a barrier to remission. Pain, functional disability, depression, and fibromyalgia have all been associated with higher patient PtGA-VAS rankings.[64,65] Pain in particular can be a driver of elevated PtGA-VAS scores in non-white patients.[66] Patient confusion regarding the domains queried by the PtGA-VAS was reflected in the poor correlation between the PtGA and the discriminant function score in the initial study validating the disease activity score.[67] The crafters of the DAS formula recognized the limitations of the PtGA-VAS and devised a formula that gave minimal weight to the PtGA-VAS. The maximum contribution of the PtGA-VAS to the DAS is 1.4, which in contradistinction to more recent remission criteria would allow a patient to be classified in remission if the SJC, TJC, and evaluator global assessment (EGA) are low. The low profile of the PtGA-VAS in the DAS is consistent with its role in the ACR 20/50/70 criteria because these criteria allow for a classification of improved disease control even if the PtGA-VAS is unchanged.[68] Given these extraneous influences on the PtGA-VAS and ambiguity regarding what the PGA is measuring, it is not surprising that a wealth of research has shown that the PtGA-VAS is often the sole variable that keeps patients' RA from being classified in a state of remission using the newer criteria.[9,10,69]

Temporal confusion is another potential issue for patients with LHL and LEP. The patient is asked to "consider all the ways arthritis has affected you." This question can easily be interpreted to recall disappointments in the even distant past regarding RA's negative impact on parenting, employment, relationships, and recreational opportunities. These issues might not be resolved *today* even if the patient is experiencing less joint swelling.

The PtGA-VAS' high numeracy demands also increase the complexity of the health care encounter for LHL and LEP patients. Patients are responsible for mapping their PtGA score onto the line somewhere between 0 and 10. This request seems straightforward to health care professionals familiar with such instruments, but less literate and numerate persons encountering it may have questions.[70] Is the scale linear or logarithmic? Logarithmic conceptualization of number scales is more common in younger persons and in cultures with less access to education.[71] Difficulty with numerical concepts is not limited to developing countries: more than 50% of US residents have basic or no quantitative numeracy skills.[34] Innumerate patients have difficulty understanding self-administered written tools.[72] The validity of VAS scales in patients with lower levels of educational attainment has been questioned because their VAS scores concentrate in the middle of the scale.[73] An additional challenge with response to the far left and far right of the scale is inverse interpretation of the VAS.[74] Although the double anchors are intended to cue patients that zero is very well and 100 equates with very poor, this is a counterintuitive concept in Western societies, and the PtGA-VAS is often completed incorrectly in an inverse fashion.[74]

There are many potential negative consequences of the complexity that the PtGA-VAS introduces to the rheumatology visit for patients with LEP or LHL. Patients with limited literacy and HL skills frequently experience shame and embarrassment when literacy-related stumbling blocks are placed in their way[38]; this is not how patients should begin their visits. The information presented above makes clear that the PtGA-VAS often fails to capture or captures inaccurately the perspective of some of the most vulnerable patients. The PtGA-VAS also can introduce dissatisfaction or confusion to an encounter. If proper communication does not occur, a patient with no swollen joints who marks their PtGA-VAS at 8 cm due to low back pain might be confused and frustrated that this score does not result in a change in their RA management. It is likely that rheumatologists base their therapeutic decisions on more objective measures such as the SJC and inflammatory indices, but overtreatment is possible with strict adherence to treat-to-target strategies. Rheumatologists who care for high proportions of LHL and LEP patients may also be inappropriately penalized for not meeting RA national quality measures for failing to assess disease activity.[75]

HOW CAN WE BETTER CAPTURE OUR MOST VULNERABLE PATIENTS' PERSPECTIVE REGARDING THEIR RHEUMATOID ARTHRITIS DISEASE ACTIVITY?

One could argue that routine measures of disease activity need to be fully tested among vulnerable patients. There are many possible changes that could be made to make the PtGA-VAS and other PROs both less complex to patients and more valuable to providers. These changes are displayed in **Box 7**. Essentially, options are to improve the PtGA-VAS, capture the PtGA in nonwritten formats, or abandon the use of the PtGA altogether.

The PtGA-VAS could be improved through consensus regarding the wording of the question, its anchors, the VAS line format, and explanations provided to patients regarding the domains the PtGA-VAS is intended to measure.[5,76] The various versions of the PtGA-VAS were not developed with patient input and not validated with the systematic rigor that has helped forge the more recently developed PROM.[60] The lack of uniformity regarding its English-language wording, anchors, and instructions for providers and patients are major weakness that likely explain its poor validity and reproducibility.[4] Given these obstacles with the English-language versions of the PtGA, it is not surprising that there are no publications regarding the validation of

Box 7
Potential strategies to improve capture of patient global assessment in rheumatoid arthritis patients with limited health literacy and limited English proficiency

- Ensure that a validated version of the instrument is available in the patients' primary language
- Use validated lower literacy versions of PROs
- Exploration of capturing the PtGA through nonwritten formats, including verbally and using computers, tablets, and smartphones
- Comprehensive standardization of all aspects of the PTGA-VAS and explanations provided to patients regarding domains being queried with potential use of model disease states
- Ongoing efforts to solicit input of diverse patient groups regarding the design and validation of PROM
- Consideration of abandonment of PtGA question in composite RA disease activity indices and substitution of standardized and validated PROM

the translation the PtGA into other languages as has been done with other PROM in underserved populations.[61] There are also no validated lower literacy versions of the PtGA such as have been developed for other PROM.[77,78] Model disease states, if validated, could help guide patients regarding how to rate the activity of their inflammatory symptoms.[79] The VAS line itself is in need of standardization: patient input and additional research needs to be done regarding the whether the patients' written response should be placed on an unmarked 10-cm line, a 10-cm line with hash marks every 5 mm, or through filling in 1 of 21 circles spaced 5 mm apart.[80] Patient input is needed in all aspects of the PtGA: most participants at 2 recent OMERACT (Outcome Measures in Rheumatology) committees thought that the PtGA-VAS needed to be further investigated.[63]

Obtaining the PtGA through nonwritten formats is one possible solution to some, but not all, of the above issues for patients with LHL and LEP. Presumably, the PtGA is often currently obtained in this fashion for such patients and those with poor vision or limited ability to complete forms due to neurologic or arthritic disease.[57] Caution is advised, however, until additional standardization and validation of verbal versions of the PtGA are performed. Research regarding verbally obtained pain scores has performed suboptimally in patients with limited literacy and inflammatory arthritis.[81] The author attempted to validate a verbal version of the PtGA at Denver Health recently with disappointing results. Correlation between the verbally obtained PtGAs and PtGA-VAS was not strong and approximately one-third of subjects provided verbal responses that were discrepant by more than 2 standard deviations from their PtGA-VAS.[57]

As nearly two-thirds of Americans have smartphones, the possible use of more advanced technology to obtain patients' PtGA scores is of great interest.[82] PtGA scores as captured by computer use, handheld devices, and touch-screen computer have shown high intraclasss correlational coefficients with the PtGA-VAS.[83–85] The National Institutes of Health Patient-Reported Outcomes Measurement Information System (PROMIS) has developed multiple item banks that are relevant to rheumatology that can be administered via computerized adaptive tests (CAT).[77] PROMIS items are available in validated versions in multiple languages, written at grade school level, and vetted by diverse populations including patients with limited literacy.[77] The PtGA is not included in the PROMIS item bank, but CAT is more patient-centric and better validated than the written PtGA-VAS.[77]

The PtGA's suspect validity impacts all patients and research subjects and not only those with LHL and LEP.[86] That the decision has been made in the past to "grandfather" the PtGA-VAS into key composite indices for RA disease activity does not mean that this should be the status quo ad infinitum. The question of whether the PtGA-VAS should be replaced in such indices by an instrument designed with both more patient input and rigorous validation according to current standards, such as the Rheumatoid Arthrits Impact of Disease (RAID), is a question that demands an answer.[87] Including the perspective of all patients including those with LEP and LHL is more desirable than composite indices that omit PROMs, such as the Modified DAS or DAS28-CRP(3).[88]

SUMMARY

LHL and LEP are widely prevalent and contribute to disparities in RA health care.[42,43] Progress is being made to ensure that PRO are comprehensible by all and both linguistically and culturally appropriate.[42,77,78] One essential PRO that is included in all RA disease activity composite indices, the PtGA-VAS, was devised before the era of systematic validation and standardization.[42,60] The PtGA-VAS introduces additional complexity to the care of LEP and LHL RA patients.[42,57] The PtGA-VAS should either be extensively retooled or be replaced by more modern and better validated instruments. Until that time, the PtGA-VAS should be used as a tool to improve patient communication.[76] Rheumatology providers should take the time to understand why their patients placed the "X" on the line where they did and then focus on treating the noninflammatory conditions that may inappropriately drive the PtGA. Optimally, this communication would take place using plain language and techniques that enhance recall and comprehension.[89] Compassionate practitioners are obligated to do no less.

REFERENCES

1. Aga AB, Lie E, Uhlig T, et al. Time trends in disease activity, response and remission rates in rheumatoid arthritis during the past decade: results from the NOR-DMARD study 2000-2010. Ann Rheum Dis 2015;74(2):381–8.
2. Singh JA, Furst DE, Bharat A, et al. 2012 update of the 2008 American College of Rheumatology recommendations for the use of disease-modifying antirheumatic drugs and biologic agents in the treatment of rheumatoid arthritis. Arthritis Care Res (Hoboken) 2012;64(5):625–39.
3. Greenberg JD, Spruill TM, Shan Y, et al. Racial and ethnic disparities in disease activity in patients with rheumatoid arthritis. Am J Med 2013;126(12):1089–98.
4. Anderson J, Caplan L, Yazdany J, et al. Rheumatoid arthritis disease activity measures: American College of Rheumatology recommendations for use in clinical practice. Arthritis Care Res (Hoboken) 2012;64(5):640–7.
5. Felson DT, Smolen JS, Wells G, et al. American College of Rheumatology/European League Against Rheumatism provisional definition of remission in rheumatoid arthritis for clinical trials. Arthritis Rheum 2011;63(3):573–86.
6. Barton JL, Imboden J, Graf J, et al. Patient-physician discordance in assessments of global disease severity in rheumatoid arthritis. Arthritis Care Res (Hoboken) 2010;62(6):857–64.
7. Hirsh JM, Boyle DJ, Collier DH, et al. Health literacy predicts the discrepancy between patient and provider global assessments of rheumatoid arthritis activity at a public urban rheumatology clinic. J Rheumatol 2010;37(5):961–6.
8. Khan NA, Spencer HJ, Abda EA, et al. Patient's global assessment of disease activity and patient's assessment of general health for rheumatoid arthritis activity assessment: are they equivalent? Ann Rheum Dis 2012;71(12):1942–9.
9. Masri KR, Shaver TS, Shahouri SH, et al. Validity and reliability problems with patient global as a component of the ACR/EULAR remission criteria as used in clinical practice. J Rheumatol 2012;39(6):1139–45.
10. Studenic P, Smolen JS, Aletaha D. Near misses of ACR/EULAR criteria for remission: effects of patient global assessment in Boolean and index-based definitions. Ann Rheum Dis 2012;71(10):1702–5.
11. Bruce B, Fries JF, Murtagh KN. Health status disparities in ethnic minority patients with rheumatoid arthritis: a cross-sectional study. J Rheumatol 2007;34(7):1475–9.
12. Barton JL, Trupin L, Schillinger D, et al. Racial and ethnic disparities in disease activity and function among persons with rheumatoid arthritis from university-affiliated clinics. Arthritis Care Res (Hoboken) 2011;63(9):1238–46.
13. Schmajuk G, Trivedi AN, Solomon DH, et al. Receipt of disease-modifying antirheumatic drugs among patients with rheumatoid arthritis in Medicare managed care plans. JAMA 2011;305(5):480–6.

14. Suarez-Almazor ME, Berrios-Rivera JP, Cox V, et al. Initiation of disease-modifying antirheumatic drug therapy in minority and disadvantaged patients with rheumatoid arthritis. J Rheumatol 2007;34(12):2400–7.
15. Kim SC, Yelin E, Tonner C, et al. Changes in use of disease-modifying antirheumatic drugs for rheumatoid arthritis in the United States during 1983-2009. Arthritis Care Res (Hoboken) 2013;65(9):1529–33.
16. Li X, Sundquist J, Sundquist K. Socioeconomic and occupational risk factors for rheumatoid arthritis: a nationwide study based on hospitalizations in Sweden. J Rheumatol 2008;35(6):986–91.
17. Harrison MJ, Farragher TM, Clarke AM, et al. Association of functional outcome with both personal- and area-level socioeconomic inequalities in patients with inflammatory polyarthritis. Arthritis Rheum 2009;61(10):1297–304.
18. Putrik P, Sokka T, Ramiro S, et al. Impact of socioeconomic gradients within and between countries on health of patients with rheumatoid arthritis (RA): lessons from QUEST RA. Best Pract Res Clin Rheumatol 2012;26(5):705–20.
19. Sokka T, Toloza S, Cutolo M, et al. Women, men, and rheumatoid arthritis: analyses of disease activity, disease characteristics, and treatments in the QUEST-RA study. Arthritis Res Ther 2009;11(1):R7.
20. Massardo L, Pons-Estel BA, Wojdyla D, et al. Early rheumatoid arthritis in Latin America: low socioeconomic status related to high disease activity at baseline. Arthritis Care Res (Hoboken) 2012;64(8):1135–43.
21. Ryan C. Language use in the United States: 2011 American community survey reports. Washington, DC: United States Cesus Bureau and Department of Commerce; 2013. Ref Type: Pamphlet.
22. Karliner LS, Napoles-Springer AM, Schillinger D, et al. Identification of limited English proficient patients in clinical care. J Gen Intern Med 2008;23(10):1555–60.
23. Institute of Medicine (US) Committee on Quality of Health Care in America. Crossing the quality chasm: a new health system for the 21st century. Washington, DC: National Academy Press; 2001. Ref Type: Pamphlet.
24. Parsons JA, Baker NA, Smith-Gorvie T, et al. To 'Get by' or 'get help'? A qualitative study of physicians' challenges and dilemmas when patients have limited English proficiency. BMJ Open 2014;4(6):e004613.
25. Lopez L, Rodriguez F, Huerta D, et al. Use of interpreters by physicians for hospitalized limited English proficient patients and its impact on patient outcomes. J Gen Intern Med 2015;30(6):783–9.
26. Fiscella K, Franks P, Doescher MP, et al. Disparities in health care by race, ethnicity, and language among the insured: findings from a national sample. Med Care 2002;40(1):52–9.
27. Fox SA, Stein JA. The effect of physician-patient communication on mammography utilization by different ethnic groups. Med Care 1991;29(11):1065–82.
28. Crane JA. Patient comprehension of doctor-patient communication on discharge from the emergency department. J Emerg Med 1997;15(1):1–7.
29. Carrasquillo O, Orav EJ, Brennan TA, et al. Impact of language barriers on patient satisfaction in an emergency department. J Gen Intern Med 1999;14(2):82–7.
30. Manson A. Language concordance as a determinant of patient compliance and emergency room use in patients with asthma. Med Care 1988;26(12):1119–28.
31. Barton JL, Trupin L, Tonner C, et al. English language proficiency, health literacy, and trust in physician are associated with shared decision making in rheumatoid arthritis. J Rheumatol 2014;41(7):1290–7.

32. Barton JL, Schmajuk G, Trupin L, et al. Poor knowledge of methotrexate associated with older age and limited English-language proficiency in a diverse rheumatoid arthritis cohort. Arthritis Res Ther 2013;15(5):R157.
33. Ratzan CS, Parker RM. Introduction. In national library of medicine current bibliographies in medicine: health literacy. Washington, DC: National Institutes of Health (US) Department of Health and Human Services; 2000. Ref Type: Pamphlet.
34. Rudd RE. Mismatch between skills of patients and tools in use: might literacy affect diagnoses and research? J Rheumatol 2010;37(5):885–6.
35. Kutner M, Greenberg E, Jin Y, et al. The health literacy of America's adults: results from the 2003 National Assessment of Adult Literacy. Washington, DC: U.S. Department of Education; 2006.
36. Kiechle ES, Bailey SC, Hedlund LA, et al. Different measures, different outcomes? A systematic review of performance-based versus self-reported measures of health literacy and numeracy. J Gen Intern Med 2015;30(10):1538–46.
37. Williams MV, Parker RM, Baker DW, et al. Inadequate functional health literacy among patients at two public hospitals. JAMA 1995;274(21):1677–82.
38. Wolf MS, Williams MV, Parker RM, et al. Patients' shame and attitudes toward discussing the results of literacy screening. J Health Commun 2007;12(8):721–32.
39. Loke YK, Hinz I, Wang X, et al. Impact of health literacy in patients with chronic musculoskeletal disease–systematic review. PLoS One 2012;7(7):e40210.
40. Morris NS, MacLean CD, Chew LD, et al. The single item literacy screener: evaluation of a brief instrument to identify limited reading ability. BMC Fam Pract 2006;7:21.
41. Hirsh JM. Can shared decision making help eliminate disparities in rheumatoid arthritis outcomes? J Rheumatol 2014;41(7):1257–9.
42. Caplan L, Wolfe F, Michaud K, et al. Strong association of health literacy with functional status among rheumatoid arthritis patients: a cross-sectional study. Arthritis Care Res (Hoboken) 2014;66(4):508–14.
43. Hirsh JM, Boyle DJ, Collier DH, et al. Limited health literacy is a common finding in a public health hospital's rheumatology clinic and is predictive of disease severity. J Clin Rheumatol 2011;17(5):236–41.
44. Kim SH. Health literacy and functional health status in Korean older adults. J Clin Nurs 2009;18(16):2337–43.
45. Paasche-Orlow MK, Wolf MS. The causal pathways linking health literacy to health outcomes. Am J Health Behav 2007;31(Suppl 1):S19–26.
46. Goekoop-Ruiterman YP, de Vries-Bouwstra JK, Allaart CF, et al. Comparison of treatment strategies in early rheumatoid arthritis: a randomized trial. Ann Intern Med 2007;146(6):406–15.
47. Kim SP, Knight SJ, Tomori C, et al. Health literacy and shared decision making for prostate cancer patients with low socioeconomic status. Cancer Invest 2001; 19(7):684–91.
48. Quinzanos I, Hirsh JM, Bright C, et al. Cross-sectional correlation of single-item health literacy screening questions with established measures of health literacy in patients with rheumatoid arthritis. Rheumatol Int 2015;35(9):1497–502.
49. van der Vaart R, Drossaert CH, Taal E, et al. Impact of patient-accessible electronic medical records in rheumatology: use, satisfaction and effects on empowerment among patients. BMC Musculoskelet Disord 2014;15:102.
50. Arthur SA, Geiser HR, Arriola KR, et al. Health literacy and control in the medical encounter: a mixed-methods analysis. J Natl Med Assoc 2009;101(7):677–83.

51. Schillinger D, Bindman A, Wang F, et al. Functional health literacy and the quality of physician-patient communication among diabetes patients. Patient Educ Couns 2004;52(3):315–23.
52. Sudore RL, Landefeld CS, Perez-Stable EJ, et al. Unraveling the relationship between literacy, language proficiency, and patient-physician communication. Patient Educ Couns 2009;75(3):398–402.
53. Gordon MM, Hampson R, Capell HA, et al. Illiteracy in rheumatoid arthritis patients as determined by the Rapid Estimate of Adult Literacy in Medicine (REALM) score. Rheumatology (Oxford) 2002;41(7):750–4.
54. Martin RW, McCallops K, Head AJ, et al. Influence of patient characteristics on perceived risks and willingness to take a proposed anti-rheumatic drug. BMC Med Inform Decis Mak 2013;13:89.
55. Wong PK, Christie L, Johnston J, et al. How well do patients understand written instructions?: health literacy assessment in rural and urban rheumatology outpatients. Medicine (Baltimore) 2014;93(25):e129.
56. Quinlan P, Price KO, Magid SK, et al. The relationship among health literacy, health knowledge, and adherence to treatment in patients with rheumatoid arthritis. HSS J 2013;9(1):42–9.
57. Hirsh JM, Davis LA, Quinzanos I, et al. Health literacy predicts discrepancies between traditional written patient assessments and verbally administered assessments in rheumatoid arthritis. J Rheumatol 2014;41(2):256–64.
58. Aletaha D, Smolen JS. Joint damage in rheumatoid arthritis progresses in remission according to the Disease Activity Score in 28 joints and is driven by residual swollen joints. Arthritis Rheum 2011;63(12):3702–11.
59. Bellamy N. Critical review of clinical assessment techniques for rheumatoid arthritis trials: new developments. Scand J Rheumatol Suppl 1989;80:3–16.
60. French T, Hewlett S, Kirwan J, et al. Different wording of the Patient Global Visual Analogue Scale (PG-VAS) affects rheumatoid arthritis patients' scoring and the overall Disease Activity Score (DAS28): a cross-sectional study. Musculoskeletal Care 2013;11(4):229–37.
61. Wallen GR, Middleton KR, Rivera-Goba MV, et al. Validating English- and Spanish-language patient-reported outcome measures in underserved patients with rheumatic disease. Arthritis Res Ther 2011;13(1):R1.
62. Adams J, Chapman J, Bradley S, et al. Literacy levels required to complete routinely used patient-reported outcome measures in rheumatology. Rheumatology (Oxford) 2013;52(3):460–4.
63. van Tuyl LH, Smolen JS, Wells GA, et al. Patient perspective on remission in rheumatoid arthritis. J Rheumatol 2011;38(8):1735–8.
64. Ranzolin A, Brenol JC, Bredemeier M, et al. Association of concomitant fibromyalgia with worse disease activity score in 28 joints, health assessment questionnaire, and short form 36 scores in patients with rheumatoid arthritis. Arthritis Rheum 2009;61(6):794–800.
65. Smedstad LM, Kvien TK, Moum T, et al. Correlates of patients' global assessment of arthritis impact. A 2-year study of 216 patients with RA. Scand J Rheumatol 1997;26(4):259–65.
66. Ward MM, Leigh JP. The relative importance of pain and functional disability to patients with rheumatoid arthritis. J Rheumatol 1993;20(9):1494–9.
67. van der Heijde DM, van 't Hof MA, van Riel PL, et al. Judging disease activity in clinical practice in rheumatoid arthritis: first step in the development of a disease activity score. Ann Rheum Dis 1990;49(11):916–20.

68. Felson DT, Anderson JJ, Boers M, et al. American College of Rheumatology. Preliminary definition of improvement in rheumatoid arthritis. Arthritis Rheum 1995; 38(6):727–35.
69. Kuriya B, Sun Y, Boire G, et al. Remission in early rheumatoid arthritis—a comparison of new ACR/EULAR remission criteria to established criteria. J Rheumatol 2012;39(6):1155–8.
70. Joyce CR, Zutshi DW, Hrubes V, et al. Comparison of fixed interval and visual analogue scales for rating chronic pain. Eur J Clin Pharmacol 1975;8(6):415–20.
71. Dehaene S, Izard V, Spelke E, et al. Log or linear? Distinct intuitions of the number scale in Western and Amazonian indigene cultures. Science 2008;320(5880): 1217–20.
72. Master VA, Johnson TV, Abbasi A, et al. Poorly numerate patients in an inner city hospital misunderstand the American Urological Association symptom score. Urology 2010;75(1):148–52.
73. Vasconcelos J, Pedro S, Marques S, et al. VAS scales might not be appropriate to measure RA outcomes among patients with low education levels. Arthritis Rheum 2009; Suppl 60:S370. Ref Type: Abstract.
74. Hernandez-Cruz B, Cardiel MH. Intra-observer reliability of commonly used outcome measures in rheumatoid arthritis. Clin Exp Rheumatol 1998;16(4): 459–62.
75. Desai SP, Yazdany J. Quality measurement and improvement in rheumatology: rheumatoid arthritis as a case study. Arthritis Rheum 2011;63(12):3649–60.
76. Studenic P, Radner H, Smolen JS, et al. Discrepancies between patients and physicians in their perceptions of rheumatoid arthritis disease activity. Arthritis Rheum 2012;64(9):2814–23.
77. Khanna D, Krishnan E, Dewitt EM, et al. The future of measuring patient-reported outcomes in rheumatology: Patient-Reported Outcomes Measurement Information System (PROMIS). Arthritis Care Res (Hoboken) 2011;63(Suppl 11):S486–90.
78. Petkovic J, Epstein J, Buchbinder R, et al. Toward ensuring health equity: readability and cultural equivalence of OMERACT patient-reported outcome measures. J Rheumatol 2015;42(12):2448–59.
79. Lati C, Guthrie LC, Ward MM. Comparison of the construct validity and sensitivity to change of the visual analog scale and a modified rating scale as measures of patient global assessment in rheumatoid arthritis. J Rheumatol 2010;37(4): 717–22.
80. Pincus T, Bergman M, Sokka T, et al. Visual analog scales in formats other than a 10 centimeter horizontal line to assess pain and other clinical data. J Rheumatol 2008;35(8):1550–8.
81. Englbrecht M, Tarner IH, van der Heijde DM, et al. Measuring pain and efficacy of pain treatment in inflammatory arthritis: a systematic literature review. J Rheumatol Suppl 2012;90:3–10.
82. Smith A. The Smartphone Difference. Pew Research Center, April, 2015. Available at: http://www.pewinternet.org/2015. Accessed January 6, 2016.
83. Athale N, Sturley A, Skoczen S, et al. A web-compatible instrument for measuring self-reported disease activity in arthritis. J Rheumatol 2004;31(2):223–8.
84. Greenwood MC, Hakim AJ, Carson E, et al. Touch-screen computer systems in the rheumatology clinic offer a reliable and user-friendly means of collecting quality-of-life and outcome data from patients with rheumatoid arthritis. Rheumatology (Oxford) 2006;45(1):66–71.

85. Heiberg T, Kvien TK, Dale O, et al. Daily health status registration (patient diary) in patients with rheumatoid arthritis: a comparison between personal digital assistant and paper-pencil format. Arthritis Rheum 2007;57(3):454–60.
86. Studenic P, Stamm T, Smolen J, et al. Reliability of patient-reported outcomes in rheumatoid arthritis patients: an observational prospective study. Rheumatology (Oxford) 2016;55(1):41–8.
87. Gossec L, Paternotte S, Aanerud GJ, et al. Finalisation and validation of the rheumatoid arthritis impact of disease score, a patient-derived composite measure of impact of rheumatoid arthritis: a EULAR initiative. Ann Rheum Dis 2011;70(6): 935–42.
88. Baker JF, Conaghan PG, Smolen JS, et al. Development and validation of modified disease activity scores in rheumatoid arthritis: superior correlation with magnetic resonance imaging-detected synovitis and radiographic progression. Arthritis Rheumatol 2014;66(4):794–802.
89. Schillinger D, Piette J, Grumbach K, et al. Closing the loop: physician communication with diabetic patients who have low health literacy. Arch Intern Med 2003; 163(1):83–90.

Challenges and Opportunities in Using Patient-reported Outcomes in Quality Measurement in Rheumatology

Elizabeth R. Wahl, MD[a], Jinoos Yazdany, MD, MPH[b,*]

KEYWORDS

- Patient-reported outcomes • Quality measures • Performance measures
- Outcome measures • Health care quality • Rheumatology

KEY POINTS

- The health care landscape in the United States is likely shifting to a model in which health systems will be reimbursed for the quality of care they provide, and developing valid, responsive, and meaningful patient-centered measures is key.
- How best to incorporate patient-reported outcome measures (PROs) in assessments of health care quality in rheumatology is underexplored.
- Experiences with widespread use of PROs in Sweden and the United Kingdom, and in smaller health systems within the United States, provide valuable lessons about challenges and opportunities in using PROs to assess quality.
- Major challenges include developing sufficient information technology infrastructure to collect data from diverse medical records and diverse patients; need for better understanding of PRO reliability, validity, and responsiveness; determining that PROs are responsive to changes in the health care environment; clarifying the role of case-mix adjustment; and understanding how measures should be summarized and reported to stakeholders.

Conflicts of interest: Neither Dr E. Wahl nor Dr J. Yazdany has any commercial or financial conflicts of interest to disclose.
Funding sources: J. Yazdany is supported by NIAMS K23 AR060259, the Russell/Engleman Rheumatology Research Center, and the Robert L. Kroc Endowed Chair in Rheumatic and Connective Tissue Diseases at the University of California, San Francisco. E. Wahl supported by a VA Quality Scholars Fellowship through the VA Office of Academic Affiliations.
[a] VA Quality Scholars Program, Division of Rheumatology, San Francisco Veterans Affairs Medical Center, 4150 Clement Street, Building 1, Room 207-1, San Francisco, CA 94121, USA; [b] Division of Rheumatology, Department of Internal Medicine, University of California, San Francisco, 1001 Potrero Avenue, Building SFGH 30, Room 3301, Box 0811, San Francisco, CA 94110, USA
* Corresponding author.
E-mail address: jinoos.yazdany@ucsf.edu

Rheum Dis Clin N Am 42 (2016) 363–375
http://dx.doi.org/10.1016/j.rdc.2016.01.008 rheumatic.theclinics.com
0889-857X/16/$ – see front matter

INTRODUCTION

Quality measures provide important insight into variability or problems within structures of care, processes of care, or outcomes of care.[1–3] Patient-reported outcomes (PROs) provide valuable information on patients' health-related quality of life, and can be used to facilitate shared decision making in the clinical setting, for comparative effectiveness research, for adverse event reporting, and in quality assessment.[1,2,4–6] However, use of PRO measures as indicators of health care quality and accountability is a new, and growing, area in the United States.

Following passage of the Patient Protection and Affordable Care Act in 2010, there has been a growing emphasis on improving performance and accountability of health care systems and individuals.[7–9] Recent legislation, the Medicare Access and CHIP (Children's Health Insurance Program) Reauthorization Act of 2015, supports a shift in physician reimbursement via a merit-based incentive payment system (MIPS), in which physicians and systems will be judged and reimbursed partly based on the quality of care they provide. Appropriate selection of measures that define quality, particularly measures that matter to beneficiaries of care, will be critical to the success of MIPS.[8,10]

Given increased recognition that patient engagement and inclusion of the patient's voice are critical to the success of a high-quality, affordable health system,[4,7,8,11] incorporating measures that reflect the patient's direct report about how they feel and function into measures that evaluate quality of care is essential. However, there are several challenges to using PRO measures to assess performance and accountability,[7,12–16] and how best to do this in rheumatology has yet to be defined.

This article discusses the role of structure, process, and outcome measures of health care quality using PROs, reviews European countries' experiences collecting and evaluating national PRO data to assess quality of care, describes the current use of PROs as quality measures in rheumatology, and frames an agenda for future work supporting the development of meaningful quality measures based on PROs.

STRUCTURE, PROCESS, AND OUTCOME: PATIENT-REPORTED OUTCOME MEASURES AS INDICATORS OF HEALTH CARE QUALITY

The ability to understand the quality of health care, defined by the Institute of Medicine as "the degree to which health care services for individuals and populations increase the likelihood of desired health outcomes and are consistent with current professional knowledge,[17]" is fundamentally linked to how quality is defined and measured. Quality measures that use PROs can address health care structures, processes, and outcomes, and there are important strengths and limitations to measuring each of these categories.

PRO outcome measures attempt to evaluate the ultimate impact of care provided, and thus are sought-after metrics of health care quality.[1,18] Outcomes can be measured at the individual level or aggregated by provider, practice, institution, organization, or region. Aggregating PRO outcomes data at the level of the health care system could theoretically identify poor performers and makes it possible for individuals to compare performance between health systems, driving accountability. However, with each level of aggregation, information about the processes and environments of care that contributed to a high or low score may become more difficult to identify.

Although outcome-based quality measures are preferred by the Centers for Medicare and Medicaid Services, they provide limited information about the processes of care that lead to an outcome. PRO outcome measures might therefore show what needs to be improved, not how to do so. By contrast, process measures using PROs (eg, whether a PRO was completed and scored, or shared with a patient) may be more actionable, and, as such, more conducive to iterative quality improvement strategies.[19] However, process measures may not map well to outcomes. This finding often reflects the presence of unmeasured factors that affect outcomes, such as socioeconomic determinants of health, which can be difficult to account for but are also often more difficult to change. The complex relationship between processes and outcomes does not invalidate process measures; it indicates the value in measuring both to understand quality and drive quality improvement. Thus, PROs are critically important in that they bring patients' voices to the fore, but inherently problematic in that clinicians do not measure or fully understand all the potentially modifiable processes of care that affect these outcomes.

The movement to use PROs as metrics of health care quality is underway. The National Quality Forum recently defined a new category of performance measures "based on PRO data aggregated for an accountable health care entity"[7] called PRO performance measures (PRO-PMs), and delineated a pathway for their endorsement.[4] Although use of PRO-PMs has gained some initial traction in oncology and mental health,[4] evidence directly linking collection of PRO measures to improvements in provider performance is conflicting or lacking.[12,15,16,20] In addition, little is understood about the relationship between PROs and the processes of care that modulate them.

NATIONAL HEALTH SYSTEMS AND PATIENT-REPORTED OUTCOMES MEASUREMENT: EXPERIENCES AND LESSONS LEARNED FROM SWEDEN AND THE UNITED KINGDOM

Sweden

National quality registers (NQRs), population-level clinical quality databases, have existed in Sweden since 1975. With the creation of NQRs, the infrastructure to collect population-level data to better understand the connection between health care processes and disease was created.[21–23] Data from NQRs are aggregated and publicly reported for use in benchmarking and to develop guidelines and patient information. Most (87%) NQRs collect PRO data, and about 20% of these report using patient-reported data for local quality improvement work.[21] PRO data from NQRs have been used to support patient-centered continuous process improvement, but participation in NQRs is voluntary and hospitals are not remunerated on the basis of PRO measure data.

The experience of the Swedish Rheumatology Quality Registry, created in 1995, highlights several important practical challenges and successes in using PRO data to improve the care of patients with rheumatoid arthritis (RA).[22,23] Between 1995 and 2009, iterative improvement cycles were used to facilitate widespread use of the quality register, with 29,000 patients from 60 clinics registered by 2009.[22] Initially, paper forms were used for data collection, and data collected were redundant with data from the health record. Providers were frustrated with the time required to complete information for the register, which detracted from patient care. With improvements in technology and work flow, the process was streamlined: patients complete an electronic questionnaire assessing self-reported health (pain, global health, daily function, and tender and swollen joints). This information is then given to the clinician, updated during the encounter, and returned to the patient. Thus, the physician and the patient see and analyze changes in disease activity together. Patient and provider satisfaction have improved, as have providers' understanding of patients' medication-taking behaviors, because patients have been more forthcoming about medication adherence while reviewing trends in disease activity.[22]

Data on PROs are aggregated at the provider, clinic, and hospital level, and are publicly reported.[23] Thus data are used to understand which hospitals in Sweden have the lowest or highest PRO disease activity measures, which hospitals have the greatest decrease in PRO disease activity measures over defined time periods, and how certain PRO measures change over time.[23] Data are also aggregated regionally to stimulate comparisons and create and open conversation about health care cost, although no data yet support the efficacy of this strategy.

Because of the breadth and depth of PRO data collected, Sweden is uniquely positioned to understand how PRO measures change over time, and, specifically, how much variation in measurement is related to patient or health system factors, or reflects natural variation, and thus, the extent to which these measures are valid indicators of health system performance. It is critical that this kind of work be done in a system in which evaluation is separate from remuneration. However, lessons about aggregate PRO data may be specific to the Swedish health care system and population, and less applicable to countries with lower literacy levels, greater racial and ethnic diversity, and multiple languages spoken.

United Kingdom

In contrast with Sweden, where formation of NQRs and collection of PROs are voluntary, gathering PRO data in United Kingdom is a government mandate.[8,10] In 2010, the National Health Service (NHS) unveiled an outcomes framework outlining a performance model emphasizing health outcomes, in which PRO measures are used to facilitate comparison of providers, improve accountability, and motivate improvements in quality.[4,7,8,11] PROs are also being used to help align patient and physician goals of care and treatment plans, such as the use of serial PRO measures in patients considering hip replacement.[8] Engaging in shared decision making and providing value-aligned care are processes that indicate high-quality care. However, a provider's aggregated PRO measure does not indicate whether value-aligned care is being provided.

Several unique challenges have arisen in the United Kingdom as a result of widespread mandatory implementation of PRO data collection. For example, the logistic burden and cost of creating the information technology infrastructure to support PRO data collection and analysis are significant. Furthermore, different patient populations may be less responsive to Web-based questionnaires, such as those who are elderly.[24] Capturing a broad spectrum of patients with a wide range of PRO responses is critical to ensuring measure validity, thus including both the sickest and most vulnerable patients, as well as patients who are most healthy but do not interact with the health care system, will be key.[8]

Because the United Kingdom is using PRO data to make determinations about the quality of care with financial repercussions, there have been specific challenges related to the ability (or failure) to attribute PROs to the quality of care provided.[8,11] Difficulties understanding when PRO variability reflects true change and when it reflects normal variation, understanding how best to use case-mix adjustment, how to define the reporting period, how to aggregate and report the data to different stakeholders, how to decide what constitutes unacceptable performance, and how to avoid misuse or misinterpretation of data are additional challenges. Therefore, the work to date suggests that far more experience with these measures is needed before they create value for patients and for the NHS.[8,25]

QUALITY REGISTRIES IN RHEUMATOLOGY: THE UNITED STATES EXPERIENCE WITH PATIENT-REPORTED OUTCOMES AS QUALITY MEASURES

Based on our systematic review of the literature (detailed in Appendix 1), evidence supporting the use of PRO measures in rheumatic disease care in the United States is scarce. However, the experience at Geisinger Health System shows that collection of PROs in a busy rheumatology clinic is feasible, is associated with high-quality processes of care, and may improve outcomes.[26]

In a recent evaluation of an electronic health record (EHR) optimized for rheumatology practice, Newman and colleagues[26] tracked 14 clinicians, nearly 6700 patients, and data from almost 20,000 encounters over a 2-year period within the Geisinger Health System in eastern Pennsylvania. The EHR, Rheum-PACER (Patient-Centered Electronic Redesign), captures, aggregates, and displays patient-reported measures of disease activity, physical function, and pain. Although the primary aim of the study was to evaluate the impact of the software on physician productivity and efficiency, the investigators also reported a modest but significant correlation (r = 0.59) between physicians' use of the software and disease control in patients with RA, defined as Clinical Disease Activity Index (CDAI), a composite outcome measure that includes a patient-reported component, of less than or equal to 10. In addition, they showed a small (3%) but significant trend of increasing numbers of patients with controlled disease (CDAI $\leq$10) over time. Use of the EHR was associated with process improvements (chart review and documentation time decreased and productivity increased); patient adherence, activation, and satisfaction scores were high at baseline and did not change.

Building infrastructure to collect PRO data from a large and diverse network of rheumatology practices in the United States will help create large data sets that will yield important information about the opportunities and challenges of using PROs for quality measurement in clinical settings. The American College of Rheumatology (ACR) national registry, Rheumatology Informatics System for Effectiveness (RISE), the Veterans Affairs Rheumatoid Arthritis registry, and quality networks like the Pediatric Rheumatology Clinical Outcomes and Improvement Network have made progress in building this infrastructure and accumulating data on PROs will continue to support and inform future quality measurement efforts.

NATIONAL QUALITY FORUM–ENDORSED QUALITY MEASURES IN RHEUMATOLOGY

The National Quality Forum (NQF) now endorses many musculoskeletal quality measures; although 9 measures included in the NQF Quality Positioning System[27] address self-reported changes in basic mobility, these are all intended to assess rehabilitation following injury, surgery, or facility admission. There are 4 NQF-endorsed RA quality measures, 2 of which include PROs: an annual recorded measure of disease activity, and an annual recorded measure of physical function. All disease activity measures include a patient-reported component. Some include only PROs (Routine Assessment of Patient Index Data 3 [RAPID3]), Patient Activity Scale (PAS, PASII), whereas others incorporate physician-reported information such as tender and swollen joint counts (CDAI), and laboratory data (Simplified Disease Activity Index and Disease Activity Score). Functional status measures require administration of a validated tool, such as the Multidimensional Health Assessment Questionnaire, Health Assessment Questionnaire II, or Patient Reported Outcomes Measurement Information System (PROMIS) Physical Function (PF-10a, PF-20, or computer adaptive test [CAT]) forms.

Both NQF-endorsed quality measures, documenting disease activity and physical function annually in patients with RA, incorporate PROs. These measures calculate the proportion of patients seen by a given clinician in a fixed time period who have the measure recorded as a score in the EHR and thus reflect structure (whether the particular system is structured to facilitate collection of these data) and process (whether providers collect these data) of care. In addition, both of these measures require that the resulting disease activity or functional status score appear in the EHR, so although the disease activity metric and the physical function metric are not outcome measures, they do allow aggregation of outcomes by practice and provider, and RISE allows national benchmarking of scores against other practices. For example, all of the disease activity measures have validated cut-points for remission, and low, moderate, and high disease activity.[28,29] This system allows aggregate benchmarking by the registry regardless of which measure clinicians use.

EXISTING UNITED STATES GUIDANCE FOR USE OF PATIENT-REPORTED OUTCOMES IN PERFORMANCE MEASUREMENT

As the health care system in the United States moves toward a new funding model in which accountability and performance are evaluated by both measures of process and outcome, ensuring that PRO measures used to evaluate performance and quality are relevant to the population, reliable, valid, interpretable, culturally and linguistically appropriate and understandable, and are not burdensome is critical. The NQF endorses measures that meet these standards, and has established a pathway for PRO performance measure endorsement.[7,13] The Technical Expert Panel (TEP) assembled from the Physician Consortium for Performance Improvement expanded on NQF guidelines and outlined 9 best practices.[30] Recommendations from NQF and the TEP are summarized in **Table 1**. A hypothetical PRO measure that could be used as a performance measure in rheumatology, conforming to NQF recommendations and the TEP best practices, is also presented in **Table 1**.

FUTURE DIRECTIONS

Challenges

- There remain significant challenges with implementation of PROs. The United States is a large and racially/ethnically, linguistically, and culturally diverse country, and has many EHRs that do not yet communicate with each other, making widespread implementation of PROs (for any purpose) challenging. However, multilingual tools, such as many PROMIS measures, are becoming available, and some EHR vendors, such as Epic Systems, are beginning to include functionality that enables more seamless collection and recording of PROs in the EHR. Moreover, technological innovations, such as the RISE registry, are aggregating data across practices with different EHRs, thereby offering a solution to some of the interoperability issues that been barriers to PRO data aggregation.
- Using PROs to assess provider quality will continue to pose challenges. Rheumatologic diseases have a long trajectory, making it potentially difficult to attribute quality of care based on PROs to a single provider or even health system over a short time period. Evidence supporting a relationship between PRO data collection and improved provider performance is not strong, but the need to improve patient-centered care is.
- More data are needed to understand whether changes in PRO outcome measures reflect changes in health care process and environment, to ensure measures are valid and reliable, and to understand whether case-mix adjustment is appropriate.
- More work is needed to understand how PRO information should be summarized and presented to various stakeholders (patients/purchasers of health care, physicians, and accountable care organizations).

Table 1
Best practices for developing and evaluating proposed PRO-PMs

Best Practices (TEP)	NQF Measure Evaluation Criteria	Hypothetical Example of Future PRO-PM for Rheumatology
1. Describe a rationale for measuring the outcome (what is knowledge gap? Does use of a PRO specifically address the gap? Are patients the most appropriate source of information?)	Evidence Performance gap Impact: importance to measure and report (evidence of value to patient/person, amenable to change)	Rationale: published cross-sectional data suggest high rates of symptomatic fatigue in patients with RA, which represents a symptomatic and potentially modifiable problem because recent data suggest that feedback from wearable devices may improve physical activity level and reduce RA-associated fatigue
2. Describe and justify the intended context of use (how will information inform change in practice to improve performance in the intended setting?)	Evidence Performance gap Impact: importance to measure and report Comparison to Related or Competing Measures	Purpose: to understand whether there are variable rates of RA-associated fatigue between practices that might be improved through feedback of rates to providers
3. Measure should have data to support its meaningfulness and importance to patients as well as adequate psychometric properties in the setting in which it will be used	Reliability and validity/scientific acceptability of measure properties	The PROMIS-Fatigue CAT instrument has been tested in patients with RA in clinical trial settings, but is not yet widely used in the clinical setting
4. Measure should have shown sensitivity to change and yield of clinically actionable information in the setting in which it will be used	Feasibility Usability and use	Studies to assess the sensitivity of PROMIS-Fatigue CAT to clinically meaningful changes in patients with RA are underway
5. Implementation strategy for measure should exist in the setting in which it will be used	Feasibility	In this hypothetical example, PROMIS-Fatigue CAT would be integrated into the electronic medical record for all practices participating in the Rheumatology RISE registry, an existing quality-reporting network. The measure would be administered, at baseline and every 3 mo for 12 mo

(*continued on next page*)

Table 1
(*continued*)

Best Practices (TEP)	NQF Measure Evaluation Criteria	Hypothetical Example of Future PRO-PM for Rheumatology
6. An analysis plan should be determined in advance that includes a risk-adjustment strategy (if appropriate), approach to missing data, and power calculation	Reliability and validity/scientific acceptability of measure properties	The proportion of patients with a PROMIS-Fatigue score >50 (US population mean) at any time during follow-up will be measured. The mean PROMIS-Fatigue score for patients in each accountable care organization (ACO) at baseline and in each rolling 3-month period will be measured. Mean within-person change in each ACO will be calculated. Sample size needs to be determined based on existing data. Exploratory risk adjustment for age, race/ethnicity, insurance status, comorbidities, baseline quality of life, and so forth will be performed
7. A framework should exist to identify and interpret clinically meaningful results	Reliability and validity/scientific acceptability of measure properties	Significant work understanding the responsiveness and minimally important difference (and relevant reporting time period) of the PROMIS-Fatigue CAT is needed before undertaking this work
8. An approach to reporting, sharing, and disseminating results should be planned and described	Usability and use	Results will be fed back to practices with a planned strategy to address recognition and management of RA-associated fatigue for sites with the lowest performance
9. An evidence-based approach should be taken to assess the impact of the measure	Comparison with related and competing measures	Regular follow-up assessments of all practices to understand trends and undertake continuous process improvement strategies locally. Until clear validity and responsiveness (and impact) of the measure is established, systems should not be evaluated using the metric

Adapted from Basch E, Spertus J, Dudley RA, et al. Methods for developing patient-reported outcome-based performance measures (PRO-PMs). Value Health 2015;18:493–504; and National Quality Forum. Patient Reported Outcomes (PROs) in Performance Measurement. National Quality Forum 2013. Available at: http://www.qualityforum.org/Publications/2012/12/Patient-Reported_Outcomes_in_Performance_Measurement.aspx. Accessed September 28, 2015.

- Much planning is needed to address competing priorities of different stakeholders when PROs are used for different purposes (patients, providers, accountable care organizations, and benchmarking organizations).

Opportunities

- Building infrastructure to develop widespread PRO collection with harmonized measures is valuable not just for quality improvement but for comparative effectiveness research as well.
- Routinely measuring PROs may help shift rheumatology care toward being even more symptom driven and better align patient and provider goals.
- Aggregating PROs at the population level may help clinicians to elucidate disparities in health. At the bedside, the role of PROs might be to facilitate incorporating the patient's voice, helping patients monitor their own progress, and ensuring that key symptoms are addressed.

RECOMMENDATIONS AND FUTURE DIRECTIONS

- Decide on the measures, with input from patients about what is most important to them, but also with input from experts about what is reliable, valid, and responsive. The ACR's RA quality measures that incorporate PROs, disease activity, and functional status, are examples of measures developed with at least some patient input.
- Develop and test a viable implementation strategy and formally test both measure implementation and its effect on downstream outcomes. Implementation of the RA PROs in EHRs around the country; formal testing of the feasibility, validity, and reliability of these early implementation strategies; and subsequent scaling of efforts to the national registry (RISE) are examples of development and testing of a PRO process measure.
- Continue foundational work necessary for use of PRO outcome performance measures. Decide on the appropriate level of aggregation (at the population or health system level rather than the individual provider level). Develop clear and consistent clinical and administrative definitions of patients who represent the population of interest, the reporting period, and the period at risk. Perform extensive study to understand the relationship between elements of care (structure, process, outcome) and PROs to clarify outcome attribution and case-mix adjustment. Use balancing measures to monitor unintended consequences at the health system level.
- Interpret aggregated PRO measures thoughtfully; if PRO measures are consistently low in safety-net settings, this could reflect poor-quality care or could represent a population of vulnerable patients with more comorbidities or barriers to care who need access to more substantial resources.
- Develop adequate information technology infrastructure to capture PRO data from diverse rheumatology practices across the United States to understand measure variability in urban and rural settings, from safety net, private practice, academic, and Veterans Affairs health systems, and in patients with different rheumatic diseases.
- Think broadly and creatively about the role of PROs in clinical care; the most effective use of PROs in clinical care may be not performance measurement at the individual physician or even practice level, but to assess how rheumatologists are caring for patients at a population level, and to elucidate disparities in health. At the bedside, the role of PROs might be to facilitate incorporating the patient's

voice, helping patients monitor their own progress, and ensure that key symptoms are addressed.

As rheumatology develops clinical practice guidelines and quality measures,[9,31–35] PROs should be considered and evaluated as candidate measures. Moving forward, standardized and routine collection of PRO measures will likely be required. Being able to evaluate this information across different rheumatologic diseases and across health care systems will allow richer understanding of the relationship between patients' health-related quality of life and the quality of rheumatologic care received, and, ideally, will promote development of novel strategies to address gaps that exist.

REFERENCES

1. Krumholz HM. Outcomes research: generating evidence for best practice and policies. Circulation 2008;118:309–18.
2. Donabedian A. The quality of care. How can it be assessed? JAMA 1988;260: 1743–8.
3. Yazdany J, MacLean CH. Quality of care in the rheumatic diseases: current status and future directions. Curr Opin Rheumatol 2008;20:159–66.
4. Basch E. New frontiers in patient-reported outcomes: adverse event reporting, comparative effectiveness, and quality assessment. Annu Rev Med 2014;65: 307–17.
5. Greenhalgh J. The applications of PROs in clinical practice: what are they, do they work, and why? Qual Life Res 2009;18:115–23.
6. Snyder CF, Aaronson NK, Choucair AK, et al. Implementing patient-reported outcomes assessment in clinical practice: a review of the options and considerations. Qual Life Res 2012;21:1305–14.
7. National Quality Forum. Patient reported outcomes (PROs) in performance measurement. National Quality Forum, ed. qualityforumorgProjectsn-rPatient-Reported_OutcomesPatient-Reported_Outcomesaspx 2013. Available at: http://www.qualityforum.org/Publications/2012/12/Patient-Reported_Outcomes_in_Performance_Measurement.aspx. Accessed September 28, 2015.
8. Black N. Patient reported outcome measures could help transform healthcare. BMJ 2013;346:f167.
9. Desai SP, Yazdany J. Quality measurement and improvement in rheumatology: rheumatoid arthritis as a case study. Arthritis Rheum 2011;63:3649–60.
10. Rosenthal MB. Physician payment after the SGR–the new meritocracy. N Engl J Med 2015;373:1187–9.
11. Valderas JM, Fitzpatrick R, Roland M. Using health status to measure NHS performance: another step into the dark for the health reform in England. BMJ Qual Saf 2012;21:352–3.
12. Fung CH, Lim Y-W, Mattke S, et al. Systematic review: the evidence that publishing patient care performance data improves quality of care. Ann Intern Med 2008;148: 111–23.
13. Cella D, Hahn E, Jensen S, et al. Methodological issues in the selection, administration, and use of patient-reported outcomes in performance measurement in health care settings. Commissioned Paper #1. Washington, DC: National Quality Forum. Available at: https://www.qualityforum.org/Projects/n-r/Patient-Reported_Outcomes/Commissioned_Paper_1.aspx. Accessed September 28, 2015.
14. Harman JS, Scholle SH, Ng JH, et al. Association of Health Plans' Healthcare Effectiveness Data and Information Set (HEDIS) performance with outcomes of enrollees with diabetes. Med Care 2010;48:217–23.

15. Boyce MB, Browne JP. The effectiveness of providing peer benchmarked feedback to hip replacement surgeons based on patient-reported outcome measures–results from the PROFILE (Patient-Reported Outcomes: feedback Interpretation and Learning Experiment) trial: a cluster randomised controlled study. BMJ Open 2015;5:e008325.
16. Kotronoulas G, Kearney N, Maguire R, et al. What is the value of the routine use of patient-reported outcome measures toward improvement of patient outcomes, processes of care, and health service outcomes in cancer care? A systematic review of controlled trials. J Clin Oncol 2014;32:1480–501.
17. Institute of Medicine (IOM). Crossing the Quality Chasm: A New Health System for the 21st Century. Washington, DC: National Academy Press; 2001.
18. Chassin MR, Loeb JM, Schmaltz SP, et al. Accountability measures–using measurement to promote quality improvement. N Engl J Med 2010;363:683–8.
19. Bilimoria KY. Facilitating quality improvement: pushing the pendulum back toward process measures. JAMA 2015;314:1333–4.
20. Boyce MB, Browne JP. Does providing feedback on patient-reported outcomes to healthcare professionals result in better outcomes for patients? A systematic review. Qual Life Res 2013;22:2265–78.
21. Nilsson E, Orwelius L, Kristenson M. Patient-reported outcomes in the Swedish National Quality Registers. J Intern Med 2016;279:141–53.
22. Ovretveit J, Keller C, Hvitfeldt Forsberg H, et al. Continuous innovation: developing and using a clinical database with new technology for patient-centred care–the case of the Swedish quality register for arthritis. Int J Qual Health Care 2013;25:118–24.
23. Nelson EC, Hvitfeldt H, Reid R, et al. Using Patient-Reported Information to Improve Health Outcomes and Health Care Value: Case Studies From Dartmouth, Karolinska and Group Health. Lebanon, NH: The Dartmouth Institute for Health Policy and Clinical Practice; 2012. Available at: http://tdi.dartmouth.edu/images/uploads/tdi_tr_pri_ia_sm.pdf. Accessed September 28, 2015.
24. Rolfson O, Salomonsson R, Dahlberg LE, et al. Internet-based follow-up questionnaire for measuring patient-reported outcome after total hip replacement surgery-reliability and response rate. Value Health 2011;14:316–21.
25. Van Der Wees PJ, Nijhuis-Van Der Sanden MWG, Ayanian JZ, et al. Integrating the use of patient-reported outcomes for both clinical practice and performance measurement: views of experts from 3 countries. Milbank Q 2014;92:754–75.
26. Newman ED, Lerch V, Billet J, et al. Improving the quality of care of patients with rheumatic disease using patient-centric electronic redesign software. Arthritis Care Res (Hoboken) 2015;67:546–53.
27. NQF Quality Positioning System. National quality forum. Available at: http://www.qualityforum.org/ProjectMeasures.aspx?projectID=73845. Accessed September 29, 2015.
28. Singh JA, Furst DE, Bharat A, et al. 2012 update of the 2008 American College of Rheumatology recommendations for the use of disease-modifying antirheumatic drugs and biologic agents in the treatment of rheumatoid arthritis. Arthritis Care Res (Hoboken) 2012;64:625–39.
29. Anderson J, Caplan L, Yazdany J, et al. Rheumatoid arthritis disease activity measures: American College of Rheumatology recommendations for use in clinical practice. Arthritis Care Res (Hoboken) 2012;64:640–7.
30. Basch E, Spertus J, Dudley RA, et al. Methods for developing patient-reported outcome-based performance measures (PRO-PMs). Value Health 2015;18:493–504.

31. Saag KG, Yazdany J, Alexander C, et al. Defining quality of care in rheumatology: the American College of Rheumatology white paper on quality measurement. Arthritis Care Res (Hoboken) 2011;63:2–9.

32. Yazdany J, Panopalis P, Gillis JZ, et al. A quality indicator set for systemic lupus erythematosus. Arthritis Rheum 2009;61:370–7.

33. Khanna D, Kowal-Bielecka O, Khanna PP, et al. Quality indicator set for systemic sclerosis. Clin Exp Rheumatol 2011;29:S33–9.

34. Petersson IF, Strömbeck B, Andersen L, et al. Development of healthcare quality indicators for rheumatoid arthritis in Europe: the eumusc.net project. Ann Rheum Dis 2014;73:906–8.

35. Stoffer MA, Smolen JS, Woolf A, et al. Development of patient-centred standards of care for osteoarthritis in Europe: the eumusc.net-project. Ann Rheum Dis 2015;74:1145–9.

APPENDIX 1: SYSTEMATIC REVIEW

The authors performed a systematic review of the literature to assess current practices, guidelines, and evidence for use of PRO measures in quality assessment in rheumatology. Specifically, the authors focused on how PROs were used in the clinical setting to promote quality improvement strategies, whether and how PRO data were aggregated, and whether these data were used to assess the quality of care delivered.

With the assistance of a professional librarian, the authors searched 3 electronic databases (MEDLINE, Web of Science, GoogleScholar), from database inception to September 2015; MeSH (medical subject headings) terms and strategy are listed in **Table 2**. The authors evaluated gray literature, including proceedings from major rheumatology meetings (ACR and the European League Against Rheumatism [EULAR]

Table 2
MeSH terms used

Search Strategy	Search Terms
1	"Patient-Reported Outcome" OR "Patient Reported Outcomes" OR "Patient Reported Outcome Measure" OR "Patient Reported Outcome Measures" OR "PRO-PM" OR ("Self Report"[MeSH] AND "Outcome Assessment (Health Care)"[MeSH])
2	"Guideline Adherence"[MeSH] OR "Outcome and Process Assessment (Health Care)"[MeSH] OR "Benchmarking"[MeSH] OR "Quality Improvement"[MeSH] OR "Quality Indicators, Health Care"[MeSH Terms] OR "quality indicator" OR "quality indicators" OR "quality measure" OR "quality measures" OR "performance indicator" OR "performance measure" OR "performance measures" OR "NQF" OR "NHS"
3	"Rheumatic Diseases"[MeSH] OR "Spondylarthropathies"[MeSH] OR "Lupus Erythematosus, Systemic"[MeSH] OR "Scleroderma, Systemic"[MeSH] OR "Vasculitis"[MeSH] OR "Myositis"[MeSH] OR "Mixed Connective Tissue Disease"[MeSH] OR "rheumatic disease" OR "lupus" OR "scleroderma" OR "vasculitis" OR "myositis" OR "ankylosing spondylitis" OR "psoriatic arthritis" OR "reactive arthritis" OR "rheumatoid arthritis" OR "juvenile arthritis"
MEDLINE	1 and 2
Web of Science	1 and 2 and 3
Google Scholar	

from 2010 to 2015), and conducted hand searches of reference lists of retrieved articles.

Studies evaluating use of PROs in a clinical trial or in comparative effectiveness research were excluded, as were articles describing use of PROs in evaluating orthopedic management of musculoskeletal conditions, such as total joint arthroplasty for osteoarthritis.

Of 534 titles identified by the literature search, 1 publication was identified that described initiatives in which PROs were explicitly used or studied in quality initiatives related to rheumatic disease care in the United States.[26] An additional case from Sweden[23] was identified by reviewing reference lists of articles related to PRO measures and quality initiatives not specific to rheumatic disease. Twenty-four abstracts from available ACR and EULAR proceedings related to PROs, and none specifically addressed quality indicators or quality measures.

Both studies identified focused on disease activity measure, pain, and physical function PROs for patients with RA. In both studies, PRO data were collected and fed back to patients and providers in real time. PRO data were used for improvement at the level of individuals (decision to escalate therapy) and aggregated at the level of providers to evaluate the relationship between collection of PRO data and health outcomes (disease activity). In the Swedish study,[23] PRO data were also aggregated by clinic and used for both national benchmarking and identification of opportunities for improvement, but there was no explicit discussion on whether this strategy led to improvements in quality of care.

This article shows the dearth of published literature evaluating PRO measures as candidate tools to evaluate quality of care in the rheumatic diseases, particularly in the United States.

The Promise of Patient-Reported Outcomes Measurement Information System—Turning Theory into Reality

A Uniform Approach to Patient-Reported Outcomes Across Rheumatic Diseases

James P. Witter, MD, PhD

KEYWORDS

• PROMIS • Patient assessment • Validation • Universal

KEY POINTS

- The Patient-Reported Outcomes Measurement Information System (PROMIS) implements modern measurement theory and techniques to advance self- and proxy assessment of symptoms and health-related quality-of-life concepts.
- PROMIS enables improved measurement precision with less respondent burden by embracing item-response theory and computer-adaptive testing.
- PROMIS focuses on measuring universally relevant domains of health and disease to allow agnostic assessments across diseases and clinical settings facilitating meaningful cross-disease comparisons.
- By standardizing patient-reported outcome assessments, PROMIS supports the accumulation of data across settings, which enables meta-analysis and increases the amount of information that can be brought to the interpretation of the scores.

PROMIS® (a registered trademark of the US Department of Health and Human Services)—the Patient-Reported Outcomes Measurement Information System—is helping to facilitate an evolution in the science of patient/person self-assessment of experiences during health or disease. PROMIS represents a cooperative research

---

Disclosure Statement: The author has nothing to disclose. Opinions in this article are those of the author and not the National Institutes of Health/National Institute of Arthritis and Musculoskeletal and Skin Diseases.

Rheumatic Diseases Clinical Program, National Institute of Arthritis and Musculoskeletal and Skin Diseases, One Democracy Plaza, 6701 Democracy Boulevard, Suite 800, Bethesda, MD 20892-4872, USA
E-mail address: james.witter@nih.gov

Rheum Dis Clin N Am 42 (2016) 377–394
http://dx.doi.org/10.1016/j.rdc.2016.01.007
0889-857X/16/$ – see front matter Published by Elsevier Inc.
rheumatic.theclinics.com

program involving multiple academic medical centers, private research organizations, and numerous Institutes across the National Institutes of Health (NIH). It was designed to bring the most advanced measurement science to the development, evaluation, and standardization of item banks to measure patient-reported outcomes (PROs) of health-related quality of life (HRQL) across medical conditions. This system is the result of adopting and implementing concepts like item response theory (IRT) and standard setting (bookmarking), commonly used in educational testing, to measure and interpret health-related outcomes. PROMIS measures are applicable to be used as primary, secondary, or exploratory outcome measures in both adult and pediatric clinical research as well as to provide assessments of HRQL in patient care settings. This evolution in the assessment of PROs is occurring in many fields of medicine, not the least of which is rheumatology.[1]

The PROMIS initiative was one of the efforts of the NIH Roadmap (later Common Fund) initiative in 2004[2] designed to re-engineer the clinical research enterprise. The funding announcement laid out a new vision by noting that, "*The clinical outcomes research enterprise would be enhanced greatly by the availability of a psychometrically validated, dynamic system to measure PROs efficiently in study participants with a wide range of chronic diseases and demographic characteristics*." As noted, it established a collaborative working group between NIH and individual research teams throughout the United States to develop a measurement system and take it through various stages of growth and maturation (see later discussion, under New Science of Patient-Reported Outcomes).

Funding for this greater than 10-year initiative resulted from the recognition at the time that there was no common PRO language and no national standardized set of PRO instruments. Rather, what existed was a "Tower of Babel" approach for assessing PROs across diseases such as rheumatoid arthritis (RA), psoriatic arthritis, or systemic lupus erythematosus (SLE). Certainly, disease-specific outcome measures, especially those that include patient self-assessments, have been demonstrated to be useful for studies within the population in whom they were developed. However, such specificity has hampered the ability to easily and meaningfully compare the level of symptoms and other burdensome aspects of compromised health that make up "health-related quality of life" from one disease to another. Arguably, this lack of a common PRO language also hinders the ability to integrate and synthesize valuable PRO data into a better understanding of common pathogenic mechanisms that drive disease and adversely impact health. Moreover, a common language is required to assess PROs for patients with multiple chronic conditions.

NEW SCIENCE OF PATIENT-REPORTED OUTCOMES

Robust qualitative and quantitative studies, using a "mixed methods approach," are essential components for PRO development and validation according to modern measurement principles and current standards.[3–5] Despite this, few of the legacy or traditional PROs currently used in clinical medicine, including rheumatology, have been developed with this degree of rigor and attention, especially the inclusion of input from those living with and impacted by the conditions under study during the instruments' development. Many of these fundamental principles, especially those that relate to establishing the content validity of a developing PRO instrument, have been delineated in the US Food and Drug Administration's (FDA) PRO Guidance Document.[4] Those principles, illustrated in **Fig. 1**, require a series of iterative steps to ensure thorough psychometric and clinically focused validation.

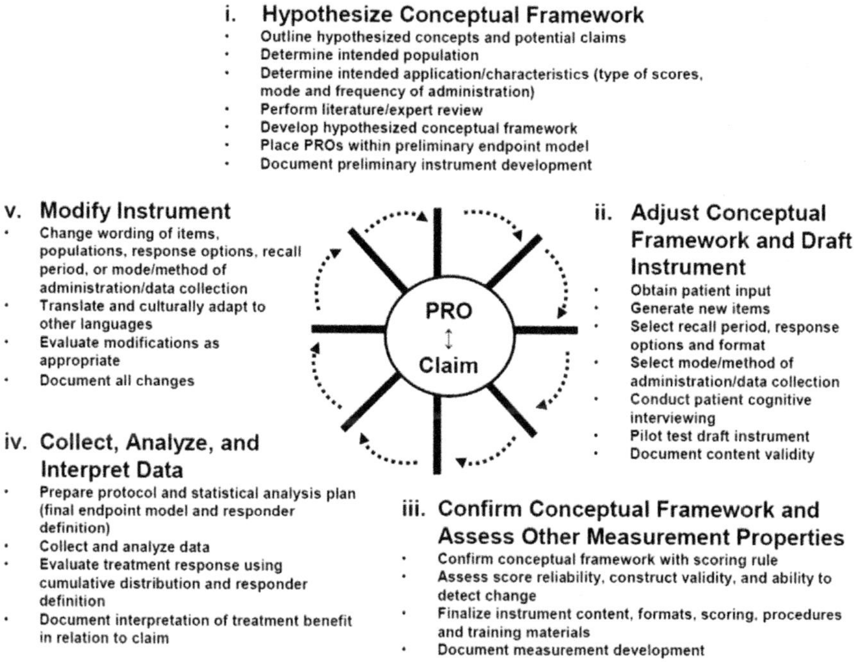

i. Hypothesize Conceptual Framework
Outline hypothesized concepts and potential claims
Determine intended population
Determine intended application/characteristics (type of scores, mode and frequency of administration)
Perform literature/expert review
Develop hypothesized conceptual framework
Place PROs within preliminary endpoint model
Document preliminary instrument development
ii. Adjust Conceptual Framework and Draft Instrument
Obtain patient input
Generate new items
Select recall period, response options and format
Select mode/method of administration/data collection
Conduct patient cognitive interviewing
Pilot test draft instrument
Document content validity
iii. Confirm Conceptual Framework and Assess Other Measurement Properties
Confirm conceptual framework with scoring rule
Assess score reliability, construct validity, and ability to detect change
Finalize instrument content, formats, scoring, procedures and training materials
Document measurement development
iv. Collect, Analyze, and Interpret Data
Prepare protocol and statistical analysis plan (final endpoint model and responder definition)
Collect and analyze data
Evaluate treatment response using cumulative distribution and responder definition
Document interpretation of treatment benefit in relation to claim
v. Modify Instrument
Change wording of items, populations, response options, recall period, or mode/method of administration/data collection
Translate and culturally adapt to other languages
Evaluate modifications as appropriate
Document all changes
PRO
Claim

Fig. 1. FDA PRO guidance wheel. (*From* U.S. Department of Health and Human Services FDA/CDER/CBER/CDRH. Guidance for industry: patient-reported outcome measures: use in medical product development to support labeling claims. US Department of Health and Human Services, 2009. Available at: http://www.fda.gov/downloads/drugs/guidancecomplianceregulatoryinformation/guidances/ucm193282.pdf. Accessed March 01, 2016.)

Even though PROMIS began years before the release of this PRO guidance, these fundamental principles for the development and validation of PROs shepherded the maturation of PROMIS from its beginning into what it is today. In fact, PROMIS has established a maturity model to standardize this process for extant, and future, PROMIS measures (http://www.nihpromis.org/Documents/PROMISStandards_Vers%202.0_MaturityModelOnly_508.pdf).

One truly unique feature of PROMIS is that it is based in IRT. IRT was developed in the educational testing fields to measure academic content in a standardized manner that would enable the enhancement of measurement precision at all levels of ability. Although grounded in sophisticated mathematical models and principles, simply stated, IRT allows patients and items (ie, questions) to be placed on the same metric. As seen in **Fig. 2**, based in this case on participants' self-reports of their physical functioning (PF), the items and the participants likely to respond to the items throughout the scale can be ordered along a continuum by their levels of difficulty from low to high functioning. In educational testing whereby items have a "correct" answer, the difficulty of items refers to how challenging the content is. In the health care setting, item difficulty may refer to how difficult a task is (eg, in the case of PF) or how "intense" or "hard to endorse" a symptom is. For example, respondents with high levels of depressive symptoms would be likely to respond "always" to the item, "I felt hopeless."

IRT also enables computer-adaptive testing (CAT), which is a distinguishing feature between a measure developed with classical test theory and IRT. As an example, the PROMIS adult PF bank currently includes 124 items. To obtain a score with such a

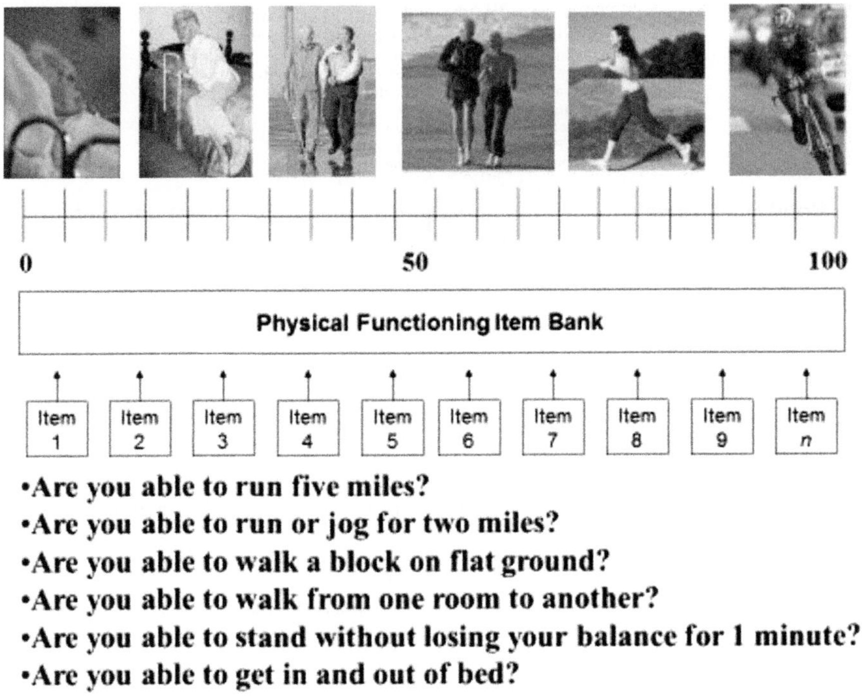
0
50
100
Physical Functioning Item Bank
Item 1
Item 2
Item 3
Item 4
Item 5
Item 6
Item 7
Item 8
Item 9
Item n
•Are you able to run five miles?
•Are you able to run or jog for two miles?
•Are you able to walk a block on flat ground?
•Are you able to walk from one room to another?
•Are you able to stand without losing your balance for 1 minute?
•Are you able to get in and out of bed?

Fig. 2. The PROMIS adult PF bank. (*Courtesy of* PROMIS Health Organization and the PROMIS Cooperative Group, Evanston, IL; with permission.)

questionnaire in a classic testing setting, patients/participants would be required to answer all 124 questions. However, with IRT and CAT, an accurate estimate of one's score on the PROMIS PF scale can be obtained by answering only a fraction of questions. CAT algorithms take advantage of this feature by administering items that are targeted at a respondent's individual level of the trait being measured. This adaptive process is depicted in **Fig. 3**. Based on how a participant answers a question, a computer-driven, mathematical algorithm selects the next best question. Using the example in **Fig. 2** of the PROMIS PF bank, it would make no sense to ask a person who reports being able to run 2 miles without difficulty whether he or she is able to get in and out of bed. Therefore, the respondent is not asked questions for which the answer is already likely known.

When a predetermined stopping criterion is met (eg, a certain level of precision around the score is obtained), the CAT stops and calculates a score (**Fig. 4**) with an explanation of what the score means. How this information is displayed to patients, researchers, and health care providers is an area of active research.[6,7] Nonetheless, a real-time assessment that can be easily accomplished and incorporated into electronic medical records records is an attractive option. CAT can result in a substantial reduction in the time and burden of capturing patient-important information. In addition to CAT versions, all PROMIS measures are available in more traditional "static" short forms. Because of the development of the short forms through IRT, scores are obtained on short forms on the same mathematical metric as those obtained through CAT. **Fig. 4** can also be used to display results from PROMIS short forms.

The metric used in PROMIS is the T score. **Fig. 5** is an idealized example of a normal (ie, Gaussian) distribution of this score with a general population mean of 50 and standard deviation of 10 points. It is idealized because PROMIS measures do not

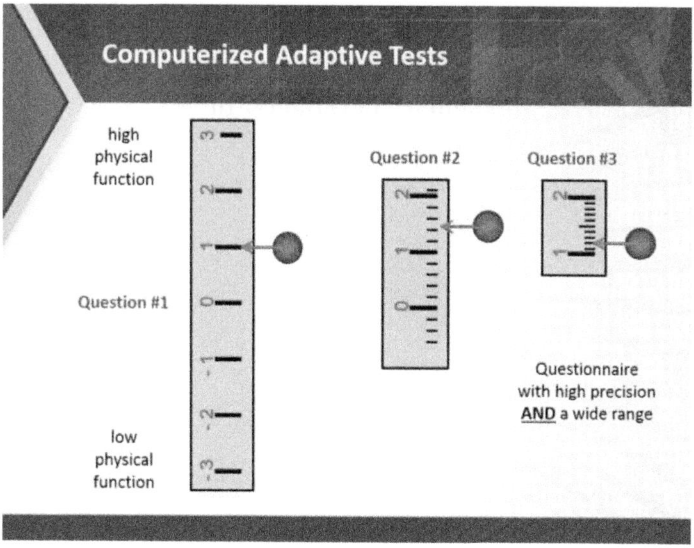

Fig. 3. An example of a PROMIS CAT. (*Courtesy of* John Ware, PhD, Watertown MA; with permission.)

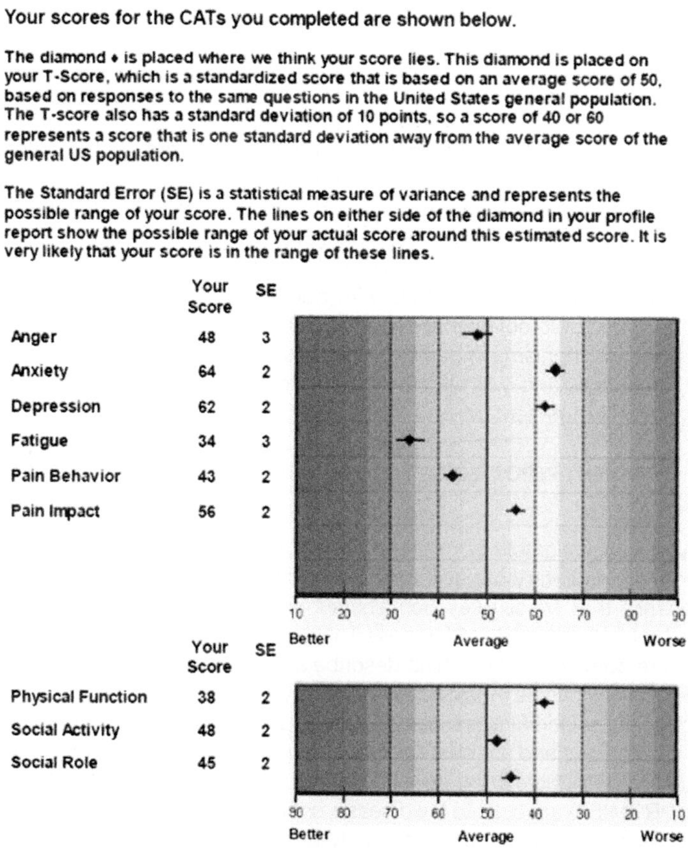

Your scores for the CATs you completed are shown below.
The diamond ♦ is placed where we think your score lies. This diamond is placed on your T-Score, which is a standardized score that is based on an average score of 50, based on responses to the same questions in the United States general population. The T-score also has a standard deviation of 10 points, so a score of 40 or 60 represents a score that is one standard deviation away from the average score of the general US population.
The Standard Error (SE) is a statistical measure of variance and represents the possible range of your score. The lines on either side of the diamond in your profile report show the possible range of your actual score around this estimated score. It is very likely that your score is in the range of these lines.
Your Score
SE
Anger 48 3
Anxiety 64 2
Depression 62 2
Fatigue 34 3
Pain Behavior 43 2
Pain Impact 56 2
10 20 30 40 50 60 70 80 90
Better
Average
Worse
Your Score
SE
Physical Function 38 2
Social Activity 48 2
Social Role 45 2
90 80 70 60 50 40 30 20 10
Better
Average
Worse

Fig. 4. An example of a PROMIS CAT display. (*Courtesy of* David Cella, PhD, Chicago, IL; with permission.)

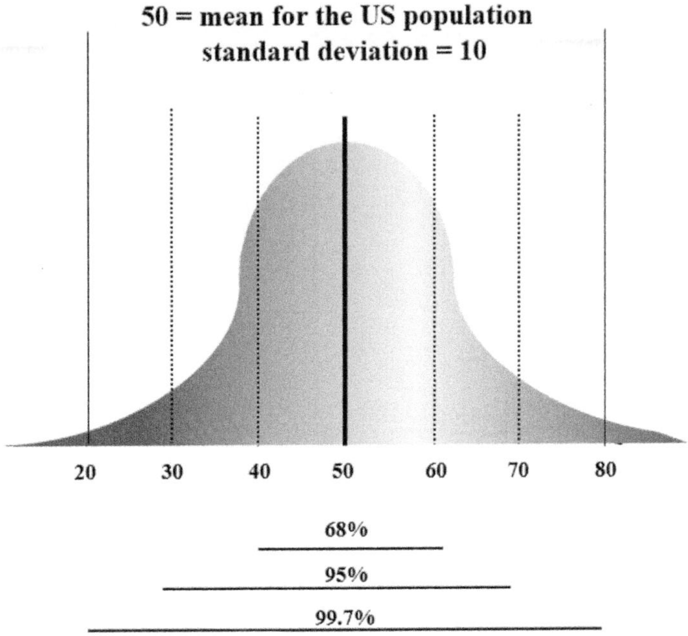

Fig. 5. The PROMIS T-score metric. (*Courtesy of* Clifton Bingham, MD, Baltimore, MD; with permission.)

necessarily exactly follow this distribution along a domain, but neither do other PRO instruments. In terms of scores, this means that values from 40 to 60 would cover 68% of the population, while scores from 20 to 80 capture 99.7%. With the explosion of "OMICs" in all facets of scientific research, PROMIS represents the contribution that "PROomics" into the OMIC family could add to the future of personalized, person-centric medicine. Integration of PROs with traditional (eg, genomics, epigenomics, metabolomics, microbiome) biomarkers of disease can lead to a better understanding of how disease mechanisms impact the domains of health, such as pain, PF, fatigue, or social interaction, and will ultimately improve the quality and generalizability of clinical research and patient care.

CONTENT OF PATIENT-REPORTED OUTCOMES MEASUREMENT INFORMATION SYSTEM MEASURES

Over the years, investigators from the PROMIS Cooperative Group have developed a robust and evolving library of psychometrically validated scales, short forms, profiles, and item banks that assess key domains/subdomains of patient-reported physical, mental, and social health. PROMIS is based on the observation that there are universally common, core domains that can help describe a person's health and disease and that these core domains can be measured in a clinically meaningful way across different diseases or conditions. Domains are latent traits, or "constructs," that represent how a patient feels or functions and are best known to the patient and ideally obtained using the patient's (or an appropriate proxy as in the case of young children) report. With a domain approach, PROMIS is agnostic to the disease, condition, and setting (eg, clinical or public health research, clinical or community-based care). Because what is being measured, the latent trait or domain, is being measured by the same instrument, the scores are instantly comparable, and no conversions are necessary.

PROMIS measures map onto the World Health Organization tripartite model of self-reported health encompassing physical, mental, and social health. This framework for adults, which is the same for pediatrics, is depicted in **Fig. 6**. The most current versions of these adult (and pediatric) instruments are accessible at the Assessment Center (http://www.assessmentcenter.net/).

Numerous options for the assessment of physical, mental, or social health were developed using PROMIS measures. The first tier of domains constitutes the PROMIS Profile measures. These Profiles, depicted in **Fig. 7**, are collections of short forms available in different lengths. The 29-, 43-, and 57-item questionnaires include 4, 6, or 8 questions from each of the 7 domains, respectively, plus a question involving pain intensity. These 7 important domains are intended to cover the range of physical, mental, and social health—a concept similar to the Short Form-36 (SF-36). As with PROs generally, longer PROMIS Profiles improve the precision of the estimate of where a patient's score is in one of these domains. Profiles also offer the option to easily include a broad range of PROMIS measures into clinical research or care without requiring the use of software. However, for considerations of maximizing precision, efficiency, and patient burden, CATs (see **Fig. 3**) may be a more attractive option than short forms in clinical settings.

PEDIATRIC PATIENT-REPORTED OUTCOMES MEASURES

In the second phase of PROMIS (eg, 2009–2014), there was a special emphasis[8] on developing and validating new pediatric (including their parent proxy) domains. The PROMIS pediatric framework was developed and additional measures were validated

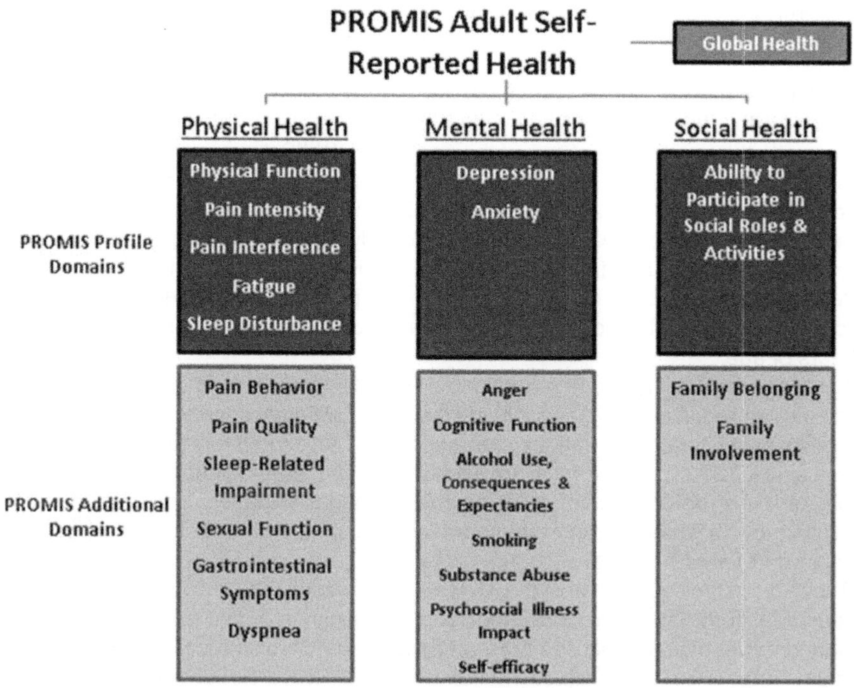

Fig. 6. Adult PROMIS domain structure. (*Courtesy of* PROMIS Health Organization and the PROMIS Cooperative Group, Evanston, IL; with permission.)

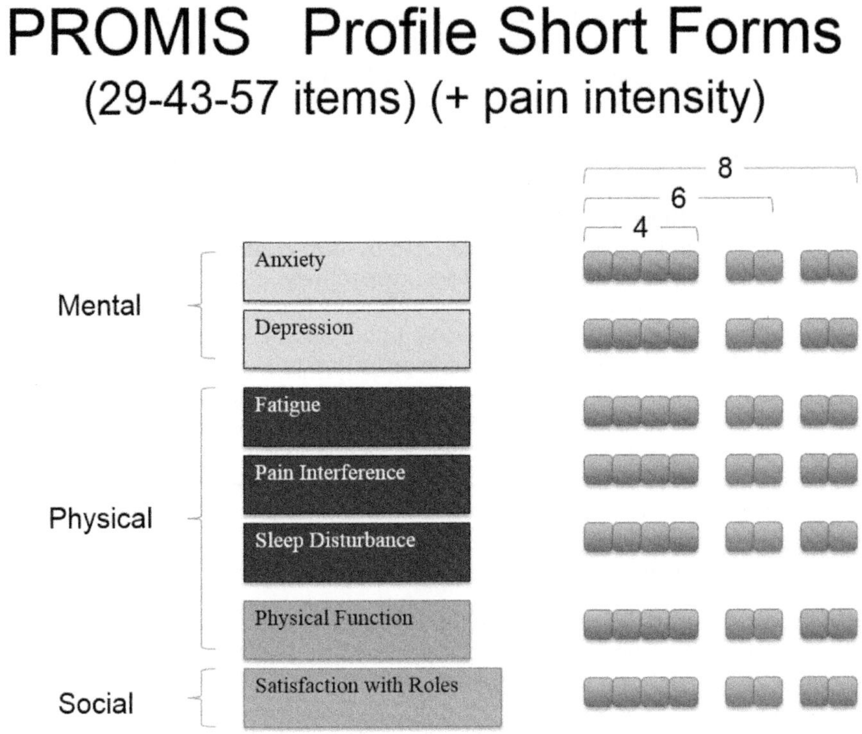

Fig. 7. The adult PROMIS profile measures. (*Courtesy of* David Cella, PhD, Chicago, IL; with permission.)

to include additional pediatric and parent or proxy domains (**Fig. 8**). Many of the domains within the pediatric framework also are measured with the PROMIS' adult framework; this is reflective of one of the goals of PROMIS, to measure across the lifespan within a domain, so that the same "latent trait" can be followed over time.

In some situations, such as with young children, traditional PROs are not possible due to the inability of children under age 8 to reliably self-report owing to their cognitive development stage. Therefore, PROMIS pediatric instruments for self-report are available for children 8 to 17 years, and parent-proxy reports are available for children aged 5 to 17 years. Currently, no PROMIS proxy measures exist for children younger than 5 years of age.

Similar to the adult banks, the top tier of PROMIS domains are included in PROMIS pediatric profiles. These domains include the 4-, 6-, or 8-item short forms of 6 domains (mobility, pain interference, fatigue, depression, anxiety, and peer relationships) along with a single item on pain intensity to yield the 25-, 37-, and 49-item versions, respectively, of these profiles. Again, owing to considerations of patient/parent burden and precision, CATs (when banks of items are available) may be a preferred option over longer short forms.[9]

The focus in the second half of the NIH PROMIS funding resulted in the new pediatric instruments (listed as in **Fig. 8** as Additional Domains). In pediatrics, the NIH-funded Validation of Pediatric Patient-Reported Outcomes in Chronic Diseases (PEPR) Consortium http://www.niams.nih.gov/Funding/Funded_Research/PEPR/default.asp will take important steps forward in clinically validating extant and newly developed PROMIS pediatric, and parent proxy instruments, for use in this often understudied population.

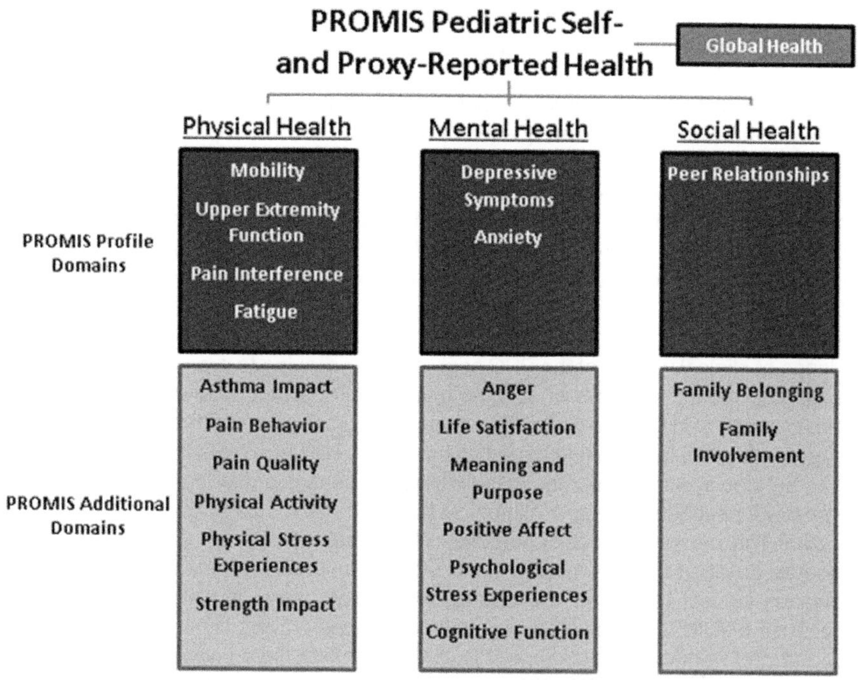

Fig. 8. PROMIS pediatric domain framework. (*Courtesy of* PROMIS Health Organization and the PROMIS Cooperative Group, Evanston, IL; with permission.)

PSYCHOMETRIC TESTING OF PATIENT-REPORTED OUTCOMES MEASUREMENT INFORMATION SYSTEM MEASURES

Validation of outcome measures is a journey, not a destination. **Fig. 9** depicts this rigorous validation journey for PROMIS measures. Foremost is ensuring that the psychometric aspects of PRO validation are adequately addressed early with psychometrically focused testing in the development of a PROMIS instrument as outlined in

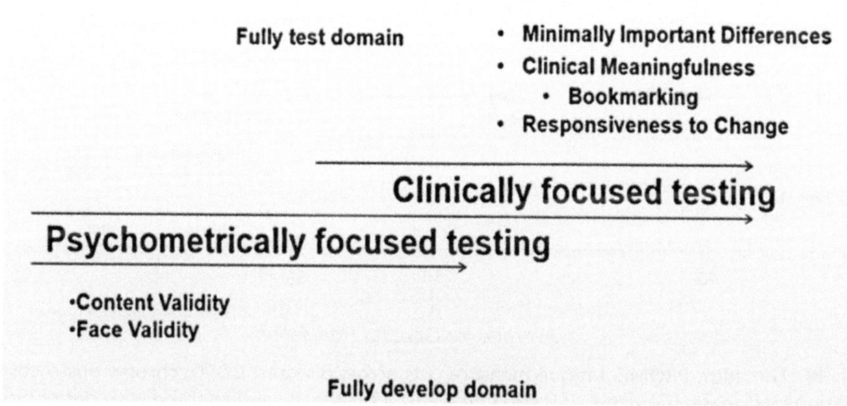

Fig. 9. The validation journey. (*Courtesy of* PROMIS Health Organization and the PROMIS Cooperative Group, Evanston, IL; with permission.)

the FDA guidance.[4] Items can be tested using qualitative techniques, such as focus groups and cognitive interviews designed to explicate the domain of interest under development. These important studies address issues such as differential item functioning, in which subgroups of respondents who are at the same level of the trait being measured answer a particular question differently. For example, the likelihood of crying is different for men and women.

Validation is a process in which evidence is collected regarding how scores on measures function for different purposes, in different contexts, and when answered by different populations. Therefore, validation of PROMIS (or any other measure) is never complete. The pertinent questions are whether the instrument is content valid for the patients under study and whether the scores are responsive to clinically meaningful changes. These more quantitative, clinically focused testing settings contribute to evidence of clinical validity of the PRO scores. When moving to practice settings, there is a need to understand both what is the minimally important difference (a property of the instrument) and what is clinically relevant change (eg, that which would inform or change health decision-making based on the result). However, with PROMIS measures that seek to be applicable across many different diseases and conditions, the issue of progressive psychometric and clinical validation is particularly germane and more complex. This complexity poses particular challenges when seeking to have PROMIS measures qualified by FDA for use in industry-sponsored trials (see later discussion, Regulatory Issues) as well as in adopting PROMIS measures in clinical practice.

Because PROMIS instruments were intended to be universally applicable to multiple adult and pediatric populations, PROMIS scientists have investigated the cross-cutting potential of adult PROMIS measures. Studies were designed to evaluate the responsiveness and sensitivity to change of PROMIS scores in varied longitudinal cohorts receiving different types of interventions. As can be seen in **Fig. 10**, the

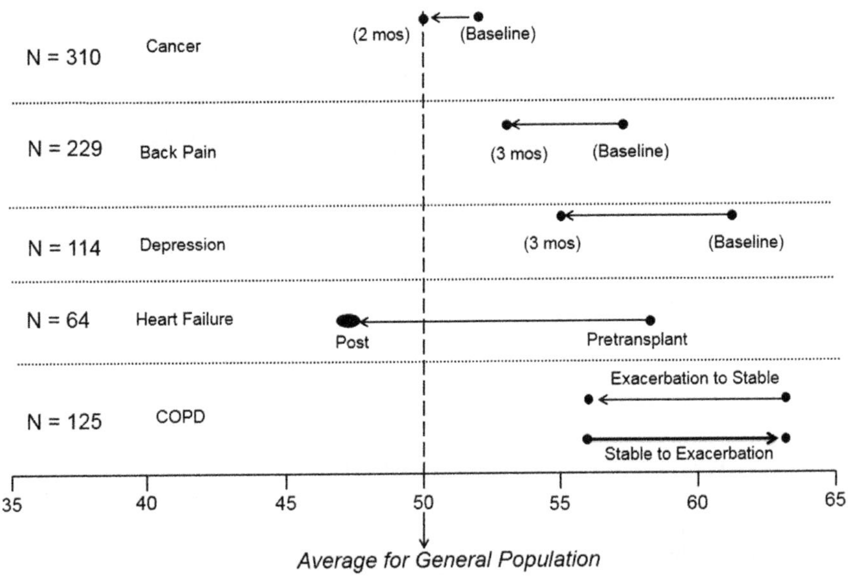

Fig. 10. The adult PROMIS fatigue measure cuts across diseases. COPD, chronic obstructive pulmonary disease. (*Courtesy of* David Cella, PhD, Chicago, IL, and adapted with permission of Peter Tugwell, MD, from Cella D, Lai JS, Jensen SE, et al. JCE series. J Clin Epidemiol. 2016 Mar 3. http://dx.doi.org/10.1016/j.jclinepi.2015.08.037. [Epub ahead of print].)

direction and generalized effect size of the changes in PROMIS fatigue offer initial proof of concept of the ability of PROMIS measures to capture change in a common domain (fatigue) caused by multiple diseases. Further details of these studies will be emerging soon.

RHEUMATOLOGY APPLICATIONS OF PATIENT-REPORTED OUTCOMES MEASUREMENT INFORMATION SYSTEM

The PROMIS PF instrument has a unique heritage emerging from the Health Assessment Questionnaire Disability Index (HAQ-DI).[10] The PROMIS PF item bank assesses one's ability to carry out activities that require physical actions, ranging from self-care (activities of daily living) to more complex activities that require a combination of skills, often within a social context. This definition is inclusive of the term disability and covers the full spectrum of PF from severe impairment to exceptional physical abilities. Because many persons with a chronic disease have more than one chronic condition and often are unable to distinguish the proportion of physical limitation attributable to each condition, the PROMIS PF items assess physical capabilities and limitations without causal attribution. The PROMIS PF bank comprises 4 related subdomains: mobility (lower extremity function), dexterity (upper extremity function), axial (neck and back function), and ability to carry out instrumental activities of daily living.

The evolution of PF/disability from the HAQ-DI to the PROMIS item bank was intended to address the so-called floor and ceiling effects seen with legacy (traditional) measures.[11] A measure with a high floor effect will miss patients who are severely disabled (eg, the bed-bound), and a measure with a low ceiling effect will miss patients who can perform daily life activities but who seek to maximize their functioning (eg, those wishing to engage in vigorous exercise). This restriction in range of measurement ultimately limits the utility of a PRO to measure a domain. Thus, the benefit of the PROMIS PF 124-item bank is that it covers a broad range of PF levels so assessing more of the trait being measured while improving its precision compared with the HAQ-DI, the SF-36 measures, or other legacy measures that informed it (**Fig. 11**). As the figure shows, the PROMIS 10-item CAT measures a greater range of PF (x-axis) with improved precision (y-axis) compared with the HAQ-DI and SF-36 measures.

It is noteworthy that the 2015 American College of Rheumatology (ACR) Guideline for the Treatment of Rheumatoid Arthritis,[12] the PROMIS PF bank, as well as the 10- and 20-item PROMIS PF short forms are mentioned as options for functional status assessment. The recommendation is to use routinely a standardized, validated measure for RA patients. The recommendation is that these measurements occur at least once per year and with greater frequency when disease is active. This ACR endorsement and recommendation will help to introduce PROMIS PF into common RA clinical research and patient care settings and enable continued clinical and psychometric validation. It remains to be seen if the ACR 20/50/70 Responder Index, which includes the HAQ-DI as one of its optional outcome measures, will adopt PROMIS PF measures instead. Such a change has been recommended by the developers of the HAQ-DI.[13,14]

PROMIS measures are being studied in a widening array of patients with rheumatic diseases in various settings. For example, the construct validity of the multidimensional PROMIS 29 profile of short forms has been studied and was recently reported in systemic sclerosis in the Scleroderma Patient-Centered Intervention Network cohort.[15] There were moderate to high correlations demonstrated between legacy measures with the correlative subdomains contained within the PROMIS 29. In

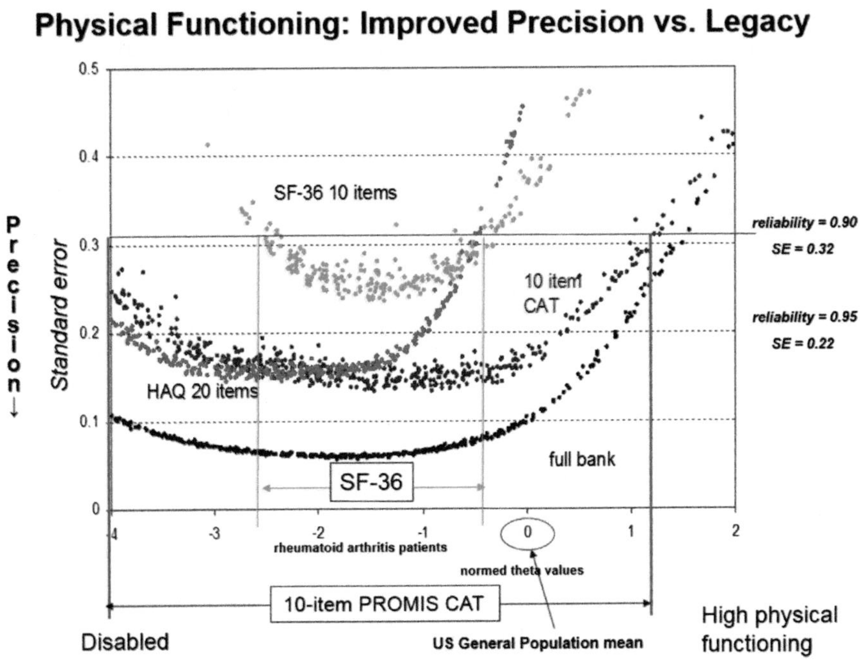

Fig. 11. PROMIS CAT and short forms compared with HAQ and SF-36. In this figure, floor versus ceiling for PF are conceptualized (x-axis) as disabled on the left-hand, bottom corner to high PF on the right-hand corner. This same PF scale is seen in **Fig. 2**. On the T-score metric (see **Fig. 5**), the average score in the US general population is centered on 0, but transformed to a score of 50 using a linear T-score transformation. Here, the US population mean is in the original metric of =0 with a possible distribution of −4 to +4. One standard deviation above or below the mean is −1 and +1, respectively, on the graph, but −10 or +10 points with the T-score transformation shown in **Fig. 5**. RA patients tend to be 1 or 2 SD lower (more disabled) compared with the US general population, which translates into a score of −1 or −2 on the graph and −40 or −30 on **Fig. 5**. The legacy SF-36, 10-item instrument captures part of this RA population; the HAQ 20-item instrument extends the floor, but not the ceiling. Both the PROMIS 10-item CAT and the full CAT (which uses the entire 124-item bank) improve not only the breadth and range of measurement but also the precision of the estimate (y-axis). The minimally important difference for the PROMIS 20-item PF short form is 2 points. SE, standard error. (*Courtesy of* Matthias Rose, PhD, MD, Berlin, Germany; with permission.)

some domains, there were floor and ceiling effects demonstrated. Because the PROMIS instruments are based on IRT-calibrated banks, additional items can be added, and their parameters can be anchored on the existing metric, making it possible to improve (iterate) existing measures without jeopardizing comparability to earlier versions.

A recent study evaluated the feasibility of using PROMIS measures in the longitudinal care of 177 patients with RA seen for routine clinical care.[16] This study demonstrated that PROMIS measures could identify the level of symptoms and impacts across a range of domains of physical, mental, and social health and across the continuum of experience from 2 standard deviations (SD) below the population mean to 2 SD above the population mean for most domains. Reliability, internal consistency, and convergent validity were demonstrated. Importantly, PROMIS measures overcame existing floor effects of legacy PROs used for RA. PROMIS measures showed known groups validity with dose-response relationships between levels of symptoms and RA disease activity measured by Clinical Disease Activity Index. Importantly, PROMIS measures were able to demonstrate the ongoing impact of RA even in patients who had achieved a target of low disease activity. The investigators of this study also recently evaluated whether PROMIS items contained within banks and short forms were relevant to people living with RA.[17] The investigators provided preliminary evidence regarding the content validity of PROMIS measures in RA patients in terms of importance and relevance of selected PROMIS domains and items to the RA experience. Additional qualitative and quantitative studies are ongoing.

PROMIS measures have also been evaluated recently in patients with psoriatic arthritis in a clinical care cohort.[18] Similar to the RA study noted above, impacts across multiple domains of physical, mental, and social health were demonstrated. PROMIS scores for pain interference, PF, sleep disturbance, sleep-related impairment, anger, and ability to participate in social roles were significantly worse in patients reporting disease flares.

Another recent study, using PROMIS CATs, assessed the feasibility and construct validity of including selected PROMIS instruments in a longitudinal cohort of patients with vasculitis.[19] PROMIS measures were found to have cross-sectional construct validity, and their scores discriminated patients with active disease from those in remission.

The feasibility of using PROMIS measures and the validity of their scores in SLE patients have been studied.[20] PROMIS CATs were successfully administered to diverse SLE patients at the point of care and remotely. Scores on PROMIS measures of many SLE-relevant domains were found to be valid, reliable, and responsive. It was particularly noteworthy that PROMIS scores did not correlate strongly with the Systemic Lupus Erythematosus Disease Activity Index (SLEDAI). The SLEDAI assesses disease activity by using a combination of clinical history, physical examination, organ-specific functional tests, and serologic studies. The lack of strong associations between objective signs and symptoms as measured by the SLEDAI and the subjective patient disease experience as measured by PROMIS highlights the crucial need to integrate PROs into clinical care to ensure optimal, personalized disease management.

The validity (known-group and ecological) and test-retest reliability of 4 PROMIS domains were evaluated in osteoarthritis (OA) patients. Short forms were compared with CATs providing initial data on the utility of PROMIS instruments for clinical and research outcomes in OA patients.[21] A task force convened by the NIH Pain Consortium drew heavily on PROMIS methodology in their recommendations for research standards on chronic lower back pain.[22] In orthopedics, as part of an initiative by the American Orthopedic Foot and Ankle Society to explore the use of CATs for patient-level reporting, the CAT version of the PROMIS PF domain has been initially validated as an excellent method for measuring PROs after injuries and treatment. The use of PROMIS PF CAT as a preferred alternative to legacy instruments, such as the SF-36, would be a paradigm shift to measure PROs in patients with foot and ankle disorders.[23]

As in adults, the PROMIS pediatric instruments have been included in a growing number of studies of children with rheumatic diseases. PROMIS pediatric assessments from both the child and the parent-proxy perspectives were included for a sample of patients with juvenile idiopathic arthritis (JIA) aged 8 to 17 years (all JIA categories) and parent proxies for ages 5 to 17 years.[24] Results demonstrated that the PROMIS pediatric short forms (8 items) were feasible to complete, responsive to JIA disease activity, and had comparable error to the full item banks for both the child and the proxy report. In a longitudinal study, 100 patients with childhood-onset lupus completed pediatric PROMIS short forms (anger, anxiety, depression, fatigue, mobility, upper extremity function, pain interference, peer relations) and accepted legacy measures.[25] The pediatric PROMIS short forms demonstrated construct validity, and scores were responsive to change in this sample, while respondent and clinician time burden were reduced relative to legacy measures. To investigate the construct validity and responsiveness to change of 7 PROMIS domains, longitudinal evaluations occurred in an outpatient chronic pain clinic and intensive pain day treatment program.[26] All 7 PROMIS domains showed responsiveness to change supporting further validation with larger and more diverse pediatric pain samples.

PATIENT-REPORTED OUTCOMES MEASUREMENT INFORMATION SYSTEM AND THE FOOD AND DRUG ADMINISTRATION

From an FDA perspective, the term qualification is a regulatory term that means the "tool" has undergone critical FDA review through the Center for Drug Evaluation and Research's Drug development Tools Qualification program.[27] Once this process is satisfied, FDA publishes these clinical outcome assessments. They are intended, as appropriate, for wider use because the process of qualification is best envisioned to occur in the precompetitive space. The FDA, NIH, and PROMIS investigators have had multiple meetings to discuss considerations in qualifying PROMIS instruments. If appropriately qualified, PROMIS measures could be included as exploratory, secondary, and eventually, primary endpoints in a wide variety of diseases in properly powered and rigorously designed industry-sponsored clinical trials. Because the PROMIS metric is the same whether measures are administered in a trial seeking FDA registration of a therapy or to patients at the point of care, meaningful comparisons of the effectiveness of a therapy can be made between scores in these very different settings.

There are currently several ongoing projects to qualify PROMIS measures as endpoints, including for industry-sponsored clinical trials. For example, the adult PROMIS fatigue measures are being looked at in myalgic encephalomyelitis/chronic fatigue syndrome/systemic exertion intolerance disease and for measurement of fatigue in adults ($\geq$18 years) with RA with mild to severe disease activity.[28] Soon to be added to this list is the adult PROMIS PF measure, which is being evaluated in adults with advanced solid tumors and sarcopenia.

As evidence accumulates from an expanding number of clinical observational studies or interventional trials supported by NIH, Patient-Centered Outcomes Research Institute, PCORI (http://www.pcori.org/), or other funding agencies both nationally and internationally that include PROMIS measures as outcomes, these data will provide important information in defining expected changes in response to various therapies. Subsets of patients can potentially be identified from such studies that are similar to those who may participate in industry-sponsored studies. However, the use of PROMIS measures as exploratory outcomes in industry-sponsored clinical trials would provide an important evidence base to further inform measure qualification.

INTERNATIONAL SCOPE

PROMIS items have been translated into more than 40 languages (http://www.nihpromis.org/measures/translations); thus, international studies are emerging as additional exciting options to advance PRO science and create unique opportunities for collaboration. An expanding PROMIS international working group (http://www.nihpromis.org/science/PROMISInternational) has developed and is executing a strategic action plan for the international spread of PROMIS. The vision for PROMIS-International is to advance the creation, evaluation, adoption, and dissemination of a cross-culturally harmonized "common metric" for measurement of person-reported health outcomes. Having valid international assessment tools is especially important for organizations such as OMERACT (Outcome Measures in Rheumatology; http://www.omeract.org/) that seek to advance patient-oriented research worldwide in rheumatic diseases, and ISOQOL (International Society for Quality of Life Research; http://www.isoqol.org/), across diseases.

FUTURE OPPORTUNITIES

PROs provide important insights into individuals' health and well-being, including the major role symptoms play in the onset and progression of disease, day-to-day function, and response to treatments. In clinical research and health care settings, robust, accurate, and feasible assessment of symptoms has the potential to greatly improve research and patient care. The current adoption and incorporation of PROMIS into large electronic health records systems such as EPIC and through projects, such as the PCORI-sponsored National Patient-Centered Clinical Research Network, PCOR-net (http://www.pcori.org/research-results/pcornet-national-patient-centered-clinical-research-network), offers new avenues and unprecedented opportunities for valuable comparative effectiveness research using "real-world" data. PROMIS can also be administered through widely used research applications, such as RedCAP (https://redcap.vanderbilt.edu/). Translation of findings from clinical trials to clinical practice would be greatly facilitated by using measures in those clinical trials that are also use in clinical practice. It is particularly encouraging and exciting that FDA acknowledges PROMIS as a means to bring patient-reported outcome measures into the era of the Precision Medicine Initiative.[29]

There is growing appreciation[16,23] in clinical medicine and patient care that PRO data, not unlike blood-derived biomarkers or advanced imaging, need to be collected routinely to support patient engagement to improve their clinical management. If this is to occur, routine PRO data collection must be viewed as beneficial to a range of stakeholders, including patients, clinicians, researchers, health care administrators, and policymakers. Additional studies are needed to determine which measures can yield reliable and valid data across settings with minimal burden, and how to coordinate resources to standardize and harmonize regional, national, and international efforts. This knowledge will be critical to successful adoption, implementation, and utility for a broad range of stakeholders. Optimal use of PROs, including PROMIS, ultimately will be the result of continued implementation into clinical care settings and sustained research funded by multiple sources, including the federal government, PCORI, and the regulated industry. Both opportunities and challenges await.

That PROMIS measures can be administered both at the time of service in clinical care (or a clinical research visit) and remotely by patients at their convenience via the Internet (such as between scheduled visits or national surveys) provides additional opportunities to examine changes in symptoms and disease impacts over time at both the individual and the population level. This access may have relevance in conditions such as RA in monitoring responses to therapy or capturing early signs of disease worsening or "flare."[30]

From its inception, PROMIS was intended to improve the ability to capture patient-centered information. PROMIS has resoundingly exceeded the goals envisioned during its idealistic beginnings in 2004,[31] but the sky is the limit for the future. The system is now operational at a national level and increasingly on an international scale. With PROMIS measures, there exists a truly unique window of opportunity for transforming national and international clinical research and improving health care. Now, more than ever, PROMIS is poised to be included in all types of pediatric and adult clinical research and patient care, including in comparative effectiveness research as well as pragmatic clinical trials, and is emerging as a potential valuable contributor to improving clinical care. Because PROMIS encompasses those aspects of health most relevant to the patient experience across diseases, it can provide useful, quantifiable information to both patients and health professionals that can be used to make more informed and shared health decisions.

Achieving the optimal potential of PROMIS will be facilitated through widespread, vigorous adoption and adaption by the clinical research and care community—such as the NIH Clinical Center.[32] Including PROMIS measures in clinical research and trials, along with appropriate disease-specific instruments, will complement and strengthen improved assessment of the patient experiences of symptoms and their HRQL. PROMIS offers the option to effectively bridge the continuum from research to population health and provide information that will truly enable precision, person-centered medicine.

REFERENCES

1. Khanna D, Krishnan E, Dewitt EM, et al. The future of measuring patient-reported outcomes in rheumatology: patient-reported outcomes measurement information system (PROMIS) [review. No abstract available]. Arthritis Care Res (Hoboken) 2011;63(Suppl 11):S486–90.
2. Available at: https://commonfund.nih.gov/promis/index. Accessed March 01, 2016.
3. Patrick DL, Burke LB, Gwaltney CJ, et al. Content validity–establishing and reporting the evidence in newly developed patient-reported outcomes (PRO) instruments for medical product evaluation: ISPOR PRO Good Research Practices Task Force report: part 2–assessing respondent understanding. Value Health 2011;14(8):978–88.
4. Available at: http://www.fda.gov/downloads/drugs/guidancecomplianceregulatoryinformation/guidances/ucm193282.pdf. Accessed March 01, 2016.
5. Kirwan JR, Bartlett SJ, Beaton DE, et al. Updating the OMERACT filter: implications for patient-reported outcomes. J Rheumatol 2014;41(5):1011–5.
6. Bantug ET, Coles T, Smith KC, et al, PRO Data Presentation Stakeholder Advisory Board. Graphical displays of patient-reported outcomes (PRO) for use in clinical practice: what makes a PRO picture worth a thousand words? [review]. Patient Educ Couns 2015. http://dx.doi.org/10.1016/j.pec.2015.10.027.
7. Brundage MD, Smith KC, Little EA, et al, PRO Data Presentation Stakeholder Advisory Board. Communicating patient-reported outcome scores using graphic formats: results from a mixed-methods evaluation. Qual Life Res 2015;24(10):2457–72.
8. Available at: http://grants.nih.gov/grants/guide/rfa-files/RFA-RM-08-023.html. Accessed March 01, 2016.
9. Available at: http://www.nihpromis.org/measures/availableinstruments. Accessed March 01, 2016.

10. Bruce B, Fries JF. The health assessment questionnaire (HAQ). Clin Exp Rheumatol 2005;23(5 Suppl 39):S14–8.
11. Fries JF, Lingala B, Siemons L, et al. Extending the floor and the ceiling for assessment of physical function. Arthritis Rheumatol 2014;66(No 5):1378–87.
12. Singh JA, Saag KG, Bridges SL Jr, et al. 2015 American College of Rheumatology guideline for the treatment of rheumatoid arthritis. Arthritis Care Res 2015. http://dx.doi.org/10.1002/acr.22783.
13. Fries JF, Krishnan E, Rose M, et al. Improved responsiveness and reduced sample size requirements of PROMIS physical function scales with item response theory. Arthritis Res Ther 2011;13(5):R147.
14. Oude Voshaar MA, Ten Klooster PM, Glas CA, et al. Relative performance of commonly used physical function questionnaires in rheumatoid arthritis and a patient-reported outcomes measurement information system computerized adaptive test. Arthritis Rheumatol 2014;66(10):2900–8.
15. Available at: http://acrabstracts.org/abstract/construct-validity-of-the-promis-29-in-systemic-sclerosis-results-from-the-scleroderma-patient-centered-intervention-network-spin-cohort/. Accessed March 01, 2016.
16. Bartlett SJ, Orbai AM, Duncan T, et al. Reliability and validity of selected PROMIS measures in people with rheumatoid arthritis. PLoS One 2015;10(9):e0138543.
17. Available at: http://acrabstracts.org/abstract/preliminary-content-validation-of-the-patient-reported-outcomes-measurement-information-system-promis-short-forms-in-people-living-with-rheumatoid-arthritis/. Accessed March 01, 2016.
18. Orbai AM, Bartlett S, Duncan T, et al. Multidimensional health related quality of life assessment using PROMIS (Patient Reported Outcome Measurement Information System) measures in psoriatic arthritis flares. Ann Rheum Dis 2014;73(Suppl 2):1048–9.
19. Available at: http://acrabstracts.org/abstract/administration-of-patient-reported-outcome-measurement-information-system-promis-instruments-by-computer-adaptive-testing-in-patients-with-systemic-vasculitis/. Accessed March 01, 2016.
20. Available at: http://acrabstracts.org/abstract/feasibility-and-validity-of-patient-reported-outcome-measurement-information-system-promis-in-sle/. Accessed March 01, 2016.
21. Broderick JE, Schneider S, Junghaenel DU, et al. Validity and reliability of patient-reported outcomes measurement information system instruments in osteoarthritis. Arthritis Care Res 2013;65(No. 10):1625–33.
22. Deyo RA, Dworkin SF, Amtmann D, et al. Report of the NIH Task Force on research standards for chronic low back pain. Pain 2014;15(6):569–85.
23. Hung M, Baumhauer JF, Latt LD, et al, National Orthopaedic Foot & Ankle Outcomes Research Network. Validation of PROMIS physical function computerized adaptive tests for orthopaedic foot and ankle outcome research. Clin Orthop Relat Res 2013;(471):3466–74.
24. Available at: http://acrabstracts.org/abstract/promis-tools-for-measurement-of-patient-reported-outcomes-in-children-with-juvenile-arthritis/. Accessed March 01, 2016.
25. Available at: http://acrabstracts.org/abstract/validation-of-patient-reported-outcomes-measurement-information-system-promis-modules-for-use-in-childhood-onset-lupus/. Accessed March 01, 2016.
26. Zuck SK, Carle A, Barnett K, et al. Longitudinal evaluation of patient reported outcomes measurement information systems (PROMIS) measures in pediatric chronic pain. Pain 2015. http://dx.doi.org/10.1097/j.pain.0000000000000378.

27. Available at: http://www.fda.gov/downloads/drugs/guidancecompliance regulatoryinformation/guidances/ucm230597.pdf. Accessed March 01, 2016.
28. Available at: http://www.fda.gov/Drugs/DevelopmentApprovalProcess/Drug DevelopmentToolsQualificationProgram/ucm450689.htm. Accessed March 01, 2016.
29. Hunter NL, O'Callaghan KM, Califf RM. Engaging patients across the spectrum of medical product development: view from the US Food and Drug Administration. JAMA 2015;314(23):2499–500.
30. Alten R, Pohl C, Choy EH, et al, The OMERACT RA Flare Definition Working Group. Developing a construct to evaluate flares in rheumatoid arthritis: a conceptual report of the OMERACT RA Flare Definition Working Group. J Rheumatol 2011; 38:1745–50. Available at: http://www.jrheum.org/content/38/8/1745.
31. Available at: http://www.nihpromis.org/Documents/PROMIS_The_First_Four_Years.pdf. Accessed March 01, 2016.
32. Bevans M, Ross A, Cella D. Patient-Reported Outcomes Measurement Information System (PROMIS): efficient, standardized tools to measure self-reported health and quality of life. Nurs Outlook 2014;62(201):339–45.

Index

Note: Page numbers of article titles are in **boldface** type.

A

ABILHAND questionnaire, 308
Activities Scale for Kids, in juvenile idiopathic arthritis, 337
Activity in Lupus to Energize and Renew study, 256–257
Affective vulnerability, in fibromyalgia, 322–323
Affordable Care Act, 364
American College of Rheumatology
  Clinical Disease Activity Measures Working Group, 223
  fibromyalgia classification of, 318
  outcome measures of, 220
  PRO data collections of, 367
  response index of, 274
American Pain Society, fibromyalgia assessment and, 319–320
American Rheumatism Association, functional classification, 206
Ankylosing spondylitis, **285–299**
Ankylosing Spondylitis Disease Activity Score (ASDAS), 287, 289, 291–294
Ankylosing Spondylitis Quality of Life questionnaire, 286–288, 290, 292
Anxiety, in fibromyalgia, 323
Arithmetical Mean of Desirability Functions, in psoriatic arthritis, 276
Arthritis
  juvenile idiopathic, **333–346**
  knee, **239–252**
  psoriatic, **265–283**
  rheumatoid. *See* Rheumatoid arthritis.
Arthritis and Rheumatism, 206
Arthritis Care and Research, 206–207
Arthritis Impact Measurement Scales, 206–207
  in psoriatic arthritis, 270
  in rheumatoid arthritis, 224
Arthritis Self-Efficacy Scales, in fibromyalgia, 324
ASDAS (Ankylosing Spondylitis Disease Activity Score), 287, 289, 291–294
Assessment of Spondyloarthritis International Society (ASAS) criteria, 286, 289
Athens Insomnia Scale, for rheumatoid arthritis, 227
Attitudes, in fibromyalgia, 323–324
Australian Rheumatoid Association, quality indicators of, 221–222
Axial spondyloarthritis, **285–299**
  history of, 286
  PROs and PROMs in
    clinical use of, 295
    measures for, 286–289
    validation of, 289–295

Rheum Dis Clin N Am 42 (2016) 395–405
http://dx.doi.org/10.1016/S0889-857X(16)30008-4

B

BASDAI (Bath Ankylosing Spondylitis Disease Activity Index), 269–272, 287–289, 291–295
Baseline Dyspnea Index, in systemic sclerosis, 306, 310
BASFI (Bath Ankylosing Spondylitis Functional Index), 287–288, 290–292
BAS-G (Bath Ankylosing Spondylitis Global) score, 287, 289
BASMI (Bath Ankylosing Spondylitis Metrology Index), 287, 290, 293
Bath Ankylosing Spondylitis Disease Activity Index (BASDAI), 269–272, 287–289, 291–295
Bath Ankylosing Spondylitis Functional Index (BASFI), 287–288, 290–292
Bath Ankylosing Spondylitis Global (BAS-G) score, 287, 289
Bath Ankylosing Spondylitis Metrology Index (BASMI), 287, 290, 293
Beck Depression Inventory
  in fibromyalgia, 322–323
  in rheumatoid arthritis, 227
Behavior, in fibromyalgia, 325
Beliefs About Pain Control Questionnaire, in fibromyalgia, 324
Beliefs, in fibromyalgia, 323–324
Boolean-based definition, in patient education, 353
Borg Dyspnea Index, in systemic sclerosis, 306, 310
Brady, Teresa, 207
Brief Pain Inventory, in fibromyalgia, 319–320, 325
British Isles Lupus Activity Disease Score, 254–255

C

Caliln, Andrei, on axial spondyloarthritis, 286
CAMPHOR (Cambridge Pulmonary Hypertension Review), in systemic sclerosis, 306, 310
Catastrophizing, in fibromyalgia, 324
Center for Epidemiologic Studies Depression Scale, in fibromyalgia, 322–323
Centers for Medicare and Medical Services, quality measures of, 364–365
Child Activity Limitations Interview-21, in juvenile idiopathic arthritis, 335–336
Child Health Questionnaire, in juvenile idiopathic arthritis, 336
Childhood and Recent Traumatic Events Scale, in fibromyalgia, 322
Childhood Health Assessment Questionnaire, in juvenile idiopathic arthritis, 335
Children's Assessment of Participation and Enjoyment, in juvenile idiopathic arthritis, 336, 338
Children's Health Insurance Program, 364
Chronic overlapping pain syndrome, 320–321
Classic test theory, 208–209
Clinical Diagnostic Criteria for Fibromyalgia, 318
Clinical Disease Activity Index, 367
Cochin Hand Function Scale, 308
Cognitive dysfunction, in fibromyalgia, 318, 321
Colombo, Realdo, on axial spondyloarthritis, 286
Complex Multi-Symptom Inventory, in fibromyalgia, 320–321
Composite PROMs
  in juvenile idiopathic arthritis, 338–339
  in psoriatic arthritis, 274–277
Composite Psoriatic Disease Activity Index, 276
Computerized adaptive testing, 367–368, 379–381, 389

in juvenile idiopathic arthritis, 339
in rheumatoid arthritis, 356
in systemic lupus erythematosus, 256
in systemic sclerosis, 310
Coping strategies, in fibromyalgia, 324
Core set of disease activity, in rheumatoid arthritis, 219

D

Depression
in fibromyalgia, 323
in rheumatoid arthritis, 227–228
in systemic sclerosis, 310
Dermatologic Life Quality Index, 268, 272–273
DFI (Dougados Functional Index), 287–288, 291, 293
Digital ulcers, in systemic sclerosis, 309–310
Disabilities of Arm, Shoulder, and Hand Questionnaire, 269, 272, 308
Disablement model, 240
Disease Activity Index for Psoriatic Arthritis, 275–276
Disease Activity Index for Reactive Arthritis, 275–276
Disease Activity Score, in psoriatic arthritis, 274–275
Domains
in PROMIS, 382–384
in rheumatic measures, 207–208
Donabedian model, quality indicators of, 221
Dougados Functional Index (DFI), 287–288, 291, 293
Dunox Hand Index, 308
Dydactic Adjustment Scale, in fibromyalgia, 325–326
Dyspnea, in systemic sclerosis, 310

E

Electronic health records
in juvenile idiopathic arthritis, 340
in quality registers, 367
English, limited proficiency in, in rheumatoid arthritis, PROMs in, **347–362**
Environmental factors, in fibromyalgia, 325
European League Against Rheumatism (EULAR)
Outcome Measures Library, 228
rheumatoid arthritis criteria of, 220–221
European Musculoskeletal Conditions Surveillance and Information Network, quality indicators of, 221
European Quality of Life Index-5 Dimensions
in psoriatic arthritis, 268, 270
in systemic lupus erythematosus, 254–255
in systemic sclerosis, 305–306

F

FACIT (Functional Assessment of Chronic Illness Therapy), in systemic sclerosis, 306, 310
Fatigue

Fatigue (*continued*)
in fibromyalgia, 318, 321
in psoriatic arthritis, 273
in rheumatoid arthritis, 220, 223, 227–228
in systemic sclerosis, 302, 310
Fibromyalgia, **317–332**
classification of, 318
clinical trials of, 326–327
comorbidities of, 320–322
definition of, 318
diagnosis of, 318–319
monitoring of, 319
phenotyping of, 319–326
Fibromyalgia Impact Questionnaire-Revised, 325
Fibrosis, in systemic sclerosis, 302
Food and Drug Administration, PROMIS and, 378, 390
Fries, James F., 206–207
Function domain, of rheumatic measures, 207–208
Functional Assessment of Chronic Illness Therapy (FACIT)
Fatigue, 269, 273
in systemic sclerosis, 306, 310
Functional status, in juvenile idiopathic arthritis, 335, 337–338

G

Galen, on axial spondyloarthritis, 286
Gastrointestinal involvement, in systemic sclerosis, 307–309
Gastrointestinal Symptoms Scale for Kids, in juvenile idiopathic arthritis, 337–338
Geisinger Health System, PRO data collection registries of, 367
General Anxiety Disorder questionnaire, 322–323
Global assessment
in psoriatic arthritis, 267
in systemic sclerosis, 305
Group for Research and Assessment of Psoriasis and Psoriatic Arthritis, 267

H

Hand involvement and disability, in systemic sclerosis, 307–308
Health Assessment Questionnaire
in ankylosing spondylitis, 288, 293
in rheumatoid arthritis, 220, 350
in systemic sclerosis, 303, 306
Health Assessment Questionnaire Disability Index, 206–209, 387
in psoriatic arthritis, 269, 272
in rheumatoid arthritis, 220, 224–225
Health care quality, definition of, 364
Health care quality, PROs and PROMs in, **363–375**
as indicators, 364–365
future of, 368, 371–372
guidelines for, 368–370
literature search for, 374–375

National Quality Forum endorsement of, 367–368
national systems for, 365–366
United States registries for, 366–367
Health literacy, limited, in rheumatoid arthritis, PROMs in, **347–362**
Health status domain, of rheumatic measures, 207–208
Health-related quality of life
in juvenile idiopathic arthritis, 338
in psoriatic arthritis, 267, 270–271
History, of patient-reported outcomes, **205–217**
beginning of, 206–207
in rheumatoid arthritis, 220–221
measures available for, 207–208
refinement of approaches for, 208–209
routine use of, 209–210
Hospital Anxiety and Depression Scale
in fibromyalgia, 322–323
in rheumatoid arthritis, 227

I

IMMPACT (Initiative on Methods, Measurement and Pain Assessment in Clinical Trials), 325–327
Independence, in rheumatoid arthritis, 223
Index-based definition, in patient education, 353
Information system. *See* PROMIS (Patient-Reported Outcomes Measurement Information System).
Initiative on Methods, Measurement and Pain Assessment in Clinical Trials (IMMPACT), in fibromyalgia, 325–327
International Classification of Functioning, Disability and Health Model, 240
International Personality Item Pool, in fibromyalgia, 323
International scope, of PROMIS, 390–391
Item response theory, 208–209, 379–380
in rheumatoid arthritis, 225

J

Juvenile Arthritis Functional Assessment Report, 337–339
Juvenile Arthritis Quality of Life Questionnaire, 336
Juvenile Arthritis Self-Report Index, 337–338
Juvenile idiopathic arthritis, PROs and PROMs in, **333–346**
categories of, 334
challenges with, 339–340
composite, 338–339
for clinical care, 340
for functional status, 335, 337–338
for medication side effects, 338
for pain, 335–336
for quality of life, 338
for research, 340–341
PROMIS, 339

K

Kelvin, Lord, 205–206
Knee Injury and Osteoarthritis Outcome Score Function in Sport and Recreation subscale, 242–247
Knee osteoarthritis, PROs and PROMs in, **239–252**
importance of, 240
Knee Injury and Osteoarthritis Outcome Score Function in Sport and Recreation subscale, 242–247
Patient Reported Outcomes Measurement Information System physical function, 247–248
psychometric properties of, 240–241
Western Ontario and Master Universities physical function subscale, 241–242
KOOS (Knee Injury and Osteoarthritis Outcome Score) Function in Sport and Recreation subscale, 242–247

L

Lansbury Systemic Index, for rheumatoid arthritis, 220
Limited health literacy and limited English proficiency, in rheumatoid arthritis, PROs and PROMs in, **347–362**
Lupus. *See* Systemic lupus erythematosus.
Lupus Patient-Reported Outcome, 257–258
Lupus Quality of Life Questionnaire, 254–258

M

McGill Pain Questionnaire, in fibromyalgia, 319
Measurement of Patient Outcome in Arthritis, 206
Measuring Health Status in Arthritis: The Arthritis Impact Measurement Scales, 206
Medical Outcome Study Sleep Measure
in fibromyalgia, 321–323
in rheumatoid arthritis, 227
Medical Outcomes Study Short Form 36
in fibromyalgia, 325
in psoriatic arthritis, 268, 270
in systemic lupus erythematosus, 254–255
Medication side effects, in juvenile idiopathic arthritis, 338
Meenan, R. F., 206
Mental Component Score, in Medical Outcomes Study Short Form 36, 270
Mental Health Inventory, for rheumatoid arthritis, 227
Merit-based incentive payment system, 364
Methotrexate Intolerance Severity Score questionnaire, 337–338
Michigan Hand Questionnaire, 308
Minimal clinical important difference, of psychometric properties, 240–241
Minimal Disease Activity, in psoriatic arthritis, 276
Mixed method approach, to PROMIS development, 378
Modified Stanford Health Assessment questionnaire, 207
Morning stiffness, in rheumatoid arthritis, 220–221
Mouth disability, in systemic sclerosis, 307–308
Mouth Handicap Scale, 308

Multidimensional Fatigue Inventory, in fibromyalgia, 321–322
Multidimensional Health Assessment Questionnaire, 223, 225, 228, 350, 367–368
Multidimensional Inventory of Subjective Cognitive Impairment, 321–322
Multiple Ability Self-Report Questionnaire, 321–322

N

Nagi model, 240
National Health Service, United Kingdom, quality indicators of, 221
National Quality Forum
performance measures of, 365
quality measures of, 367–370
National quality registers, 365–366
NEO Personality Inventory, in fibromyalgia, 323
Numerical rating scales, in juvenile idiopathic arthritis, 335

O

OMERACT. *See* Outcome Measures in Rheumatology (OMERACT).
Osteoarthritis
knee, **239–252**
PROs and PROMs in, 389
Outcome Measures in Rheumatology (OMERACT), 391
in fibromyalgia, 325–327
in psoriatic arthritis, 266–267
in rheumatoid arthritis, 220, 222–223, 356
in systemic lupus erythematosus, 254

P

Pain
in fibromyalgia, 322–324
in juvenile idiopathic arthritis, 335–336
in psoriatic arthritis, 266–267
in rheumatoid arthritis, 220, 223, 226
in systemic sclerosis, 309
Pain Beliefs and Perceptions Inventory, in fibromyalgia, 324
Pain Catastrophizing Scale, in fibromyalgia, 324
Pain Disability Index, in fibromyalgia, 325
Pain Interference Scale, in fibromyalgia, 325
painDETECT, in fibromyalgia, 320
Pathology domain, of rheumatic measures, 207–208
Patient Activity Scale, 223, 367–368
Patient global assessment, in rheumatoid arthritis, 226
Patient Global Assessment of Disease Activity, Visual Analog Scale with, in rheumatoid arthritis, 348–356
Patient Health Questionnaire
in fibromyalgia, 323
in rheumatoid arthritis, 227
Patient-Centered Electronic Redesign (Rheum-PACER), 367
Patient-Centered Outcomes Research Institute, 390–391

Patient-reported outcomes and outcome measures
challenges in, **363–375**
history of, **205–217**
in axial spondyloarthritis, **265–299**
in fibromyalgia, **317–332**
in juvenile idiopathic arthritis, **233–246**
in knee osteoarthritis, **239–252**
in psoriatic arthritis, **265–283**
in rheumatoid arthritis, **219–237, 347–362**
in systemic lupus erythematosus, **253–263**
in systemic sclerosis, **301–316**
in vulnerable populations, **347–362**
information system for, **377–394**
Patient-Reported Outcomes Measurement Information System. *See* PROMIS (Patient-Reported Outcomes Measurement Information System).
Paulus Criteria, for rheumatoid arthritis, 220
Pediatric Outcomes Data Collection Instrument, 337
Pediatric Pain Questionnaire, in juvenile idiopathic arthritis, 335–336
Pediatric patients
juvenile idiopathic arthritis in, **333–346**
PROMIS for, 383–384
Pediatric Quality of Life Inventory, in juvenile idiopathic arthritis, 335–336
Pediatric Quality of Life Scales, in juvenile idiopathic arthritis, 336
Pediatric Rheumatology Clinical Outcomes and Improvement Network, 367
Pediatric Rheumatology Quality of Life Scale, 336
Pennebaker Inventory of Limbic Languidness, 320–321
Perceived Stress Scale, in fibromyalgia, 322–323
Personality inventory, in fibromyalgia, 323
Physical Activity Index, for juvenile idiopathic arthritis, 337
Physical Activity Questionnaire, in juvenile idiopathic arthritis, 338
Physical Component Score, in Medical Outcomes Study Short Form 36, 270
Physical function domain
in rheumatic measures, 208–209
in rheumatoid arthritis, 224–226
Physician Consortium for Performance Improvement, 368
Pincus, Theodore, 209
Pittsburgh Sleep Diary, for rheumatoid arthritis, 227
Pittsburgh Sleep Quality Index, in fibromyalgia, 322
Pittsburgh Sleep Subscales, in fibromyalgia, 321
Polysomnography, for rheumatoid arthritis, 227
Porter, Michael, 221
Positive and Negative Affect Scale, in fibromyalgia, 322–323
Process, as quality indicator, in rheumatoid arthritis, 221
PROMIS (Patient-Reported Outcomes Measurement Information System), 208–209, 367–368, **377–394**
content of, 382–383
description of, 377–378
development of, 378–382
Food and Drug Administration and, 378, 390
future of, 391–392
history of, 377–378

in fibromyalgia, 321, 323
in juvenile idiopathic arthritis, 335–339
in knee osteoarthritis, 247–248
in pediatric patients, 383–384
in rheumatoid arthritis, 225–226, 229
in systemic lupus erythematosus, 256–257
in systemic sclerosis, 306–308, 310
international scope of, 390–391
rheumatology applications of, 385–390
standardization in, 378
validation of, 384–387
PROs and PROMs. *See* Patient-reported outcomes and outcome measures.
Pruritus, in systemic sclerosis, 310
PsA Quality of Life Index, in psoriatic arthritis, 268, 270
Psoriasis Symptom Inventory, 266, 269, 273
Psoriatic Arthritis Disease Activity Score, 276
Psoriatic Arthritis Impact of Disease, 266, 268, 271
Psoriatic arthritis, PROs and PROMs in, **265–283,** 389
composite, 274–277
fatigue, 273
global assessment, 267
health-related quality of life, 267, 270–271
impact of disease, 271–272
pain, 266–267
skin symptoms, 272–273
sleep disturbance, 274
work productivity, 273–274
Psoriatic Arthritis Quality of Life index, 266, 270–271
Psoriatic Arthritis Response Criteria, 276–277
Psychological domain, of rheumatic measures, 207–208
Psychometric properties, in knee osteoarthritis, 240–241
Psychometric theory, modern, 208–209
Pulmonary arterial hypertension, in systemic sclerosis, 310

Q

Quality indicators, for rheumatoid arthritis, 221–222
Quality of life domain, of rheumatic measures, 207–208
Quality of life, in juvenile idiopathic arthritis, 338
Quality of Life in Neurologic Disorders, 256
Quick-DASH, in systemic sclerosis, 308

R

RAPID (Routine Assessment of Patient Index Data), 223
Raynaud's phenomenons, in systemic sclerosis, 307–310
Regional Pain Scale, for rheumatoid arthritis, 226
Reliability, of psychometric properties, 240–241
Remission, in rheumatoid arthritis, 222–223
Research, in juvenile idiopathic arthritis, 340–341
Responsiveness, of psychometric properties, 240–241

Rheumatoid arthritis, **219–237**
PROMIS for, 387–390
PROs and PROMs in, 271
history of, 220–221
in domains, 224–227
in pain, 226
in patient global assessment, 226
in physical function domain, 224–226
in remission, 222–223
quality indicators for, 221–222
scoring systems for, 223
uses of, 221–223
with limited health literacy and limited English proficiency, **347–362**
remission in, 222–223
signs and symptoms of, 219–220
Rheumatoid Arthritis Disease Activity Index, 223, 270
Rheumatoid Arthritis Pain Scale, 226
Rheumatology Informatics System for Effectiveness, 229, 367
Rheum-PACER (Patient-Centered Electronic Redesign), 367
Routine Assessment of Patient Index Data (RAPID), 223, 270, 367–368

S

Sacroiliac joints, arthritis of, **285–299**
Scleroderma Clinical Trials Consortium Gastrointestinal Scale, 303, 308–309
Scleroderma Health Assessment Questionnaire, 303, 305
Scleroderma, PROs and PROMs in, **301–316**
Self-efficacy, in fibromyalgia, 324
Sensitivity, of psychometric properties, 240–241
Sensitivity to change, of psychometric properties, 240–241
Sexual dysfunction, in systemic sclerosis, 310
Short Test of Functional Health in Adults, 349
Short-Form Health survey, in systemic sclerosis, 305–306
Simplified Disease Activity Index, 352, 367–368
Single-Item Literacy Screening questions, 349–350
Skin symptoms, in psoriatic arthritis, 272–273
SLE Quality of Life Questionnaire, 257–258
Sleep disturbance
in fibromyalgia, 318, 321
in psoriatic arthritis, 274
in rheumatoid arthritis, 227–228
SLE-Specific quality of Life Questionnaire, 257–258
Social factors, in fibromyalgia, 325
SPARTAN (Spondyloarthritis Research and Treatment Network), 295
Spine, arthritis of, **285–299**
Spondyloarthritis Research and Treatment Network (SPARTAN), 295
Sports domain, in rheumatoid arthritis, 225
State-Trait Anxiety Inventory, in fibromyalgia, 322–323
Steinbrocker committee, 206
Steinbrocker-Blazer therapeutic score card, for rheumatoid arthritis, 220
Stress, in fibromyalgia, 322–323

Structure, as quality indicator, in rheumatoid arthritis, 221
Survey of Pain Attitudes, in fibromyalgia, 324
Swedish Rheumatology Quality Registry, 365–366
Symptom Burden Index, in systemic sclerosis, 305–306
Systemic Index, for rheumatoid arthritis, 220
Systemic lupus erythematosus, PROMs in, **253–263**
  disease-specific, 257–259
  generic, 254–257
Systemic sclerosis, PROs and PROMs in, **301–316,** 387–388

T

Technical Expert Panel, 368
Tender points, in fibromyalgia, 318
Ten-Item Personality Inventory, in fibromyalgia, 323
Therapeutic score card, for rheumatoid arthritis, 220
Transition Dyspnea Index, in systemic sclerosis, 306

U

Ulcers, digital, in systemic sclerosis, 309–310
United Kingdom, PRO data collection registries of, 366
United Kingdom Systemic Sclerosis Functional Score, 305–306

V

Validation, of PROMs, in axial spondyloarthritis, 289–295
Validity, of psychometric properties, 240–241
Veterans Affairs Rheumatoid Arthritis registry, 367
Visual analog scale
  in fibromyalgia, 319–320
  in juvenile idiopathic arthritis, 335–336
  in systemic sclerosis, 309
  Patient Global Assessment of Disease Activity with, in rheumatoid arthritis, 348–356

W

Walking domain, in rheumatoid arthritis, 225
West Haven-Yale Multidimensional Work Productivity and Activity Impairment, in fibromyalgia, 325–326
Western Ontario and Master Universities physical function subscale, in knee osteoarthritis, 241–242
Wolfe, Frederick, 209
WOMAN (Western Ontario and Master Universities) physical function subscale, in knee osteoarthritis, 241–242
Women's Health Initiative Insomnia Rating Scale, 227
Wong Baker FACES Pain Rating Scale, in juvenile idiopathic arthritis, 335–336
Work Productivity and Activity Impairment, in fibromyalgia, 325–326
Work Productivity Survey, in psoriatic arthritis, 269, 273–274
Worst Itch-Numerical Rating Scale, 266, 273

Printed and bound by CPI Group (UK) Ltd, Croydon, CR0 4YY
08/05/2025
01864684-0001